Obstetrics and Gynaecology at a Glance

Obstetrics and Gynaecology at a Glance

Errol R. Norwitz

MD, DPhil (Oxon), FACOG
Associate Professor, Yale University School of Medicine
Director of Perinatal Research
Director, Division of Maternal-Fetal Medicine
Department of Obstetrics, Gynecology & Reproductive Sciences
Yale-New Haven Hospital
New Haven, CT, USA

John O. Schorge

MD, FACOG, FACS
Associate Professor
Patricia Duniven Fletcher Professor in Gynecologic Oncology
Division of Gynecologic Oncology
Department of Obstetrics and Gynecology
University of Texas Southwestern Medical School
Dallas, TX, USA

Second edition

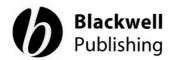

Published by Blackwell Publishing Ltd
Blackwell Publishing, Inc., 350 Main Street, Malden, Massachusetts 02148-5020, USA
Blackwell Publishing Ltd, 9600 Garsington Road, Oxford OX4 2DQ, UK
Blackwell Publishing Asia Pty Ltd, 550 Swanston Street, Carlton, Victoria 3053, Australia

First published 2001
Reprinted 2003, 2004
Second edition 2006

2   2007

Library of Congress Cataloging-in-Publication Data

Norwitz, Errol R.
    Obstetrics and gynaecology at a glance / Errol R. Norwitz, John O. Schorge.— 2nd ed.
        p.   ;   cm.
    Rev. ed. of: Obstetrics and gynecology at a glance / Errol R. Norwitz, John O. Schorge. 2001.
    Includes bibliographical references and index.
    ISBN 978-1-4051-3186-5
    1. Gynecology—Handbooks, manuals, etc.   2. Obstetrics—Handbooks, manuals, etc.
    [DNLM: 1. Genital Diseases, Female—Handbooks.   2. Pregnancy
Complications—Handbooks. WP 39 N893o 2006]   I. Schorge, John O.   II. Norwitz, Errol R. Obstetrics and gynecology at a glance.   III. Title.

RG110.N67 2006
618—dc22

                                                                    2005032551

A catalogue record for this title is available from the British Library

Set in 9/11.5pt Times by SNP Best-set Typesetter Ltd., Hong Kong
Printed and bound in Singapore by Markono Print Media Pte Ltd

Commissioning Editor: Martin Sugden
Development Editor: Geraldine Jeffers
Production Controller: Kate Charman

For further information on Blackwell Publishing, visit our website:
http://www.blackwellpublishing.com

The publisher's policy is to use permanent paper from mills that operate a sustainable forestry policy, and which has been manufactured from pulp processed using acid-free and elementary chlorine-free practices. Furthermore, the publisher ensures that the text paper and cover board used have met acceptable environmental accreditation standards.

Contents

Preface

The medical and scientific problems of this world cannot be solved by skeptics whose horizons are limited by practical realities. We need women and men who dream of things that cannot be and ask why not.

Professor Egon Diczfalusy, Karolinska Institute, Stockholm, Sweden, 1992

Medicine continues to attract the brightest and most dedicated students to its ranks. The opportunity to nurture the talented young minds that will one day rise up to lead the medical community remains the single greatest privilege for the academic clinician. Nowhere is this privilege—and challenge—more apparent than in obstetrics and gynaecology, a discipline that remains more art than science. Although clinicians in all disciplines aspire to practice rational evidence-based medicine, many basic questions in the field of obstetrics and gynaecology remain unanswered. While cardiologists measure changes in calcium flux within a single myocardial cell and nephrologists estimate changes in osmotic gradient along a single nephron, obstetrician–gynaecologists continue to debate such questions as: How is the LH surge regulated? What causes endometriosis? Why is there still no effective screening test for ovarian cancer? What triggers labour?

This text is written primarily for medical students starting their clinical rotations. It is designed to give the reader a succinct yet comprehensive review of obstetrics and gynaecology. Each chapter consists of two pages: a page of text and an accompanying set of images or algorithms that serve to complement the text. It is the sincere hope of the authors that the readers will find this book interesting, easy to read, and informative. Not all questions can be answered in a formal text format. Students should be encouraged to question and challenge their clinical teachers. Only then can the field move forward. Remember: 'We need women and men who dream of things that cannot be and ask why not.'

Errol R. Norwitz, MD, DPhil, FACOG
John O. Schorge, MD, FACOG, FACS

Acknowledgements

To my wife, Ann; my parents, Rollo and Marionne; and my children, Nicholas, Gabriella, and Sam.

E.R.N.

I would like to thank my wife, Sharon; my children, Dante, Lena, and Rocco; and my dog Kramer for their support during the completion of this book. In addition, I would like to express my deep appreciation for the mentors who inspired me during my obstetrics and gynaecology training—most notably John Repke, Kelly Molpus, Karen Lu, Ross Berkowitz, and Sam Mok.

J.O.S.

Further reading

Cunningham F.G., Leveno K.J., Bloom S.L., Hauth J.C., Gilstrap L.C. III & Wenstrom K.D. (eds) (2005) *Williams Obstetrics, 22nd edn.* McGraw-Hill, New York.

Dildy G.A. III, Belfort M.A., Saade G.R., Phelan J.P., Hankins G.D.V. & Clark S.L. (2004). *Critical Care Obstetrics, 4th edn.* Blackwell Science, Oxford.

Gabbe S.G., Niebyl J.R. & Simpson J.L. (eds) (2004). *Obstetrics: Normal and Abnormal Pregnancies, 4th edn.* Churchill Livingstone, New York.

Hoskins W.J., Perez C.A., Young R.C., Barakat R.R., Markman M. & Randall M.E. (eds) (2004) *Principles and Practice of Gynecologic Oncology, 4th edn.* Lippincott-Raven, Philadelphia.

Rock J.A. & Jones H.W. III (eds) (2003) *TeLinde's Operative Gynecology, 9th edn.* Lippincott-Raven, Philadelphia.

Speroff L. & Fritz M.A. (eds) (2004) *Clinical Gynecologic Endocrinology and Infertility, 7th edn.* Lippincott-Raven, Philadelphia.

Stenchever M.A., Droegemueller W., Herbst A.L. & Mishell D.R. Jr (eds) (2002) *Comprehensive Gynecology, 4th edn.* Mosby-Year Book Inc., St. Louis.

Strauss J.F. III & Barbieri R.L. (eds) (2004) *Yen and Jaffee's Reproductive Endocrinology, 5th edn.* Elsevier, Philadelphia.

Weiner C.P. & Buhimschi C.S. (2004) *Drugs for Pregnant and Lactating Women.* Churchill Livingstone, New York.

Table and figure acknowledgements

The following tables and figures have been redrawn from the originals and were used with permission of the publishers. Every effort has been made by the author and the publishers to contact all the copyright holders to obtain their permission to reproduce copyright material. However, if any have been inadvertently overlooked, the publisher will be pleased to make the necessary arrangements at the first opportunity.

2 Anatomy of the female reproductive tract Parts of the figure redrawn with permission from: Morrow, C.P. & Curtain, J.P. (1996) *Gynecologic Cancer Surgery*, p. 115. Churchill Livingstone, London.

5 Ectopic pregnancy Table redrawn with permission from: The American College of Obstetricians and Gynecologists. (1998) *Medical Management of Tubal Pregnancy*. ACOG practice bulletin No. 3, Washington, DC.

9 Benign disorders of the lower genital tract Parts of the figure redrawn with permission from: Netter, F.H. (1992) The Reproductive System. In: *The CIBA Collection of Medical Illustrations, Vol 2*, 9th edn, pp. 140 & 151. ICON, New Jersey.

10 Benign disorders of the upper genital tract Parts of the figure redrawn with permission from: DiSaia, P.J. & Creasman, W.T. (1997) *Clinical Gynecologic Oncology*, 5th edn, pp. 150 & 261. Mosby, St. Louis; Netter, F.H. (1992) The Reproductive System. In: *The CIBA Collection of Medical Illustrations, Vol 2*, 9th edn, p. 201. ICON, New Jersey.

11 Endometriosis and adenomyosis Parts of the figure redrawn with permission from: Ryan, K.J., Berkowitz, R.S. & Barbieri, R.L. (1995) *Kistner's Gynecology: Principles and Practice*, 6th edn, p. 254. Mosby, St Louis.

13 Sterilization Parts of the figure redrawn with permission from: Speroff, L., Glass, R.H. & Kase, N.G. (1994) *Clinical Gynecologic Endocrinology and Infertility*, 5th edn, pp. 695–697. Lippincott, Williams & Wilkins, Philadelphia.

16 Gynaecological surgery Parts of the figure redrawn with permission from: Wheeless, C.R. (1997) *Atlas of Pelvic Surgery*, 3rd edn, p. 263. Lippincott, Williams & Wilkins, Philadelphia.

19 Puberty and precocious puberty Parts of the figure redrawn with permission from: Speroff, L., Glass, R.H. & Kase, N.G. (1994) *Clinical Gynecologic Endocrinology and Infertility*, 5th edn, pp. 378–379. Lippincott, Williams & Wilkins, Philadelphia.

20 Amenorrhea Parts of the figure redrawn with permission from: Netter, F.H. (1992) The Reproductive System. In: *The CIBA Collection of Medical Illustrations, Vol 2*, 9th edn, p. 193. ICON, New Jersey.

25 Assisted reproductive technology Parts of the figure redrawn with permission from: Gershenson, D.M., DeCherney, A.H. & Curry, S.L. (1993) *Operative Gynecology*, pp. 557–564. W.B. Saunders, Philadelphia.

33 Embryology and early fetal development Parts of the figure redrawn with permission from: Moore, K.L. (1988) *The Developing Human: Clinically Orientated Embryology*, 4th edn. W.B. Saunders, Philadelphia; Moore, K.L. & Persaud, T.V.N. (1993) *The Developing Human: Clinically Orientated Embryology*, 5th edn. W.B. Saunders, Philadelphia.

34 Fetal physiology Parts of the figure redrawn with permission from: Brown, A.R. & Assali, N.S. (1968) *The Fetus and Neonate, Biology of Gestation*, p. 361. Academic Press, New York; Fox, H. & Elston, C.W. (1978) *Pathology of the Placenta*. W.B. Saunders, Philadelphia.

35 Endocrinology of pregnancy and parturition Parts of the figure redrawn with permission from: Norwitz, E.R., Robinson, J.N. & Repke, J.T. (1999) The initiation of parturition: a comparative analysis across the species. *Current Problems in Obstetrics and Gynecology and Fertility*, **22**, 41–72.

36 Maternal adaptation to pregnancy Parts of the figure redrawn with permission from: Leontic, E.A. (1977) Respiratory disease in pregnancy. *The Medical Clinics of North America*, **61**, 114; Scott, D.E. (1972) Anemia during pregnancy. *Obstetrics and Gynecology Annual*, **1**, 219. Table redrawn with permission from: Clark, S.L., Cotton, D.B., Lee, W., Bishop, C. & Hill, T. (1989) Central hemodynamic assessment of normal-term pregnancy. *American Journal of Obstetrics and Gynecology*, **161**, 1439.

37 Prenatal diagnosis Parts of the figure redrawn with permission from: Wald, N. & Cuckle, H.S. (1987) Recent advances in screening for neural tube defects. *Bailleres Clinical Obstetrics and Gynaecology*, **1**, 656. Table redrawn with permission from: Patient education bulletin. (1994) *Maternal serum screening for birth defects*. No. APO89, American College of Obstetrics & Gynecology, Washington, DC.

38 Obstetric ultrasound Parts of the figure redrawn with permission from: Romero, R., Pilu, G., Jeanty, P., Ghidini, A. & Hobbins, J.C. (1998) *Prenatal Diagnosis of Congenital Anomalies*, pp, 128–129. Appleton & Lange, New York.

44 Thyroid disease in pregnancy Parts of the figure redrawn with permission from: Fisher, D.A. & Carson, P.R. (1994) Maternal and fetal thyroid functin. *New England Journal of Medicine*, **331** (Suppl, 16), 1072–1078.

52 Multiple pregnancy Parts of the figure redrawn with permission from: Norwitz, E.R. (1998) Multiple pregnancy: trends past, present and future. *Infertility and Reproductive Medicine Clinics of North America*, **9**, (Suppl. 3), 351–69.

54 Premature labour Parts of the figure redrawn with permission from: Norwitz, E.R., Robinson, J.N. & Repke, J.T. (1999) The initiation of parturition: a comparative analysis across the species. *Current Problems in Obstetrics and Gynecology and Fertility*, **22** (Suppl. 2), 41–72. Table redrawn with permission from: Norwitz, E.R., Robinson, J.N. & Challis, J.R.G. (1999) The control of labor. *The New England Journal of Medicine*, **341** (Suppl. 9), 664.

58 Normal labour and delivery Friedman, E.A. (1978) *Labor: Clinical Evaluation and Management*, 2nd edn. Appleton-Century-Crofts, New York; Norwitz, E.R., Robinson, J.N. & Repke, J.T. The initiation and management of normal labor. In: *The Physiologic Basis of Gynecology and Obstetrics*. (eds. D.B. Seifer, P. Samuels & D.A. Kniss), p. 422. Lippincott, Williams & Wilkins, Philadelphia.

1 History taking and physical examination

LEOPOLD MANOEUVRES

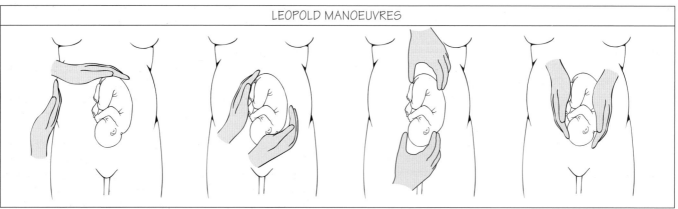

SPECULA FOR GYNAECOLOGICAL EXAMINATION

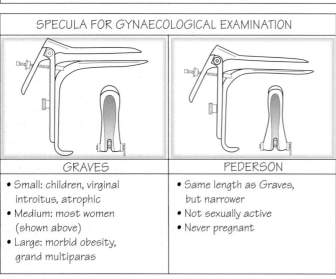

GRAVES	PEDERSON
• Small: children, virginal introitus, atrophic • Medium: most women (shown above) • Large: morbid obesity, grand multiparas	• Same length as Graves, but narrower • Not sexually active • Never pregnant

PERFORMING A PAP SMEAR

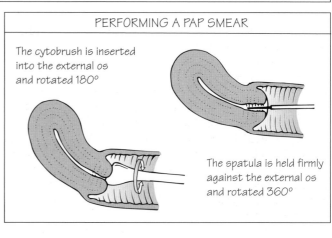

The cytobrush is inserted into the external os and rotated 180°

The spatula is held firmly against the external os and rotated 360°

PELVIC EXAMINATION

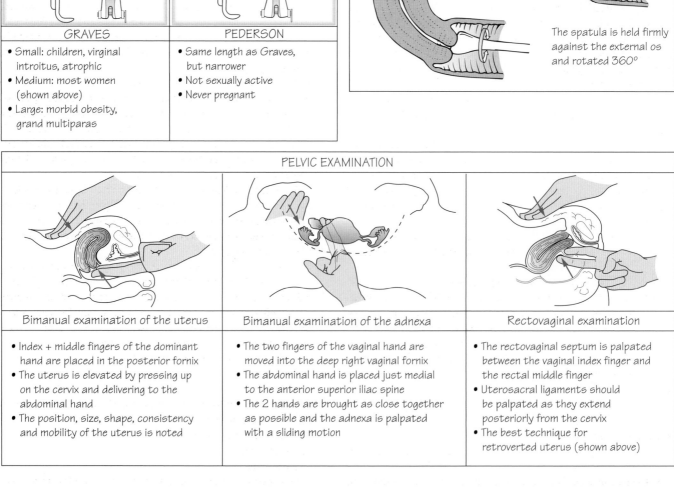

Bimanual examination of the uterus	Bimanual examination of the adnexa	Rectovaginal examination
• Index + middle fingers of the dominant hand are placed in the posterior fornix • The uterus is elevated by pressing up on the cervix and delivering to the abdominal hand • The position, size, shape, consistency and mobility of the uterus is noted	• The two fingers of the vaginal hand are moved into the deep right vaginal fornix • The abdominal hand is placed just medial to the anterior superior iliac spine • The 2 hands are brought as close together as possible and the adnexa is palpated with a sliding motion	• The rectovaginal septum is palpated between the vaginal index finger and the rectal middle finger • Uterosacral ligaments should be palpated as they extend posteriorly from the cervix • The best technique for retroverted uterus (shown above)

General comments

• Dress appropriately and conduct yourself in a professional manner at all times.

• Take a history before asking the patient to undress for her physical examination.

• Introduce yourself by name and title and then all members of your team.

• When taking a history always sit facing the patient and make direct eye contact. Address questions directly to the patient but be culturally sensitive. For example, some cultures discourage hand shaking. In other cultures, the husband or male family members will answer questions directed at the woman.

• Listening is important in developing a trusting relationship. Understand the problem from the patient's point of view and establish a management plan. Acknowledge important points in the history by verbal or non-verbal cues e.g. nodding.

History

• *Chief complaint.* Patients should be encouraged to express, in their own words, the main purpose of the visit. Pertinent open-ended questions can help clarify the details.

• *Present illness.* The interview should be comprehensive, but tailored to the patient's chief complaints.

• *Past medical and surgical history.* The patient should be asked to list any significant health problems. Current and prior medications should be listed and all allergic reactions should be noted.

• *Gynaecological history.* Pertinent aspects of her gynaecological history should include a detailed menstrual history (age of menarche/menopause, cycle length, and duration, last menstrual period), contraceptive history, prior vaginal or pelvic infections, sexual history, and previous surgical gynaecological procedures (including biopsies and other minor operations).

• *Obstetric history.* All pregnancies should be detailed including gestational ages, pregnancy-related complications, and pregnancy outcomes.

• *Family history.* A detailed family history should be taken. Serious illnesses (diabetes, cardiovascular disease, hypertension) or causes of death for each individual should be recorded, with particular attention to first-generation relatives. A family history of unexplained mental retardation or genetic syndromes may have implications for further pregnancies.

• *Social history.* The patient should be asked about her occupation and where and with whom she lives. She should be asked about cigarette smoking, illicit drug use, and alcohol use.

• *Review of systems.* A directed review of general symptoms is invaluable to uncover seemingly (to the patient) unrelated aspects of her health. Areas of importance include: constitutional (weight loss/gain, hot flushes), cardiovascular (chest pain, shortness of breath), gastrointestinal (irritable bowel syndrome, hepatitis), genito-urinary (incontinence, haematuria), neurological (numbness, decreased sensation), psychiatric (depression, suicidal ideations), and other body systems.

Physical examination

1 General examination

• A complete physical examination should be performed at the first visit with a chaperone present.

• The patient should be asked to disrobe completely and should be covered by an appropriate hospital gown.

2 Abdominal examination

• The abdomen should be carefully *inspected* for symmetry, scars, distension, and hair pattern; *palpated* for organomegaly or masses; and *ausculated* for bowel sounds.

• If a woman is pregnant, the 4 Leopold manoeuvres should be performed (*opposite*) to assess the number, lie, presentation, and well-being of the fetus(es).

3 Pelvic examination

• Pelvic examinaton should be conducted with the patient lying supine on the examining table with her legs in stirrups.

• The patient should be as relaxed as possible. This can be facilitated by explaining exactly what you plan to do before you do it and by gentle touching.

• *Inspection* of the perineum involves assessment of the hair pattern, skin, presence of lesions (vesicles, warts, pigmented nevi), evidence of trauma, haemorrhoids, and abnormalities of the perineal body. Genital prolapse can be assessed by gently separating the labia and inspecting the vagina while the patient bears down (Valsalva manoeuvre).

• *Palpation* of the labia may identify swollen or infected Bartholin's or Skene's glands.

• *Speculum examination* begins by choosing the appropriate type and size of speculum (*opposite*), making sure that it has been warmed, and then touching the tip against the patient's leg as an advance warning. Gentle spreading of the labia and downward pressure may be helpful. The speculum is then inserted by placing the blades through the introitus and guiding the tip in a downward motion toward the rectum. The blades are inserted to their full length and then opened to reveal the cervix. The vaginal canal should be examined for erythema, lesions, or discharge. The cervix should be pink, shiny, and clear.

• The *Papanicolaou (Pap) smear (opposite)* is designed to sample the transformation zone of the cervix (the junction of the squamous cells lining the vagina and the columnar cells lining the endocervical canal). The material obtained is then smeared thinly on a microscopic slide and immediately fixed by spraying. Alternatively, the spatula may be scraped to dislodge cells into a liquid-based cytology vial and prepared for cytological interpretation.

• *Bimanual examination (opposite)* allows the physician to palpate the uterus and adnexae. In the normal and non-pregnant state, the uterus is approximately 6×4 cm (the size of a fist). A normal ovary is approximately 3×2 cm in size, but is often not palpable in obese or post-menopausal women.

• A *rectovaginal examination (opposite)* may yield additional information, especially when pelvic organs are positioned in the posterior cul-de-sac. Separately, a *rectal examination* performed circumferentially with the examining finger can rule out distally located colorectal cancers. The physician may also note the tone of the anal sphincter, any other abnormalities (haemorrhoids, fissures, masses), and test a stool sample for occult blood.

Screening tests and preventative health

• Patients should routinely be counselled about the importance of screening tests, including:

(i) breast self-examinations

(ii) mammograms

(iii) Pap smears

• A discussion should also be held about healthy lifestyle changes (diet, exercise), safe sexual practices, and contraception.

2 Anatomy of the female reproductive tract

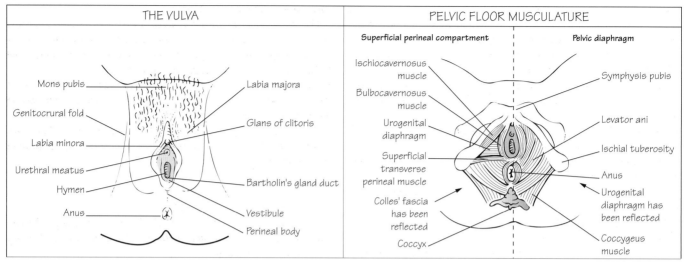

THE VULVA

Mons pubis
Genitocrural fold
Labia minora
Urethral meatus
Hymen
Anus

Labia majora
Glans of clitoris
Bartholin's gland duct
Vestibule
Perineal body

PELVIC FLOOR MUSCULATURE

Superficial perineal compartment | Pelvic diaphragm

Ischiocavernosus muscle
Bulbocavernosus muscle
Urogenital diaphragm
Superficial transverse perineal muscle
Colles' fascia has been reflected
Coccyx

Symphysis pubis
Levator ani
Ischial tuberosity
Anus
Urogenital diaphragm has been reflected
Coccygeus muscle

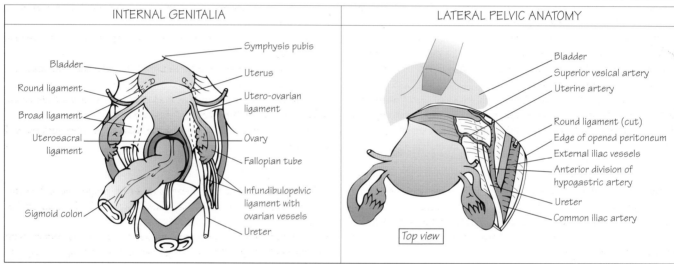

INTERNAL GENITALIA

Bladder
Round ligament
Broad ligament
Uterosacral ligament
Sigmoid colon

Symphysis pubis
Uterus
Utero-ovarian ligament
Ovary
Fallopian tube
Infundibulopelvic ligament with ovarian vessels
Ureter

LATERAL PELVIC ANATOMY

Bladder
Superior vesical artery
Uterine artery
Round ligament (cut)
Edge of opened peritoneum
External iliac vessels
Anterior division of hypogastric artery
Ureter
Common iliac artery

Top view

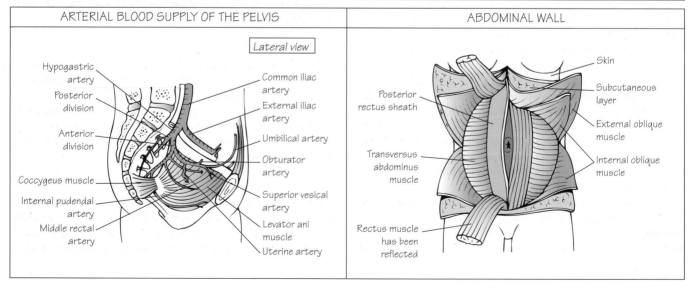

ARTERIAL BLOOD SUPPLY OF THE PELVIS

Lateral view

Hypogastric artery
Posterior division
Anterior division
Coccygeus muscle
Internal pudendal artery
Middle rectal artery

Common iliac artery
External iliac artery
Umbilical artery
Obturator artery
Superior vesical artery
Levator ani muscle
Uterine artery

ABDOMINAL WALL

Posterior rectus sheath
Transversus abdominus muscle
Rectus muscle has been reflected

Skin
Subcutaneous layer
External oblique muscle
Internal oblique muscle

The vulva and pelvic floor musculature *(opposite)*

• The *vulva* is the visible external female genitalia bounded by the mons pubis anteriorly, the anus posteriorly, and the genitocrural folds laterally.
• The *perineum* is located between the urethral meatus and the anus, including both the skin and the underlying muscle.
• The *mons pubis* consists of hair-bearing skin over a cushion of adipose tissue that lies on the symphysis pubis.
• The *labia majora* are two large, hair-bearing cutaneous folds of adipose and fibrous tissue extending from the mons pubis to the perineal body.
• The *clitoris* is a short, erectile organ with a visible glans. It is the female homologue of the male penis.
• The *labia minora* are two thin, hairless skin folds medial to the labia majora which originate at the clitoris.
• The *vestibule* is the cleft of tissue between the labia minora that is visualized when they are held apart.
• *Bartholin's glands* are situated at each side of the vaginal orifice with duct openings at 5 and 7 o'clock.
• The *superficial perineal compartment* is located between Colles' fascia and the urogenital diaphragm. Within it are found the ischiocavernosus, bulbocavernosus, and superficial transverse perineal muscles.
• The *urogenital diaphragm (perineal membrane)* is a triangular sheet of dense, fibromuscular tissue stretched between the symphysis pubis and ischial tuberosities in the anterior half of the pelvic outlet. Its primary function is to support the vagina and perineal body.
• The *pelvic diaphragm* is found above the urogenital diaphragm and forms the inferior border of the abdominopelvic cavity. It is composed of a funnel-shaped sling of fascia and muscle (levator ani, coccygeus).

Internal genitalia and lateral pelvic anatomy *(opposite)*

• The *uterus* is a fibromuscular organ whose shape, weight, and dimensions vary considerably. The dome-shaped top is termed the fundus.
• The *cervix* is connected to the uterus at the internal os. It is made up primarily of dense fibrous connective tissue. The cervical canal opens into the vagina at the external os.
• The *vagina* is a thin-walled, distensible, fibromuscular tube that extends from the vestibule of the vulva to the uterine cervix.
• The *fallopian tubes* (oviducts) are paired tubular structures that arise from the upper lateral portion of the uterus, widening in their distal third (ampulla).
• The *ovaries* are whitish-grey, almond-sized organs attached to the uterus medially by the utero-ovarian ligaments and to the pelvic sidewall laterally by a vascular pedicle, the infundibulopelvic ligament.
• The *ureters* are whitish, muscular tubes which serve as a conduit for urine from the kidney to the bladder trigone. They course over the common iliac vessels from lateral to medial at the level of the pelvic brim before passing under the uterine vessels just lateral to the cervix ('water under the bridge').
• The *bladder* is a hollow muscular organ that lies between the symphysis pubis and the uterus. The size and shape varies with the volume of urine.
• The *sigmoid colon* enters the pelvis on the left, forming the rectum at the level of the second and third sacral vertebrae and ending at the anal canal.
• The *round ligaments* are paired fibrous bands that originate at the uterine fundus and exit the pelvis through the internal inguinal ring. They provide little structural support.
• The *broad ligaments* are thin reflections of the peritoneum stretching from the pelvic sidewalls to the uterus. They provide virtually no suspensory support, but are draped over the fallopian tubes, ovaries, round ligaments, ureters, and other pelvic structures.
• The *cardinal (Mackenrodt's) ligaments* provide the major support of the uterus and cervix. They extend from the lateral aspects of the cervix and vagina to the pelvic sidewalls.
• The *uterosacral ligaments* serve a minor role in the anatomic support of the cervix. They extend from the upper cervix posteriorly to the third sacral vertebra.

Arterial blood supply of the pelvis *(opposite)*

• The *aorta* bifurcates at the fourth lumbar vertebra to form the two common iliac arteries that, in turn, divide to form the external iliac and hypogastric (internal iliac) arteries.
• The *external iliac artery* passes under the inguinal ligament to become the femoral artery.
• The *hypogastric artery* branches into anterior and posterior divisions to supply the pelvis.
• The *ovarian arteries* originate from the infrarenal aorta and reach the ovaries via the infundibulopelvic ligament.
• The *inferior mesenteric artery* arises from the aorta, 3 cm above the bifurcation, to supply the descending colon.
• The *internal pudendal artery* supplies the rectum, labia, clitoris, and perineum.

Innervation of the genital tract

• The *superior hypogastric plexus* is the main component of the autonomic nervous system providing innervation to the internal genital organs.
• The *pudendal nerve* arises from the sacral plexus and courses with the pudendal artery and vein through the pudendal (Alcock's) canal to supply both motor and sensory fibres to the muscles and skin of the perineum.

Lymphatic drainage

• The vulva and distal third of the vagina are supplied by an anastomotic series of lymphatic channels which coalesce to drain primarily into the superficial inguinal nodes.
• Lymphatic drainage of the upper two-thirds of the vagina and uterus is primarily to the obturator, external iliac, and hypogastric nodes.
• The lymphatic drainage of the ovary follows the ovarian vessels to the paraaortic lymph nodes.

Abdominal wall *(opposite)*

Layers of the abdominal wall include — from the outside to the inside — the *skin, subcutaneous layer* (Scarpa's fascia), *musculo-aponeurotic layer* (rectus sheath, external oblique muscle, internal oblique muscle, transversus abdominis muscle), *transversalis fascia*, and *peritoneum*.

The menstrual cycle

HORMONAL REGULATION OF OVULATION

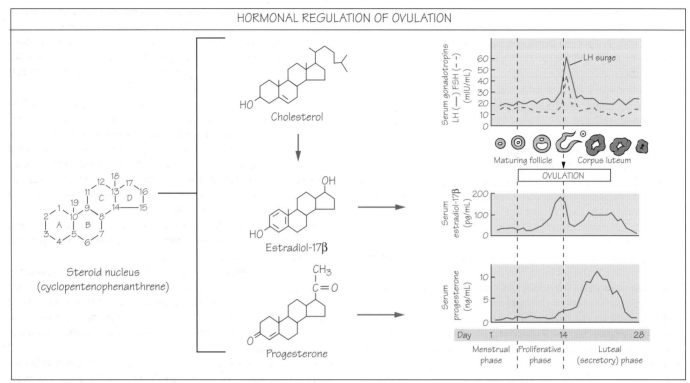

BIOLOGIC BASIS OF MENSTRUATION

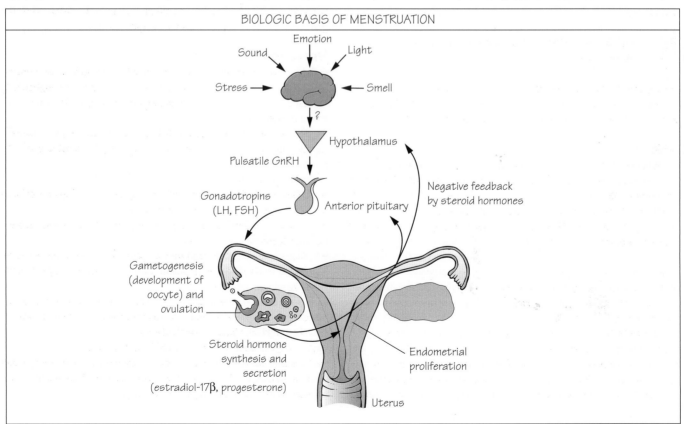

Definitions
• *Menstruation:* cyclic uterine bleeding experienced by most women of reproductive age.
• *Menarche* (the onset of menstruation) occurs at an average age of 12 years (normal range, 8–16).
• *Puberty* (Chapter 19) is a general term encompassing the entire transitional stage from childhood to sexual maturity.
• Ovulatory menstrual cycles usually last between 24 and 35 days (average, 28).
• The average duration of menstruation is 3–7 days.
• The average menstrual blood loss is 80 mL.
• *Menopause* (Chapter 26): cessation of menses.

Hormonal regulation of ovulation *(opposite)*
The cyclopentenophenanthrene ring structure is the basic carbon skeleton for all steroid hormones. Cholesterol is the parent steroid from which all the glucocorticoids, mineralcorticoids, and gonadal steroids are derived.

Phases of the menstrual cycle
• The first day of menstruation is defined as day 1 of the menstrual cycle.
• The *menstrual phase* refers to the period of shedding of the endometrial lining.
• The *proliferative phase* of the menstrual cycle begins at the end of the menstrual phase (usually day 4) and ends at ovulation (usually day 13 or 14). This phase is characterized by endometrial thickening and ovarian follicular maturation.
• The *luteinizing hormone (LH)* surge on day 13 or 14 triggers ovulation.
• The *luteal* (secretory) phase starts at ovulation and lasts through to day 28 of the menstrual cycle. The corpus luteum develops to synthesize steroid hormones.

Biological basis of menstruation *(opposite)*
Co-ordination of the menstrual cycle depends on a complex interaction between the brain, pituitary, ovaries, and endometrium.

Brain
• The *hypothalamus* acts as a transducer to convert neuronal stimuli from the cerebral cortex into pulses of neuropeptides, which travel to the anterior pituitary.
• Hypothalamic production of neuropeptides, such as gonadotropin-releasing hormone (GnRH), is modulated by *negative feedback* of steroid hormones.

Pituitary
• *Pulsatile* GnRH from the hypothalamus initiates the synthesis and secretion of the pituitary gonadotropins, LH, and follicle-stimulating hormone (FSH).
• LH and FSH production is also subject to negative feedback regulation by the steroid hormones.
• In reproductive-age women, LH and FSH levels generally remain in the 10–20 mIU/mL range. After the menopause or oophorectomy, estradiol-17β levels decline and pituitary gonadotropins are released from negative feedback, achieving circulating concentrations of more than 50 mIU/mL.

Ovaries
• Primitive germ cells (oogonia) divide by mitosis during fetal embryogenesis, peaking at around 7 million by 5 months of gestation.
• Meiotic division then begins, resulting in formation of primary oocytes. However, rapid atresia reduces the number of available follicles to 2 million at birth. At puberty, only around 300,000–400,000 follicles remain.
• Oocytes remain 'resting' in *meiotic prophase* until puberty. Resting ovarian follicles are surrounded by thecal and granulosa cells: FSH stimulates the granulosa cells and LH stimulates the thecal cells.
• Only a single 'dominant follicle' develops each menstrual cycle. When it produces enough estrogen to sustain a circulating estradiol-17β concentration of approximately 200 pg/mL for 48 hours, the hypothalamic–pituitary axis responds by secreting a surge of gonadotropins, primarily LH. This *LH surge* precedes ovulation by 24–36 hours.
• Following ovulation, the follicle collapses to form the *corpus luteum*. This endocrine organ mainly synthesizes progesterone to prepare the endometrium for pregnancy.
• If implantation does not occur the corpus luteum will degenerate, resulting in a precipitous decline in circulating steroid hormone levels and the onset of menstruation. The decreasing steroid hormone levels release the negative feedback mechanism, inducing the pituitary to increase gonadotropin secretion. As a result, a new cycle of follicular recruitment is initiated.
• If implantation does occur, the embryo will rescue the corpus luteum by producing human chorionic gonadotropin (hCG) to prevent menstruation. At 7–9 weeks of gestation, the placenta takes over the production of progesterone from the corpus luteum.

Endometrium
• Estradiol-17β production by the ovarian follicles induces endometrial proliferation. Progesterone synthesis by the corpus luteum then acts to mature the estrogen-primed endometrium in preparation for blastocyst implantation.
• Lowered steroid hormone levels in the late secretory phase cause a collapse of the endometrial vasculature, resulting in menstruation.

Premenstrual syndrome (PMS)
• *Definition:* cyclic appearance of a constellation of symptoms prior to menstruation which affect lifestyle or work.
• *Symptoms:* abdominal bloating, anxiety, breast tenderness, depression, irritability.
• *Diagnosis* does not depend on the specific symptom, but rather on the ability to chart the cyclic nature of the complaint in a predictable fashion.
• *Impact:* 40% of reproductive age women report significant problems related to their cycles, but only 1% have such severe PMS that it threatens their work and interpersonal relationships.
• *Aetiology:* the precise cause of PMS is not known.
• **Treatment** should start with supportive therapy, aerobic exercise, and diet modification. *Fluoxetine* or *sertraline* have been shown to reduce symptoms of depression, anger, and anxiety.

4 Abnormal vaginal bleeding

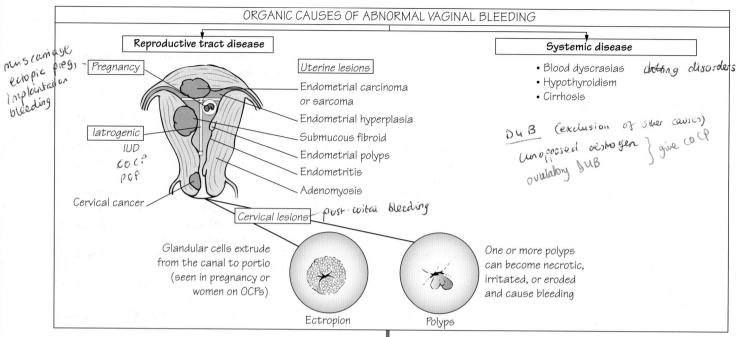

miscarriage
ectopic preg,
implantation
bleeding

ORGANIC CAUSES OF ABNORMAL VAGINAL BLEEDING

Reproductive tract disease

Pregnancy

Uterine lesions

Endometrial carcinoma or sarcoma

Endometrial hyperplasia

Submucous fibroid

Endometrial polyps

Endometritis

Adenomyosis

Iatrogenic
IUD
COC?
POP

Cervical cancer

Cervical lesions   post-coital bleeding

Glandular cells extrude from the canal to portio (seen in pregnancy or women on OCPs)

One or more polyps can become necrotic, irritated, or eroded and cause bleeding

Ectropion

Polyps

Systemic disease

- Blood dyscrasias   clotting disorders
- Hypothyroidism
- Cirrhosis

DUB (exclusion of other causes)
unopposed oestrogen } give COCP
ovulatory DUB

FURTHER EVALUATION OF THE UTERUS

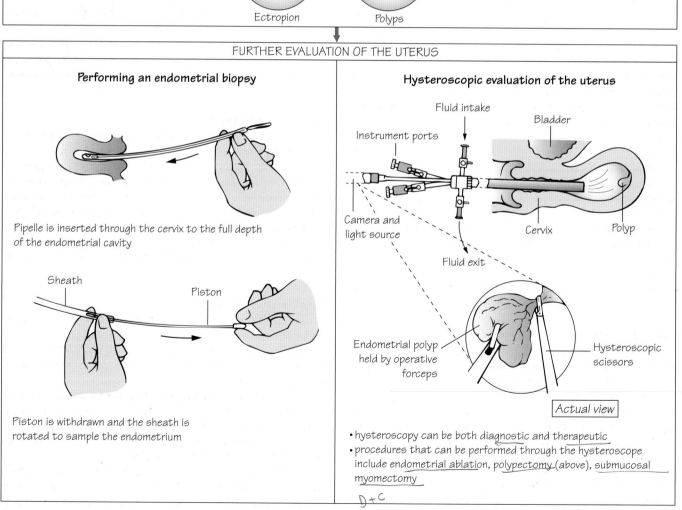

Performing an endometrial biopsy

Pipelle is inserted through the cervix to the full depth of the endometrial cavity

Sheath

Piston

Piston is withdrawn and the sheath is rotated to sample the endometrium

Hysteroscopic evaluation of the uterus

Fluid intake

Bladder

Instrument ports

Camera and light source

Cervix

Polyp

Fluid exit

Endometrial polyp held by operative forceps

Hysteroscopic scissors

Actual view

- hysteroscopy can be both diagnostic and therapeutic
- procedures that can be performed through the hysteroscope include endometrial ablation, polypectomy (above), submucosal myomectomy

D + C

Definitions

- *Menorrhagia:* prolonged (>7 days) and/or heavy (>80 mL) uterine bleeding occurring at regular intervals.
- *Metrorrhagia*: variable amounts of inter-menstrual bleeding occurring at irregular but frequent intervals.
- *Polymenorrhea*: an abnormally short interval (<21 days) between regular menses.
- *Oligomenorrhea:* an abnormally long interval (>35 days) between regular menses.

Causes of abnormal vaginal bleeding

Organic causes (opposite)

1 Reproductive tract disease
- *Pregnancy-related conditions* are the most common causes of abnormal vaginal bleeding in reproductive-age women (threatened, incomplete, and missed abortion [Chapter 15]; ectopic pregnancy [Chapter 5]; gestational trophoblastic disease [Chapter 32]). Implantation bleeding is also quite common at about the time of the 1st missed menstrual period.
- *Uterine lesions* commonly produce menorrhagia or metrorrhagia by increasing endometrial surface area, distorting the endometrial vasculature, or having a friable/inflamed surface.
- *Cervical lesions* usually result in metrorrhagia (especially post-coital bleeding) due to erosion or direct trauma.
- *Iatrogenic causes* include the intrauterine device (IUD), oral/injectable steroids for contraception or hormone replacement, and tranquilizers or other psychotropic drugs. Oral contraceptives are often associated with irregular bleeding during the first 3 months of use, if doses are missed, or if the patient is a smoker. Long-acting progesterone-only contraceptives (Depo-Provera, Implanon) frequently cause irregular bleeding. Some patients may be unknowingly taking herbal medications (St. John's wort, ginseng) that have an impact on the endometrium.

2 Systemic disease
- Blood dyscrasias such as von Willebrand's disease and prothrombin deficiency may present with profuse vaginal bleeding during adolescence. Other disorders that produce platelet deficiency (leukaemia, severe sepsis) may also present as irregular bleeding.
- Hypothyroidism is frequently associated with menorrhagia and/or metrorrhagia. Hyperthyroidism is usually not associated with menstrual abnormalities, but oligomenorrhoea and amenorrhea are possible.
- Cirrhosis is associated with excessive bleeding secondary to the reduced capacity of the liver to metabolize estrogens.

Dysfunctional (endocrinological) causes

The diagnosis of dysfunctional uterine bleeding (DUB) can be made after organic, systemic, and iatrogenic causes for abnormal vaginal bleeding have been ruled out (diagnosis of exclusion).

1 **Anovulatory DUB**
- The predominant type in the post-menarcheal and pre-menopausal years due to alterations in neuroendocrinological function.
- Characterized by continuous production of estradiol-17β without corpus luteum formation and progesterone release.
- Unopposed estrogen leads to continuous proliferation of the endometrium which eventually outgrows its blood supply and is sloughed in an irregular, unpredictable pattern.

2 **Ovulatory DUB**
- Incidence: up to 10% of ovulatory women.

- Mid-cycle spotting following the LH surge is usually physiologic. Polymenorrhoea is most often due to shortening of the follicular phase of menstruation. Alternatively, the luteal phase may be prolonged by a persistent corpus luteum.

Diagnosis

- Patient age is the most important factor in the evaluation.
- Ruling out pregnancy-related complications should be the *first priority* in all reproductive-age women.
- A complete list of medications is essential to rule out their interference with normal menstruation.
- Non-gynaecological physical findings (thyromegaly, hepatomegaly) may suggest the presence of an underlying systemic disorder. Genito-urinary (urinary infection) or gastrointestinal (haemorrhoids) bleeding may be mistakenly interpreted by the patient as vaginal bleeding.
- Pelvic examination may reveal an obvious structural abnormality (cervical polyp), but frequently additional evaluation is necessary.
- Measurement of serum haemoglobin concentration, iron levels, and ferritin levels are objective measures of the quantity and duration of menstrual blood loss. Additional laboratory tests (thyroid-stimulating hormone, coagulation profile) may be indicated.
- A *menstrual calendar* may be helpful in accurately determining the amount, frequency, and duration of the bleeding.
- Ovulation can be assessed by careful history-taking and, if necessary, *ovulation prediction kits* (Chapter 23).
- Further evaluation of the uterus (*opposite*) can be achieved in non-pregnant women by performing an *endometrial biopsy* or *hysteroscopy*. *Pelvic ultrasound* may also be indicated if the cause of bleeding cannot be confirmed.

Medical management

The majority of women with abnormal vaginal bleeding can be treated medically, particularly in the absence of a structural lesion.
- *Oral contraceptives* effectively correct the vast majority of common menstrual irregularities (anovulatory and ovulatory DUB). However, DUB can occasionally present as an acute haemorrhage requiring short-term, high-dose oral or intravenous estrogen therapy to transiently support the endometrium.
- *Non-steroidal anti-inflammatory drugs* (mefenamic acid) have been shown to reduce menstrual blood loss, particularly in ovulatory patients.

Surgical management

Structural abnormalities frequently require surgical intervention to alleviate symptoms.
- *Dilatation and curettage (D & C)* can be both diagnostic and therapeutic, especially in women with acute vaginal bleeding due to endometrial overgrowth.
- *Hysteroscopy* is an office or day-surgery procedure that can be used to diagnose and treat abnormal uterine lesions. The uterine cavity is distended with fluid, allowing direct visualization of the abnormality and use of hysteroscopic instruments. *Endometrial ablation* can dramatically reduce the amount of cyclic blood loss.
- *Hysterectomy* (Chapter 16) is usually reserved for women with structural lesions not amenable to more conservative surgery (multiple large leiomyomas, uterine prolapse). It may also be indicated in women with persistent DUB, but only if medical therapy has failed.

5 Ectopic pregnancy

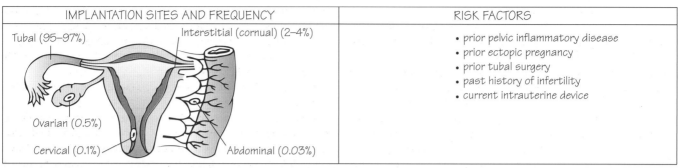

IMPLANTATION SITES AND FREQUENCY

Tubal (95–97%)
Interstitial (cornual) (2–4%)
Ovarian (0.5%)
Cervical (0.1%)
Abdominal (0.03%)

RISK FACTORS

- prior pelvic inflammatory disease
- prior ectopic pregnancy
- prior tubal surgery
- past history of infertility
- current intrauterine device

DIAGNOSIS

- history
- examination
- serial β-hCG measurements
- ultrasound
- culdocentesis
  – with upward traction on the posterior lip of the cervix, the needle is advanced into the posterior vaginal fornix

Uterus
Tenaculum
20 cc syringe with 18 gauge spinal needle
Peritoneal cavity

MEDICAL THERAPY

Criteria for receiving methotrexate	Contraindications to medical therapy

Absolute indications
  Haemodynamically stable without active bleeding or signs of hemoperitoneum
  Patient desires future fertility
  General anaesthesia poses significant risk
  Patient is able to return for follow-up care
Relative indications
  Unruptured mass <3.5 cm at its greatest dimension
  No fetal cardiac motion detected
  Patient whose β-hCG level does not exceed 6000 mIU/mL
	Absolute contraindications
	  Breast-feeding
	  Immunodeficiency
	  Alcoholism or other chronic liver disease
	  Blood dyscrasias,
	  Leukopenia, thrombocytopenia, or significant anaemia
	  Known sensitivity to methotrexate
	  Active pulmonary disease
	  Peptic ulcer disease
	  Hepatic, renal or haematologic dysfunction
	Relative contraindications
	  Gestational sac > 3.5 cm
	  Embryonic cardiac motion

Medical therapy

Surgical therapy

Definitive surgery (salpingectomy)

Conservative surgery

LAPAROSCOPIC LINEAR SALPINGOSTOMY FOR TUBAL ECTOPIC PREGNANCY

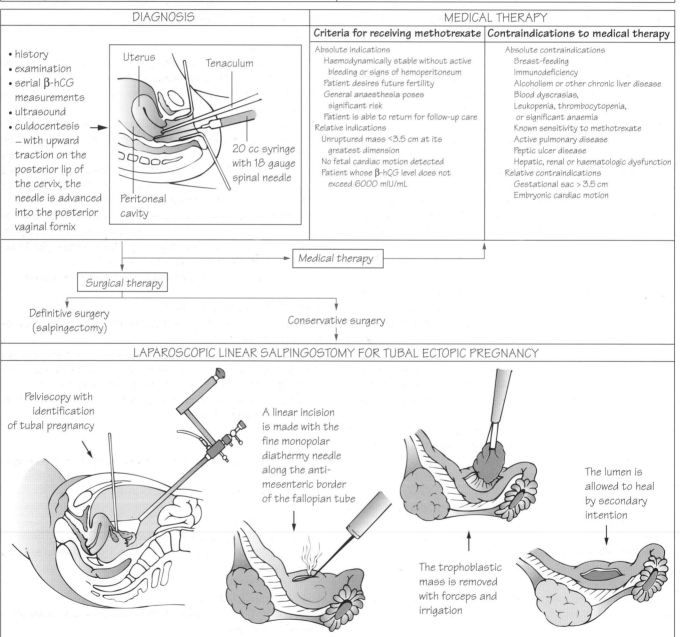

Pelviscopy with identification of tubal pregnancy

A linear incision is made with the fine monopolar diathermy needle along the anti-mesenteric border of the fallopian tube

The trophoblastic mass is removed with forceps and irrigation

The lumen is allowed to heal by secondary intention

Definition

Any gestation in which implantation occurs at a location other than the endometrial lining *(opposite)*.

Epidemiology and risk factors

• *Incidence* in the UK and USA is roughly 20/1000 conceptions.
• *Mortality:* 10% of pregnancy-related maternal deaths (most common cause of death in the first half of pregnancy).
• *Risk factors: (opposite)* past history of *pelvic inflammatory disease* (Chapter 8), especially that caused by *Chlamydia trachomatis* is most important. However, >50% of patients have no risk factors.
• *Aetiology.* The major cause of ectopic pregnancy is *acute salpingitis*: permanent agglutination of the folds of the endosalpinx can allow passage of the smaller sperm while the fertilized ovum (morula) gets trapped in blind pockets formed by adhesions. Contraception failure, hormonal alterations, and previous termination also contribute to an increased risk of ectopic pregnancy.

Symptoms and signs

Frequently the diagnosis is established before symptoms or signs develop due to the use of early serum testing and vaginal sonography.
• *Abdominal pain, absence of menses, and irregular vaginal bleeding* (usually spotting) are the main symptoms.
• Ruptured ectopic pregnancies cause shoulder pain in 10–20% of cases as a result of diaphragmatic irritation from the haemoperitoneum. Syncope also may occur due to intense, sudden pain. Other symptoms may include dizziness and an urge to defecate.
• The most common presenting sign in a woman with symptomatic ectopic pregnancy is *abdominal tenderness*. Half of women will have a palpable adnexal mass. Profound intraperitoneal haemorrhage will lead to tachycardia and hypotension.

Diagnosis *(opposite)*

A thorough history and physical examination are essential. The extent should be dictated by the severity of symptoms at presentation.
• Serial quantitative levels of the *β-subunit of human chorionic gonadotropin (β-hCG)* are important. In normal early pregnancy, serum β-hCG levels should double every 48 hours.
• *Transvaginal sonography* can detect an intrauterine gestational sac at a serum β-hCG level of 1000–1200 mIU/mL (approximately 5 weeks from LMP). ≥6000 mIU/mL is required to see an intrauterine gestational sac by trans-abdominal sonography.
• *Culdocentesis* may be performed in the office or emergency room and can quickly confirm the presence of free blood in the peritoneal cavity. When 10 mL of non-clotting blood is aspirated, the test is positive.
• *Uterine curettage* can effectively exclude an ectopic pregnancy by demonstrating pathological evidence of products of conception if the pregnancy is undesired.
• *Laparoscopy* (Chapter 16) may ultimately be indicated in some circumstances to make the diagnosis and initiate treatment.

Management

Due to earlier diagnosis, the goal of treatment has shifted from preventing mortality to reducing morbidity and preserving fertility.

Medical therapy *(opposite)*

• *Methotrexate (MTX)* (50 mg/m² intramuscular injection) is effective treatment for select patients who meet criteria. The dose is administered on day 1, but serum β-hCG levels may continue to rise for several days. An acceptable response is defined as a ≤15% decrease in serum β-hCG levels from day 4 to day 7. β-hCG levels should thereafter be followed weekly.
• Most cases will be successfully treated with one dose of MTX, but up to 25% will require two or more doses if the β-hCG level eventually plateaus or rises. Patients with a gestational sac >3.5 cm, β-hCG >6000 mIU/mL or fetal cardiac motion are at higher risk for MTX 'failure' and should be considered for surgical management.
• MTX side-effects (nausea, vomiting, bloating, transient transaminitis) are generally mild.
• Increased abdominal pain will occur in up to 75% of patients due to tubal abortion or serosal irritation as a result of haematoma stretching. Sonography can be used to rule out significant haemoperitoneum. However, all MTX patients should be closely monitored during follow-up due to the risk of rupture and haemorrhage.

Surgical therapy

• Definitive surgery (salpingectomy) is the treatment of choice for women who present *haemodynamically unstable*.
• Conservative surgery is entirely appropriate for the *haemodynamically stable* patient.
  1 *Laparoscopic linear salpingostomy (opposite)* is the most common procedure. The injection of vasopressin prior to the linear incision can be used to markedly decrease bleeding. Serum β-hCG levels must be followed until undetectable in conservatively managed patients because 5–10% will develop a *persistent ectopic pregnancy* which may require further treatment with MTX.
  2 Partial salpingectomy involves removal of the damaged portion of the fallopian tube and is indicated when there is extensive damage or continued bleeding after salpingostomy. This procedure should not be performed unless re-anastomosis is planned.
• The only indication for oophorectomy is to achieve haemostasis.

Interstitial (cornual) pregnancy

• Implantation of the embryo into the fallopian tube where it passes through the myometrium.
• Frequently associated with severe morbidity because patients become symptomatic later in gestation, are difficult to diagnose and lesions often produce massive haemorrhage when they rupture.
• Laparotomy with *cornual resection* or *hysterectomy* is often required.
• Maternal mortality rate is 2%.

Ovarian pregnancy

• Patients are usually thought to clinically have a ruptured corpus luteum cyst.
• Usually associated with profuse haemorrhage.

Cervical pregnancy

• Most occur after a previous sharp uterine curettage.
• May be successfully treated by MTX, but more advanced cases require hysterectomy.

Abdominal pregnancy

• Most occur secondary to tubal abortion with secondary implantation in the peritoneal cavity.
• Laparotomy with removal of the fetus is necessary. The placenta may be ligated and left *in situ* since it often derives its blood supply from the gastrointestinal tract and can be difficult to remove.

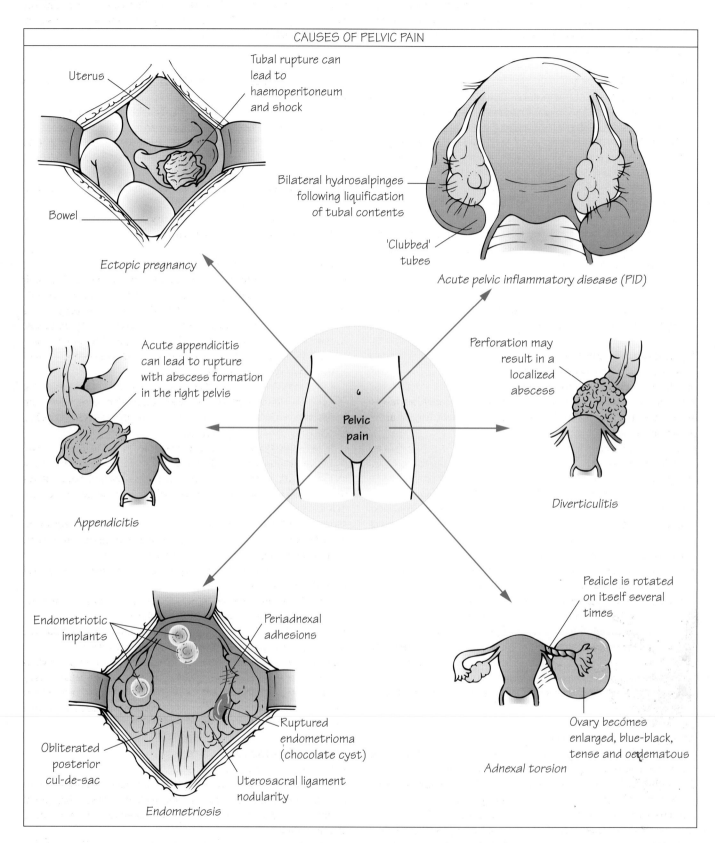

CAUSES OF PELVIC PAIN

Uterus

Tubal rupture can lead to haemoperitoneum and shock

Bowel

Ectopic pregnancy

Bilateral hydrosalpinges following liquification of tubal contents

'Clubbed' tubes

Acute pelvic inflammatory disease (PID)

Acute appendicitis can lead to rupture with abscess formation in the right pelvis

Appendicitis

Perforation may result in a localized abscess

Diverticulitis

Endometriotic implants

Periadnexal adhesions

Ruptured endometrioma (chocolate cyst)

Obliterated posterior cul-de-sac

Uterosacral ligament nodularity

Endometriosis

Pedicle is rotated on itself several times

Ovary becomes enlarged, blue-black, tense and oedematous

Adnexal torsion

Pelvic pain

- Pelvic pain is a subjective perception rather than an objective sensation, making evaluation of the patient difficult.
- Pelvic pain associated with menses is the most common gynaecological pain complaint. However, domestic discord, physical or sexual abuse, rape, alcohol, or drug abuse, or other stresses may all be expressed in the form of pain.

Evaluation strategies
- The history provides a description of the nature, intensity, and distribution of the pain. However, imprecise localization is typical with intra-abdominal processes.
- The physical examination includes a comprehensive gynaecological examination. Specific attention should be paid to reproducing the pain symptoms.
- Chlamydia/gonorrhoea cervical cultures and urinalysis with culture are frequently helpful.
- Ultrasonography and other imaging studies may be indicated.
- Specialized diagnostic studies based on the presumptive diagnosis may require consultation with other specialists in anaesthesiology, orthopaedics, neurology, or gastroenterology.

Acute pelvic pain
Acute pelvic pain requires aggressive management because of the possibility that a life-threatening condition exists.

Gynaecological causes
Most general gynaecological causes of acute pelvic pain can be divided into three categories: infection, rupture, and torsion.
- *Ectopic pregnancy* (*opposite*; Chapter 5). In all reproductive-age women, the first priority in evaluating acute pelvic pain is to rule out the possibility of a ruptured ectopic pregnancy.
- *Acute pelvic inflammatory disease* (PID) (*opposite*; Chapter 8) is an ascending bacterial infection that often presents with high fever, severe pelvic pain, nausea and evidence of cervical motion tenderness in sexually active women.
- *Rupture of an ovarian cyst.* Intra-abdominal rupture of a follicular cyst, corpus luteum, or endometrioma is a common cause of acute pelvic pain. The pain may be severe enough to cause syncope. The condition is usually self-limiting with limited intra-peritoneal bleeding.
- *Adnexal torsion* (*opposite*) is seen most commonly in adolescent or reproductive-age women. By twisting on its vascular pedicle, any adnexal mass (ovarian dermoid, hydatid of Morgagni) can cause severe pain by suddenly compromising its blood supply. The pain will frequently wax and wane with associated nausea and vomiting.
- *Threatened*, *inevitable*, or *incomplete miscarriages* are generally accompanied by midline pelvic pain, usually of a crampy, intermittent nature (Chapter 15).
- *Degenerating fibroids* or *ovarian tumours* may cause localized sharp or aching pain.

Non-gynaecological causes
- *Appendicitis* (*opposite*) is the most common acute surgical condition of the abdomen, occurring in all age groups. Classically, the pain is initially diffuse and centered in the umbilical area but, after several hours, localizes to the right lower quadrant (McBurney's point). It is often accompanied by low-grade fever, anorexia, and leucocytosis.
- *Diverticulitis* (*opposite*) occurs most frequently in older women. It is characterized by left-sided pelvic pain, bloody diarrhoea, fever, and leucocytosis.

- *Urinary tract disorders* (cystitis, pyelonephritis, renal calculi) can cause acute or referred suprapubic pain, pressure, and/or dysuria.
- *Mesenteric lymphadenitis* most often follows an upper respiratory infection in young girls. The pain is usually more diffuse and less severe than in appendicitis.

Chronic pelvic pain
Unrelieved pain that has continued to be a major, disabling condition for at least 6 months.
- 10–20% of hysterectomies are performed for this indication.
- There is often little correlation between the objective severity of abdominal disease and the amount of perceived pain: 1/3 of women who undergo laparoscopy for chronic pelvic pain will have no identifiable cause.
- Depression and sleep disturbance are commonly associated with psychological diagnoses.
- Women are much more likely to have been victims of sexual abuse.
- Difficult to cure or manage adequately.

Gynaecological causes
- *Dysmenorrhoea* is the most common cause of chronic pelvic pain. It is defined as cyclic uterine pain occurring before or during menses. Primary dysmenorrhoea is not associated with pelvic pathology, and is thought to be due to excessive prostaglandin production by the uterus. Secondary dysmenorrhoea is usually due to acquired conditions (such as endometriosis). Oral contraceptives and non-steroidal anti-inflammatory drugs are helpful.
- *Endometriosis* (*opposite*; Chapter 11) has a spectrum of pain that ranges from dysmenorrhoea to severe, intractable, continuous pain which may be disabling. The severity of pain often does not correlate with the degree of pelvic pathology.
- *Adenomyosis* (Chapter 11) is a common condition that is usually only identified by hysterectomy. Most frequently, women are asymptomatic and this is an incidental pathology finding. An enlarged, boggy uterus that is mildly tender to bi-manual palpation is suggestive of the diagnosis.
- *Fibroids* (Chapter 10) are the most frequent (benign) tumours found in the female pelvis. They may cause pain either by putting pressure on adjacent organs or by undergoing degeneration.
- *Retained ovarian syndrome* is characterized by recurrent adnexal pain after hysterectomy.
- *Genital prolapse* (Chapter 18) may lead to complaints of heaviness, pressure, a dropping sensation, or pelvic aching.
- *Chronic PID* is characterized by continued pelvic pain, usually as a result of hydrosalpinx, tubo-ovarian cyst, or pelvic adhesions.
- ***Treatment:*** nutritional supplementation, physical therapy modalities, acupuncture/acupressure, anti-depressants, surgical adhesiolysis. Hysterectomy is highly effective in improving pelvic pain, psychological symptoms, sexual dysfunction, and quality of life even if no uterine pathology can be identified.

Non-gynaecological causes
- *Adhesions* after infection or surgery.
- *Gastrointestinal disturbances* such as inflammatory bowel disease (Crohn's disease, ulcerative colitis), constipation, and faecal impaction.
- *Musculoskeletal problems* such as faulty posture, muscle strain, or disc herniation.
- *Interstitial cystitis* (a chronic inflammatory condition of the bladder).

7 Lower genital tract infections

VAGINITIS		
Bacterial vaginosis	**Candidiasis**	**Trichomoniasis**

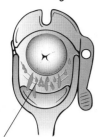

Thin, homogeneous, malodorous (fishy) white-grey vaginal discharge

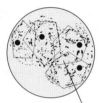

Saline wet mount

'Clue cells' with adherent coccoid bacteria, no leukocytes, absent lactobacilli

Vaginal pH > 4.5 (normal 3.8–4.2)

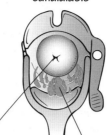

Vagina is often hyperemic and oedematous

Thick, white non-malodorous discharge that appears 'cottage cheese'-like

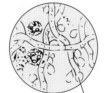

KOH wet mount

Budding yeast, hyphal forms

Vaginal pH ≤ 4.5 (usually)

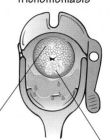

'Strawberry' appearance of cervix due to small petechial haemorrhages

Copious greenish-yellow discharge with frothy appearance

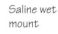

Saline wet mount

Trichomonads (mobile protozoa with four flagellae and central nucleus)

Lymphocytes >10/HPF

Vaginal pH > 4.5

INFECTIONS OF THE VULVA		
Genital warts	**Genital herpes**	**Bartholin's gland abscess**

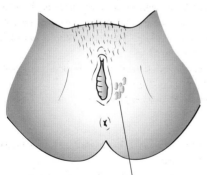

Lesions appear as multiple, exophytic painless excrescences around the labia and perineum. When numerous, they may give rise to a confluent cauliflower-like mass

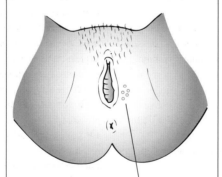

Groups of vesicles which are fragile and tend to break forming small ulcers
• major symptoms are burning pain and local pruritus

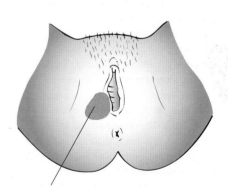

Tender, red, fluctuant mass
• occur in the labia minora/ labia majora fold at 5- or 7-o'clock
• major symptoms are fever and acute unilateral vulvar pain

Vulvovaginitis is the most common gynaecological problem for which women seek treatment. Symptoms may include vaginal discharge, vulvar pruritis and vaginal odour. The aetiological agents responsible can commonly be identified in the office by obtaining an appropriate sample of the vaginal discharge for microscopic examination.

Bacterial vaginosis (BV) *(opposite)*
• *Aetiology:* overgrowth of several bacterial species in the vagina — specifically a decrease in lactobacilli and an increase in anaerobic organisms.
• *Incidence:* the most common cause of vaginitis in young women.
• *Symptoms:* non-pruritic vaginal discharge with a "fishy" odour, but 50% of women are asymptomatic.
• *Diagnosis:* positive KOH whiff test, pH >4.5, clue cells on saline wet-mount, homogeneous discharge (need 3 out of 4 clinical criteria).
• *Treatment:* oral/intravaginal metronidazole or clindamycin.

Candidiasis *(opposite)*
• *Aetiology:* over 200 strains of *Candida albicans* can colonize and cause vaginitis. It is unknown why *Candida* is pathogenic in some women, but not in others.
• *Incidence:* the second most common cause of symptomatic vaginitis.
• *Symptoms:* intense pruritus and vulvovaginal erythema.
• *Diagnosis:* KOH wet-mount to see the presence of branched and budding hyphae. Culture in Sabouraud's medium may be indicated for selected cases.
• *Treatment:* topical clotrimazole (Canestin) or oral fluconazole (Diflucan).

Trichomoniasis *(opposite)*
• *Aetiology: Trichomonas vaginalis* is an anaerobic protozoan and humans are the only known host.
• *Incidence:* this common sexually transmitted disease (*STD*) affects 180 million women worldwide.
• *Symptoms:* profuse malodorous vaginal discharge, post-coital bleeding, vulvovaginal erthyema.
• *Diagnosis:* trichomonads seen on saline wet-mount are pathognomonic. Other features include an abundance of leucocytes and pH >4.5. Organisms may be evident on a Pap smear in asymptomatic women.
• *Treatment:* oral metronidazole.

Chlamydial cervicitis
• *Aetiology: Chlamydia trachomatis* is an obligate intracellular bacterial parasite of columnar epithelial cells.
• *Incidence:* the most prevalent *STD* in the UK and USA. 30% of infections are associated with gonorrhoea.
• *Symptoms:* purulent or mucoid discharge, post-coital bleeding and vaginitis, but many asymptomatic women are identified through screening or contact tracing.
• *Diagnosis:* DNA probe test or enzyme-linked immunosorbent assay.
• *Treatment:* oral azithromycin or doxycycline.

Gonococcal cervicitis/vaginitis
• *Aetiology: Neisseria gonorrhoeae* is a gram-negative aerobic diplococcus.
• *Incidence:* common but less prevalent *STD* than chlamydia.
• *Symptoms:* profuse, odourless, non-irritating, creamy white or yellow vaginal discharge, but may also be asymptomatic. 10–20% of women develop acute salpingitis with fever and pelvic pain. 5%

exhibit disseminated gonorrhoea infection with chills, fever, malaise, asymmetric polyarthralgias, and painful skin lesions.
• *Diagnosis:* a positive culture on selective media such as modified Thayer–Martin agar. 20% of patients will have detectable infection at multiple sites (pharynx, rectum).
• *Treatment:* oral ciprofloxacin (USA practice favours intramuscular ceftriaxone or oral cefixime).

Genital warts (condyloma acuminatum) *(opposite)*
• *Aetiology: Human papillomavirus* (HPV) infection is transmitted by skin-to-skin contact.
• *Incidence:* the most common viral *STD*.
• *Symptoms:* uncomplicated cases are asymptomatic.
• *Diagnosis:* usually clinical inspection is sufficient, but colposcopy and/or biopsy may be required.
• *Treatment:* office cryotherapy or other less common options depending on the extent: outpatient laser surgery, local cytotoxic agents (trichloroacetic acid, podofilox).

Genital herpes *(opposite)*
• *Aetiology: Herpes simplex virus* (HSV) type 1 (15%) or type 2 (85%).
• *Incidence:* this *STD* is the most common cause of genital ulcers.
• *Symptoms:* first episode primary HSV infection is characterized by systemic symptoms, including malaise and fever. However, genital herpes is a recurrent infection with periods of active infection separated by periods of latency.
• *Diagnosis:* usually clinical inspection is sufficient, but viral isolation by tissue culture is also very reliable.
• *Treatment:* oral acyclovir or valacyclovir (topicals are not effective).

Syphilis
• *Aetiology:* The spirochete *Treponema pallidum*.
• *Incidence:* an endemic *STD* in Europe in the 15th century, but its prevalence has declined dramatically.
• *Symptoms:* a systemic disease with myriad clinical presentations. Primary infection is marked by a painless, solitary ulcer at the site of acquisition. Secondary symptoms include a facial-sparing rash with involvement of the palms and soles. The classic skin lesion of late syphilis is the solitary gumma nodule.
• *Diagnosis:* dark-field examination of scrapings from a lesion and/or serologic screening (rapid plasma reagin test).
• *Treatment:* intramuscular benzathine penicillin.

Other infections
• *Bartholin's gland abscess (opposite). **Treatment:*** surgical incision and placement of a Word catheter.
• *Pediculosis pubis* (scabies) is an intensely pruritic *STD* caused by the crab louse. ***Treatment:*** lindane (Kwell).
• *Molluscum contagiosum* is an asymptomatic, papular *STD* of the vulva caused by the poxvirus. Most cases resolve without treatment.
• *Necrotizing fasciitis* is a rapidly progressive, frequently fatal infection. ***Treatment:*** immediate wide surgical debridement and parenteral antibiotics.
• *Hydradenitis suppurativa* is a staphylococcal or streptococcal infection of the vulvar apocrine glands. ***Treatment:*** excision.
• Rare vulvar STDs include: *lymphogranuloma venereum* (caused by *Chlamydia trachomatis*), *chancroid* (caused by *Haemophilus ducreyi*), *donovanosis/granuloma inguinale* (caused by *Calymmatobacterium granulomatis*).

8 Pelvic inflammatory disease (PID)

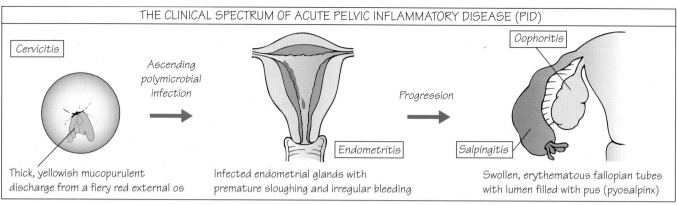

THE CLINICAL SPECTRUM OF ACUTE PELVIC INFLAMMATORY DISEASE (PID)

Cervicitis

Ascending polymicrobial infection

Oophoritis

Endometritis

Salpingitis

Thick, yellowish mucopurulent discharge from a fiery red external os

Infected endometrial glands with premature sloughing and irregular bleeding

Swollen, erythematous fallopian tubes with lumen filled with pus (pyosalpinx)

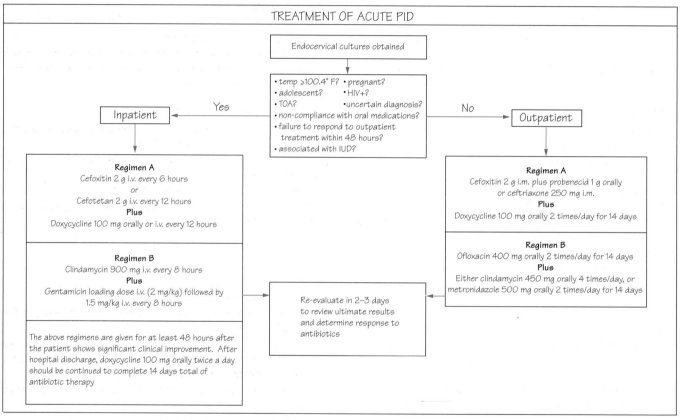

TREATMENT OF ACUTE PID

Endocervical cultures obtained

- temp ≥100.4° F? • pregnant?
- adolescent? • HIV+?
- TOA? • uncertain diagnosis?
- non-compliance with oral medications?
- failure to respond to outpatient treatment within 48 hours?
- associated with IUD?

Inpatient ← Yes | No → **Outpatient**

Regimen A
Cefoxitin 2 g i.v. every 6 hours
or
Cefotetan 2 g i.v. every 12 hours
Plus
Doxycycline 100 mg orally or i.v. every 12 hours

Regimen B
Clindamycin 900 mg i.v. every 8 hours
Plus
Gentamicin loading dose i.v. (2 mg/kg) followed by 1.5 mg/kg i.v. every 8 hours

The above regimens are given for at least 48 hours after the patient shows significant clinical improvement. After hospital discharge, doxycycline 100 mg orally twice a day should be continued to complete 14 days total of antibiotic therapy

Re-evaluate in 2–3 days to review ultimate results and determine response to antibiotics

Regimen A
Cefoxitin 2 g i.m. plus probenecid 1 g orally or ceftriaxone 250 mg i.m.
Plus
Doxycycline 100 mg orally 2 times/day for 14 days

Regimen B
Ofloxacin 400 mg orally 2 times/day for 14 days
Plus
Either clindamycin 450 mg orally 4 times/day, or metronidazole 500 mg orally 2 times/day for 14 days

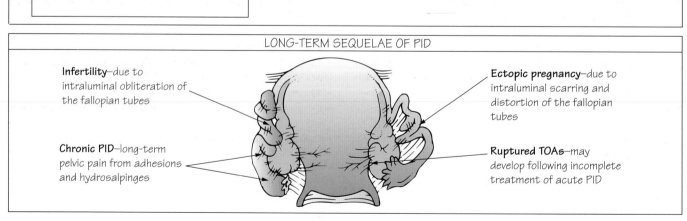

LONG-TERM SEQUELAE OF PID

Infertility–due to intraluminal obliteration of the fallopian tubes

Ectopic pregnancy–due to intraluminal scarring and distortion of the fallopian tubes

Chronic PID–long-term pelvic pain from adhesions and hydrosalpinges

Ruptured TOAs–may develop following incomplete treatment of acute PID

The most common gynaecological disorder necessitating hospitalization for reproductive-age women in the USA and UK.

Definition
• A clinical spectrum of infection *(opposite)* that may involve the cervix, endometrium, fallopian tubes, ovaries, uterus, broad ligaments, intra-peritoneal cavity, and perihepatic region.
• Acute PID (acute salpingitis) refers to the acute clinical syndrome of ascending infection.
• Chronic PID is an outdated term that refers to the long-term sequelae.

Aetiology
• The pathogenesis is incompletely understood, but involves a polymicrobial infection ascending from the bacterial flora of the vagina and cervix.
• *Chlamydia trachomatis* and/or *Neisseria gonorrhoeae* are detectable in >50% of women. These pathogens are probably responsible for the initial invasion of the upper genital tract, with other organisms becoming involved secondarily.
• 15% of cases follow a surgical procedure (endometrial biopsy, intrauterine device (IUD) placement) which breaks the cervical mucous barrier and directly transmits vaginal bacteria to the upper genital tract.

Risk factors
• Classically, the highest risk woman is a menstruating teenager who has multiple sexual partners, does not use contraception and lives in an area with a high prevalence of *STDs*.
• The incidence decreases with advancing age: 75% of patients are <25 years.
• Having multiple partners increases the risk by 5-fold.
• Frequent vaginal douching increases the risk by 3-fold.
• Pre-menarchal, pregnant or post-menopausal women rarely contract PID.
• Women who have an IUD are at increased risk, but barrier (condom, diaphragm) and oral contraceptives decrease the risk.
• Previous PID is a risk factor for future episodes: 25% of women will develop another infection.

Symptoms and signs
• Pain in the lower abdomen and pelvis is the most common complaint. However, many women experience minimal or no discernible symptoms.
• 75% of women have a mucopurulent cervical discharge.
• Abnormal vaginal bleeding, especially metrorrhagia, is common.
• One-third present with a fever ≤38°C.
• Nausea and vomiting are usually late symptoms.
• 5% of women will present with *Fitz–Hugh–Curtis syndrome* (perihepatic inflammation and adhesions). This condition is characterized by pleuritic upper quadrant pain, and is often mistakenly diagnosed as pneumonia or acute cholecystitis.

Diagnosis
• The clinical features of PID are often enigmatic, making diagnosis difficult.

• Women meeting the clinical and laboratory criteria for PID may have a separate pathological process (appendicitis, endometriosis, rupture of an adnexal mass) or a normal pelvis in up to 50% of cases.
• Endocervical cultures for chlamydia and gonorrhoea should be obtained at presentation.
• Ultrasonographic detection of an abscess, purulent fluid on culdocentesis, and/or an elevated erythrocyte sediment rate may be helpful.
• The most accurate method of diagnosis of acute PID is direct visualization during laparoscopy.

Treatment of acute PID *(opposite)*
• Antibiotic treatment should be started as soon as possible.
• 75% of women can be managed as outpatients.
• Tuboovarian abscesses (TOAs) should be drained immediately.
• Management should include treatment of male partners and education for the prevention of re-infection.

Surgical management
• Indicated for patients with either a ruptured TOA or a TOA that does not respond to conservative therapy.
• Every effort should be made to preserve the reproductive organs if future fertility is desired. However, bilateral salpingo-oophorectomy with hysterectomy may be required.

Long-term sequelae of PID *(opposite)*
• *Infertility* occurs in 10% of women with a single episode of acute PID and depends on the severity of the infection.
• *Chronic PID* is a recurrent pain syndrome that develops in 20% of women as a result of inflammation.
• *Ectopic pregnancy* is increased 6- to 10-fold.
• *Ruptured TOAs* have a 5–10% risk of death due chiefly to the development of adult respiratory distress syndrome.

Rare causes of pelvic inflammatory disease
Actinomycosis
• A rare cause of upper genital tract infection.
• *Actinomyces israelii* is an anaerobic, gram-positive, non-acid-fast pleomorphic bacterium.
• The diagnosis should be suspected if such organisms are identified on cervical gram stain or if an endometrial biopsy shows 'sulphur granules.' However definitive diagnosis requires a positive culture.
• *Treatment:* high-dose parenteral penicillin plus oral doxycycline for 6 weeks.

Pelvic tuberculosis
• Rarely identified in developed countries, but is a common cause of chronic PID and infertility in the Third World.
• *Mycobacterium tuberculosis* is the causative agent.
• Definitive diagnosis requires histological evidence of granulomas, giant cells, and caseous necrosis.
• *Treatment:* multiple antituberculosis drugs for 18–24 months.

9 Benign disorders of the lower genital tract

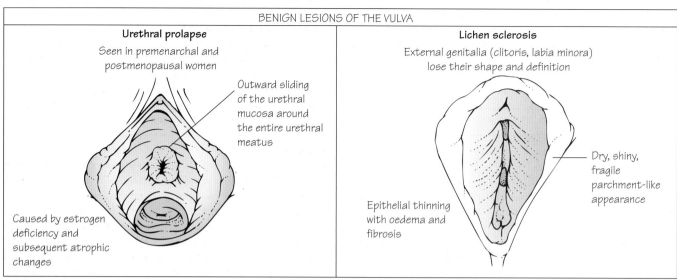

BENIGN LESIONS OF THE VULVA

Urethral prolapse

Seen in premenarchal and postmenopausal women

Outward sliding of the urethral mucosa around the entire urethral meatus

Caused by estrogen deficiency and subsequent atrophic changes

Lichen sclerosis

External genitalia (clitoris, labia minora) lose their shape and definition

Dry, shiny, fragile parchment-like appearance

Epithelial thinning with oedema and fibrosis

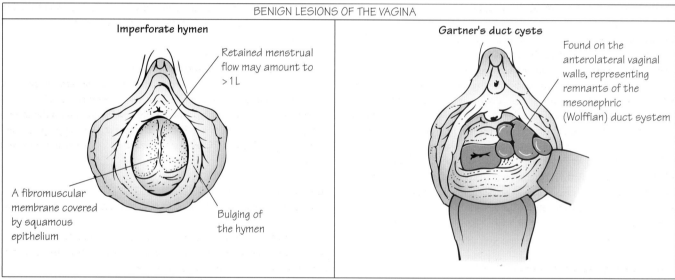

BENIGN LESIONS OF THE VAGINA

Imperforate hymen

Retained menstrual flow may amount to >1 L

A fibromuscular membrane covered by squamous epithelium

Bulging of the hymen

Gartner's duct cysts

Found on the anterolateral vaginal walls, representing remnants of the mesonephric (Wolffian) duct system

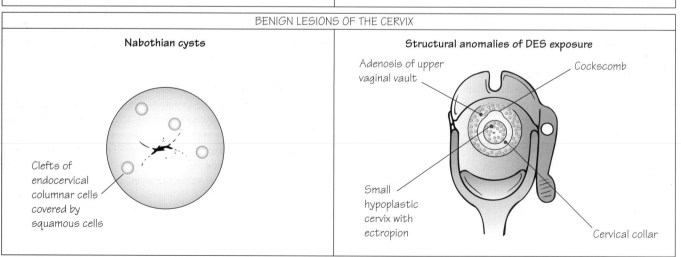

BENIGN LESIONS OF THE CERVIX

Nabothian cysts

Clefts of endocervical columnar cells covered by squamous cells

Structural anomalies of DES exposure

Adenosis of upper vaginal vault

Cockscomb

Small hypoplastic cervix with ectropion

Cervical collar

Vulvar lesions
Urethral disorders
• *Urethral prolapse (opposite)* may cause dysuria, but often is asymptomatic. *Treatment:* topical estrogen cream; hot sitz baths and antibiotics may reduce inflammation and infection; surgical excision is rarely needed.
• *Urethral diverticulum* is a sac or pouch that may cause dysuria, urgency, or haematuria. *Treatment:* excision with layered closure or marsupialization.

Vulvar cysts and benign tumours
• *Bartholin cysts* result from occlusion of the excretory duct. *Treatment:* most will resolve spontaneously, but marsupialization is performed for recurrent lesions.
• *Hernias (hydroceles, cysts) of the canal of Nuck* are abnormal dilatations of the peritoneum that accompany the round ligament through the inguinal canal and into the labia majora. *Treatment:* excision of the hernia sac.
• *Epidermal inclusion cysts* are formed when a focus of epithelium is buried beneath the skin surface and becomes encysted. *Treatment:* excision if symptomatic or if the diagnosis is unclear.

Non-neoplastic epithelial disorders
• *Lichen sclerosis (opposite)* is an atrophic change that usually occurs in post-menopausal women. The main symptom, if any, is pruritus. Diagnosis can often be made by inspection alone, but biopsy is confirmatory. *Treatment:* topical testosterone or corticosteroids.
• *Squamous cell hyperplasia* is a diagnosis of exclusion that represents a chronic reaction to fungal vulvitis, allergies, or unknown stimuli. Pruritus and excoriations are often evident. Pathological findings are non-specific. *Treatment:* management of the inciting cause and/or topical corticosteroids.
• *Lichen planus* is a chronic inflammatory dermatitis of unknown aetiology. It is characterized by multiple, small, shiny, purple cutaneous papules. *Treatment:* vaginal corticosteroid suppositories.
• *Psoriasis* is an incurable inflammatory dermatitis that may involve the vulva. Diagnosis is made by inspection and biopsy is confirmatory. *Treatment:* ultraviolet light or topical corticosteroids.

Other benign vulvar lesions
• *Vulvar vestibulitis* is a poorly understood inflammatory process that may be suggested on physical examination by reproducible exquisite pinpoint pressure tenderness. *Treatment:* topical agents or surgical excision.
• *Idiopathic vulvodynia* (vulvar pain) is a diagnosis of exclusion without specific physical findings. *Treatment:* tricyclic antidepressants.

Vaginal lesions
Congenital anomalies
• *Müllerian agenesis* (Chapter 20) results from abnormal development of the distal Müllerian ducts, and is usually associated with absence of the uterus and vagina. *Treatment:* progressive vaginal dilatation or surgical creation of a neovagina.
• *Imperforate hymen (opposite)* is a distal failure of vaginal vault canalization during embryogenesis. A *transverse vaginal septum* is a more proximal failure of vaginal vault canalization. Diagnosis is usually made at menarche when patients present with cyclic abdominal pain due to retained menstrual flow. *Treatment:* surgical excision.

Vaginal cysts and benign tumours
• *Epithelial inclusion cysts* are the most common cystic structures in the vagina, usually resulting from birth trauma or gynaecological surgery. *Treatment:* surgical excision.
• *Gartner's duct cysts (opposite)* or other embryonic epithelial remnants may be multiple and are usually an incidental finding on routine physical examination. *Treatment:* surgical excision.

Other vaginal lesions
• *Vaginal lacerations* occur most commonly secondary to sexual intercourse. Other causes include blunt trauma (straddle) injuries and penetration injuries by foreign objects. *Treatment:* surgical repair.
• *Atrophic vaginitis* is a disorder of post-menopausal women. Lack of estrogen causes the vaginal mucosa to become thin, causing dryness and bleeding. *Treatment:* oral or topical estrogen.
• *Fistulae* from the bladder, urethra, ureter, and small or large bowel may occur in any part of the vaginal canal. *Treatment:* surgical repair.
• *Foreign bodies* (retained tampons, pessaries) can lead to ulceration and infection of the vagina. *Treatment:* removal and local care.

Cervical lesions
Cervical cysts and benign tumours
• *Nabothian cysts (opposite)* are so common that they are considered a normal feature of the adult cervix. *Treatment:* none is needed.
• *Polyps* are the most common benign neoplastic growths of the cervix. They usually originate due to inflammation with focal hyperplasia and localized proliferation. *Treatment:* removal by twisting the stalk and gently pulling.

Cervical stenosis
• Acquired causes include cervical surgery, radiation, infection, neoplasia, or atrophic changes.
• Symptoms in pre-menopausal women may include dysmenorrhoea, sub-fertility, abnormal vaginal bleeding, and amenorrhoea. Post-menopausal women are usually asymptomatic.
• Complications may include development of a hydrometra (clear fluid in the uterus), haematometra (blood), or pyometra (pus). *Treatment* (if needed): cervical dilation to re-establish the patency of the canal.

Diethylstilbestrol exposure
• Diethylstilbestrol (DES) is a synthetic estrogen that was administered between the 1940s and 1970s to prevent miscarriage in some women with high-risk pregnancies.
• Women who were exposed to DES *in utero* frequently have extension of glandular epithelium on the ectocervix (ectropion) and upper vagina (vaginal adenosis). *Treatment:* none is needed.
• Structural anomalies of DES exposure *(opposite)* include *transverse ridges, collars, hoods, cockscombs, hypoplasia,* and *pseudopolyps.*

10 Benign disorders of the upper genital tract

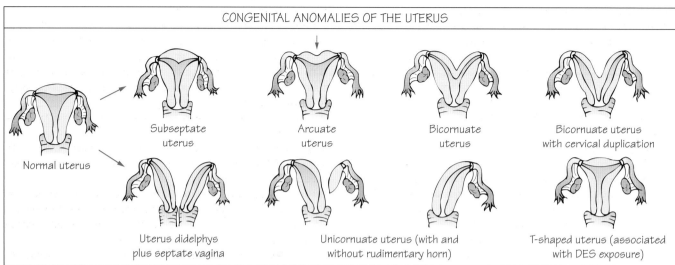

CONGENITAL ANOMALIES OF THE UTERUS

Normal uterus

Subseptate uterus

Arcuate uterus

Bicornuate uterus

Bicornuate uterus with cervical duplication

Uterus didelphys plus septate vagina

Unicornuate uterus (with and without rudimentary horn)

T-shaped uterus (associated with DES exposure)

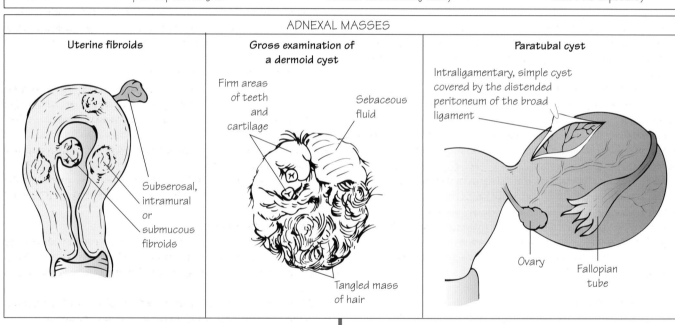

ADNEXAL MASSES

Uterine fibroids

Subserosal, intramural or submucous fibroids

Gross examination of a dermoid cyst

Firm areas of teeth and cartilage

Sebaceous fluid

Tangled mass of hair

Paratubal cyst

Intraligamentary, simple cyst covered by the distended peritoneum of the broad ligament

Ovary

Fallopian tube

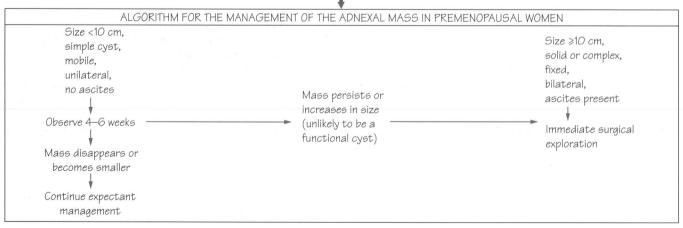

ALGORITHM FOR THE MANAGEMENT OF THE ADNEXAL MASS IN PREMENOPAUSAL WOMEN

Size <10 cm, simple cyst, mobile, unilateral, no ascites

↓

Observe 4–6 weeks → Mass persists or increases in size (unlikely to be a functional cyst) →

↓

Mass disappears or becomes smaller

↓

Continue expectant management

Size ≥10 cm, solid or complex, fixed, bilateral, ascites present

↓

Immediate surgical exploration

Uterine lesions

Congenital anomalies (opposite)
• Normal Müllerian duct fusion during embryogenesis results in a triangular-shaped uterine cavity and canalized upper vagina. Incomplete fusion results in a variety of congenital anomalies.
• *Uterine didelphys* is the most extreme form of incomplete fusion with two separate uteri and cervices and a septate upper vagina. Partial fusion is more common, resulting in an *arcuate*, *bicornuate* or *septate* uterus. A *unicornuate* uterus arises from one Müllerian duct and its attached tube; the other Müllerian duct may be rudimentary or absent.

Fibroids (leiomyomas, myomas) (opposite)
The most common neoplasm of the female pelvis.
• *Aetiology*. Uterine fibroids are benign proliferations of smooth muscle and fibrous connective tissue that originate from a single cell. They are usually multiple, range in diameter from 1mm to >20cm, and are surrounded by a pseudocapsule of compressed smooth muscle fibres. Fibroids typically arise after menarche and regress after menopause, implicating estrogen as a growth promoter.
• *Classification*. All fibroids begin within the myometrium. Continued growth in one direction will ultimately determine how the fibroid will be classified.
• *Symptoms*. Most patients are asymptomatic. The most common symptom is abnormal vaginal bleeding (usually menorrhagia). Pelvic pain or pressure and a variety of reproductive disorders (infertility, recurrent spontaneous abortion) may occur.
• *Diagnosis*. Palpation of an enlarged, irregular uterus on bi-manual examination is suggestive. Ultrasound may be used to confirm the diagnosis.
• *Expectant management*. Most patients do not require any treatment.
• *Medical management*. Gonadotropin-releasing hormone (GnRH) agonists can effectively shrink fibroids and improve symptoms by inducing a hypoestrogenic state. GnRH agonists can be used for up to 6 months unless combined with 'add-back' hormones.
• *Surgery*. Fibroids are the most common indication for hysterectomy. Conservative surgery (myomectomy) preserves fertility while achieving effective relief of symptoms. Uterine artery embolization can provide good short-term relief of bulk-related symptoms as well as a reduction in menstrual flow.

Endometrial polyps
Localized overgrowths of endometrial glands and stroma that usually arise at the uterine fundus. The majority are asymptomatic, but some present with abnormal vaginal bleeding.

Adnexal masses
Age is the most important factor for determining the potential for malignancy. 5–10% of women will have surgery for an adnexal mass during their lifetime.

Benign ovarian cystic masses
The sonographic appearance of irregular borders, ascites, papillations, or septations within an ovarian cyst should increase concern about malignancy (Chapter 31).
• *Functional cysts* are the most common clinically detectable enlargements of the ovary occurring during the reproductive years. The majority will resolve spontaneously within 4–6 weeks.
• *Dermoids (benign cystic teratomas; opposite)* represent 25% of all ovarian neoplasms. They vary in size from a few millimetres to 25 cm in diameter, and are bilateral in 10–15% of cases. They are usually complex cystic structures that contain elements from all three germ cell layers (endoderm, mesoderm, and ectoderm). 1–2% will undergo malignant transformation.
• *Serous cystadenomas* are common uni- or multilocular cysts. 10–20% are bilateral.
• *Mucinous cystadenomas* are multilocular, lobulated, and smooth-surfaced. Bilateral lesions are rare. These lesions may become huge, occasionally weighing >50kg.
• *Ovarian endometriomas* ('chocolate cysts') are cystic areas of endometriosis that are usually bilateral and may reach 15–20cm in size. On bimanual examination, the adnexa are often tender and immobile due to associated inflammation and adhesions.
• *Theca-lutein cysts* result from overstimulation of the ovaries by excessive amounts of human chorionic gonadotropin (hCG). These cysts may occur in association with complete molar pregnancies (Chapter 32), and are usually bilateral.

Benign ovarian solid neoplasms
• *Ovarian fibromas* are the most common benign solid ovarian neoplasms. They are slow-growing and vary widely in size. *Meig's syndrome* refers to the clinical triad of an ovarian fibroma, ascites, and hydrothorax.
• *Brenner tumours* are rare, smooth, fibro-epithelial ovarian tumours. 10% are bilateral.
• *Serous adenofibromas and cystadenofibromas* are partially solid tumours with a predominance of connective tissue. 25% are bilateral.

Fallopian tube lesions
• *Paratubal cysts (opposite)* are usually asymptomatic and discovered incidentally. The cysts are thin-walled and filled with clear fluid. They are remnants of the embryonic Wolffian (mesonephric) duct system.
• *Hydrosalpinges* are abnormally dilated fallopian tubes that represent sequelae of previous pelvic inflammatory disease (Chapter 8).

Management of the adnexal mass
NOTE: any woman with a solid ovarian neoplasm should have surgery to exclude the possibility of malignancy.
• *Pre-menopausal women: opposite.*
• *Post-menopausal women*. All adnexal masses (except simple cysts) should be considered malignant until proven otherwise by surgical evaluation.
• The overwhelming majority of adnexal masses are benign, regardless of patient age.

COMMON SITES OF ENDOMETRIOSIS

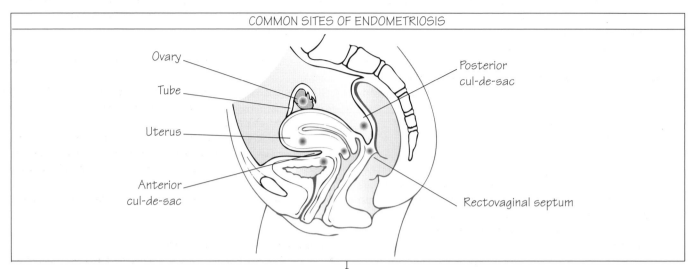

AMERICAN FERTILITY SOCIETY (AFS) CLASSIFICATION OF ENDOMETRIOSIS

Points assigned for each lesion visualized at surgery

		Endometriosis	<1 cm	1–3 cm	>3 cm
Peritoneum		Superficial	1	2	4
		Deep	2	4	6
Ovary	R	Superficial	1	2	4
		Deep	4	16	20
	L	Superficial	1	2	4
		Deep	4	16	20

Posterior cul-de-sac obliteration	Partial		Complete
	4		40

		Adhesions	<1/3 enclosure	1/3–2/3 enclosure	>2/3 enclosure
Ovary	R	Filmy	1	2	4
		Dense	4	8	16
	L	Filmy	1	2	4
		Dense	4	8	16
Tube	R	Filmy	1	2	4
		Dense	4	8	16
	L	Filmy	1	2	4
		Dense	4	8	16

Stage I (minimal) 1–5 points

Stage II (mild) 6–15 points

Superficial implants

Deep implants

Filmy adhesions

Stage III (moderate) 16–40 points

Stage IV (severe) >40 points

Dense adhesions

Complete obliteration of the posterior cul-de-sac

LAPAROSCOPIC EXCISION OF OVARIAN ENDOMETRIOMA

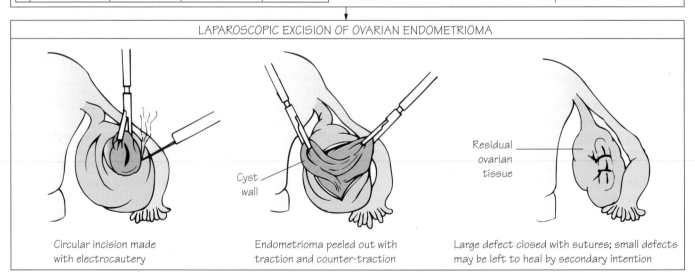

Circular incision made with electrocautery

Cyst wall

Endometrioma peeled out with traction and counter-traction

Residual ovarian tissue

Large defect closed with sutures; small defects may be left to heal by secondary intention

Endometriosis

- *Definition*: functional endometrial glands and stroma outside the uterine cavity *(opposite)*.
- *Incidence*: 5–10% of reproductive-age women and 30% of infertile women are believed to have evidence for endometriosis. However the true incidence is unknown.
- *Age* at first diagnosis averages 27 years.
- *Pathogenesis* is unclear. Theories include retrograde menstruation, coelomic metaplasia, and haematogenous or lymphatic spread. Endometriosis is usually not found prior to menarche and characteristically regresses after the menopause.

Symptoms and signs

- The most common symptoms are *pelvic pain* and *infertility*, but many patients are asymptomatic.
- *Cyclic pain* is the hallmark of endometriosis, including secondary dysmenorrhoea (begins with menstruation and is maximal at the time of maximal flow), deep dyspareunia (pain with intercourse), and sacral backache with menses. Symptoms can also arise from rectal, ureteral, or bladder involvement.
- The severity of symptoms does not necessarily correlate with the degree of pelvic disease. Indeed, many women with minimal endometriosis complain of severe pelvic pain.
- Infertility may result from anatomical distortion of the pelvic architecture due to extensive endometriosis and adhesions, but also occurs in women with minimal disease for unknown reasons.
- Common physical findings include a fixed, retroverted uterus, nodularity of the uterosacral ligaments, and enlarged, tender adnexa.

Diagnosis

- Pelvic ultrasonography may suggest the presence of one or more *endometriomas* (blood-filled ovarian cysts) which are commonly adherent to the surrounding pelvic structures due to recurrent leakage and fibrotic reaction.
- History and physical examination may suggest the presence of endometriosis, but a definitive diagnosis can only be made by direct visualization of endometriotic lesions and pathological examination of biopsy specimens.
- Endometriotic lesions vary in appearance. Early lesions on the peritoneal surface are small and vesicular, and contain clear fluid which becomes brown due to recurrent bleeding. Later lesions have a typical 'powder-burn' appearance which refers to a puckered, black area surrounded by a stellate scar.
- Endometriotic lesions may occur anywhere in the body. The most common site is the ovary. Lesions occur less commonly outside the abdomen (lungs, vulva).

Classification

- The American Fertility Society classification system *(opposite)* is based on surgical findings with points subjectively assigned to each lesion depending on its size and depth. The presence and extent of adhesions are also scored.
- Most women present with stage I or II disease.

Medical management

- Empirical medical treatment with oral contraceptives is recommended for symptomatic women.
- Symptomatic relief for dysmenorrhoea, dyspareunia, and/or pelvic pain is usually successful with medication, although relief may be short-lived.
- The *primary goal* of medical management is suppression of ovulation and induction of amenorrhoea. This will allow the implants to become dormant and fibrotic.
- *Treatment:*
  (i) *Oral contraceptives* will usually relieve mild to moderate pelvic pain.
  (ii) *Progestins* alone may provide significant pain relief, but side-effects include breakthrough bleeding (60%) and worsening depression (10%).
  (iii) *Gonadotropin-releasing hormone (GnRH) agonists* are very effective in creating a 'medical oophorectomy.' Treatment is usually limited to 6 months unless combined with 'add-back' hormonal therapy (oestrogen ± progestin).
- Narcotic dependence is a frequent problem in women with chronic pain unresponsive to treatment.

Conservative surgery *(opposite)*

- Pelvic adhesions and large (>2 cm) endometriomas are best treated surgically rather than medically.
- Goal: to excise or destroy as much of the endometriosis as possible while restoring normal anatomy and salvaging as much normal ovarian tissue as possible.
- Can improve pregnancy rates in women with moderate to severe endometriosis.
- *Presacral neurectomy* and/or *uterosacral nerve ablation* may benefit selected patients.

Definitive surgery

- Hysterectomy with bilateral salpingo-oophorectomy is the most definitive treatment.
- One or both ovaries may be retained with a 20% risk of another operation for continued pain.
- Hormone replacement therapy (Chapter 26) should be considered postoperatively if both ovaries are removed. There is a theoretical benefit of combination estrogen and progesterone to prevent malignant transformation of any residual endometriotic implants.
- Pelvic pain may be unrelieved despite definitive surgery.

Adenomyosis

- *Definition:* presence of endometrial glands and stroma within the myometrium.
- *Incidence:* estimated to occur in 20% of women.
- *Symptoms and signs:* dysmenorrhoea, menorrhagia, a smoothly enlarged boggy uterus on pelvic examination.
- *Diagnosis* may be suggested by pelvic ultrasonography and/or magnetic resonance imaging, but adenomyosis is a histopathological diagnosis.
- *Treatment:* there is no effective medical treatment. Hysterectomy is curative for symptomatic women.

12 Contraception

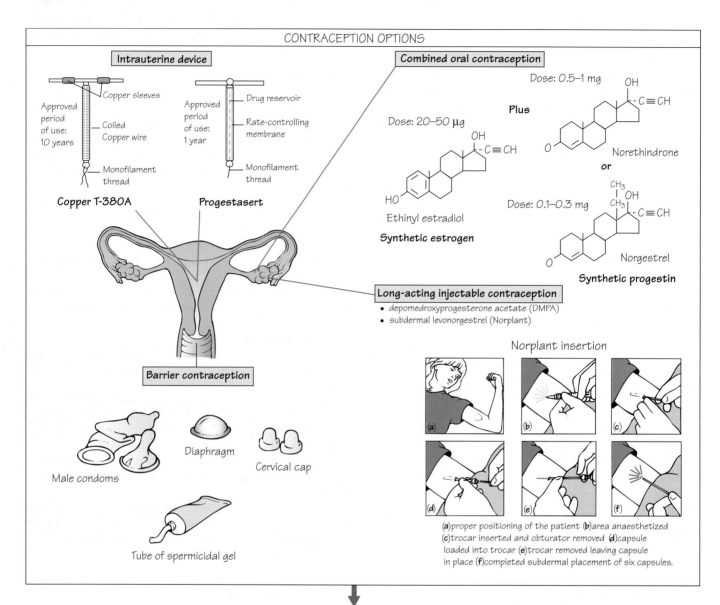

CONTRACEPTION OPTIONS

Intrauterine device

Approved period of use: 10 years — Copper sleeves, Coiled Copper wire, Monofilament thread

Copper T-380A

Approved period of use: 1 year — Drug reservoir, Rate-controlling membrane, Monofilament thread

Progestasert

Combined oral contraception

Dose: 0.5–1 mg

Norethindrone

Dose: 20–50 µg

Ethinyl estradiol
Synthetic estrogen

Plus

or

Dose: 0.1–0.3 mg

Norgestrel
Synthetic progestin

Long-acting injectable contraception
- depomedroxyprogesterone acetate (DMPA)
- subdermal levonorgestrel (Norplant)

Norplant insertion

(a) proper positioning of the patient (b) area anaesthetized (c) trocar inserted and obturator removed (d) capsule loaded into trocar (e) trocar removed leaving capsule in place (f) completed subdermal placement of six capsules.

Barrier contraception

Male condoms

Diaphragm

Cervical cap

Tube of spermicidal gel

FAILURE RATES FOR VARIOUS CONTRACEPTIVE METHODS

Method	Percentage of women becoming pregnant within 1 year	
	Perfect use	Typical use
None	-	85
Oral contraceptives	0.1	5
Condoms	5	15
Diaphragm	5	20
Spermicides	5	25
IUD	-	1–2
DMPA	-	<1
Norplant	-	<1

- *Definition:* the voluntary prevention of pregnancy.
- *Contraceptive options (opposite)* depend primarily on the motivation of the user, but none are 100% effective, easy to use, readily reversible, and without side-effects.

Oral contraceptive pills (OCPs)

The most popular method of reversible contraception.

- *Composition.* Most are combination OCPs, containing both a synthetic estrogen (ethinyl estradiol) and a progestin. The progestin-only pill ('minipill') is much less popular since it is associated with a higher incidence of irregular bleeding and is less effective than combined OCPs in preventing pregnancy.
- *Administration.* For simplicity, the first OCP is taken on the first day of menstruation or on day 5 of the menstrual cycle. Thereafter, one tablet is taken every day for 21 days, followed by 7 days without exogenous hormone. An anovulatory (withdrawal) bleed will occur within 3–5 days of stopping exogenous hormone. Most OCP preparations contain 28 tablets (the last 7 tablets are placebo) which allow a woman to take a tablet each day throughout the cycle. Alternative contraception (such as barrier contraception) should be used for the first month when OCPs may not be fully protective.
- *Mechanism of action.* OCPs prevent pregnancy by (i) preventing ovulation through central inhibition of the mid-cycle LH surge, (ii) acting peripherally to decrease oviductal function and (iii) thickening the cervical mucus.
- *Health benefits.* OCPs reduce menstrual cramps and decrease uterine bleeding. They protect against benign breast disease, prevent formation of ovarian cysts and reduce the incidence and severity of PID. In addition, OCPs reduce the risk of endometrial and ovarian cancer.
- *Side-effects:* irregular breakthrough bleeding (especially if doses are missed). Estrogen-induced side-effects include nausea, headache, elevated blood pressure, weight gain and breast pain.
- *Absolute contraindications:* thromboembolic disease, chronic liver disease, undiagnosed uterine bleeding, pregnancy and estrogen-dependent neoplasia.
- *Relative contraindications:* smoking in women >35 years, migraine headaches, cardiac disease, diabetic complications.

Long-acting injectable contraception

Depomedroxyprogesterone acetate (DMPA)

- *Dosing:* 150 mg intramuscularly every 12 weeks.
- *Mechanism:* prevents ovulation by blocking the mid-cycle LH surge.
- *Side-effects:* markedly irregular vaginal bleeding, amenorrhoea, weight gain, alopecia, reduced libido, depression.

Sub-dermal etonogestrel (Implanon) or levonorgestrel (Norplant)

- *Dosing:* six capsules inserted beneath the skin of the upper arm are effective for 3 (Implanon) to 5 (Norplant) years.
- *Mechanism:* prevention of ovulation. Secondary mechanisms include impaired oocyte maturation and thickened cervical mucus.
- *Side-effects:* similar to DMPA. Removal usually takes longer than placement and may be mildly uncomfortable due to fibrosis.

Barrier contraception

Male condoms (prophylactics)

Covers the penis during coitus and prevents deposition of semen in the vagina. Condoms are disposable, convenient to use, inexpensive, readily available and prevent the spread of sexually transmitted diseases (STDs) (Chapter 7).

Intravaginal devices

- The *diaphragm* is a circular patch of latex rubber held in place by a collapsible metal frame. It prevents passage of sperm into the cervical canal, but must be removed several hours after coitus.
- The *cervical cap* is smaller than the diaphragm, fitting tightly over the cervix. Although it may be left in place for several days after coitus, the cervical cap is more difficult to place and has a higher failure rate than the diaphragm.
- The *female condom* fits loosely inside the vagina and covers the perineum. It is used infrequently.

Spermicides

- *Nonoxynol-9,* a non-toxic detergent that destroys the cell membrane of sperm, is the main active ingredient.
- Spermicides are available without prescription as foam, cream, or suppositories. They can be used alone or with a barrier device.

Intrauterine device (IUD)

The most commonly used reversible contraceptive worldwide. Most useful for women at low risk of STDs and requires no daily maintenance.

- *Dosing:* may be inserted at any time in the menstrual cycle once a pre-existing pregnancy has been excluded. Uterine perforation may occur at the time of insertion, but is rare. The expulsion rate is 5% in the first year.
- *Mechanism:* prevents fertilization and implantation by inducing a local, sterile, inflammatory reaction that is hostile to the oocyte, sperm, and zygote.
- *Side-effects:* menorrhagia and dysmenorrhoea are the primary reasons for early removal of the copper T-380A IUD. Conversely, the levonorgestrel intrauterine system (Mirena) reduces menstrual blood flow and cramping.

Emergency contraception (morning-after pill)

- Commonly requested due to failure of a barrier method (condom) or failure to use any method.
- The risk of pregnancy can be reduced by 75% if taken within 72 hours of unprotected intercourse.
- *Dosing:* single dose of 1.5 mg levonorgestrel (UK standard) or two pills (each: 0.05 mg ethinyl estradiol, 0.25 mg levonorgestrel) followed by a second dose 12 hours later (USA standard).

Failure rates (opposite)

The *rhythm method* (periodic abstinence), *coitus interruptus* (withdrawal of the penis prior to ejaculation), *postcoital douching*, and *prolonged breast-feeding* are unreliable methods of contraception with high failure rates.

13 Sterilization

FEMALE STERILIZATION

MINILAPAROTOMY TECHNIQUES
Pomeroy tubal ligation

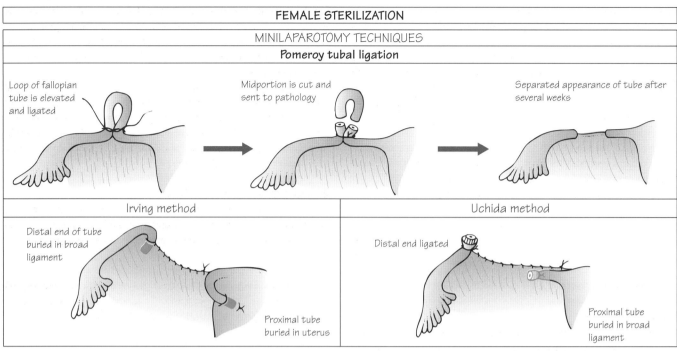

Loop of fallopian tube is elevated and ligated

Midportion is cut and sent to pathology

Separated appearance of tube after several weeks

Irving method	Uchida method
Distal end of tube buried in broad ligament	Distal end ligated
Proximal tube buried in uterus	Proximal tube buried in broad ligament

LAPAROSCOPIC TECHNIQUES

Mechanical occlusion devices	Bipolar cautery

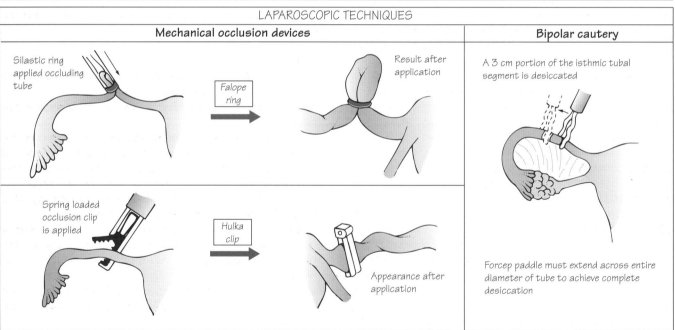

Silastic ring applied occluding tube

Falope ring

Result after application

A 3 cm portion of the isthmic tubal segment is desiccated

Spring loaded occlusion clip is applied

Hulka clip

Appearance after application

Forcep paddle must extend across entire diameter of tube to achieve complete desiccation

10–YEAR FAILURE RATES

Minilaparotomy		Laparoscopy	
Pomeroy	7 per 1000	Bipolar cautery	20 per 1000
Irving	nil	Falope ring	15 per 1000
Uchida	nil	Hulka clip	30 per 1000
		Filshie clip	30 per 1000

- *Definition:* a surgical procedure that is aimed at permanently blocking or removing part of the female or male genital tracts to prevent fertilization.
- *Frequency:* the most common method of family planning worldwide. More than 220 million couples use surgical sterilization for contraception, 90% of whom live in developing countries. The ratio of female to male sterilization is 3:1.
- *Risks:* all patients undergoing surgical sterilization should be aware of the nature, efficacy, safety, and complications of the operation as well as alternative methods of contraception. Many couples are under the false impression that sterilization procedures are easily reversed. It is the responsibility of the surgeon to make it clear that such procedures are intended to be permanent.
- *Regret:* the strongest indicator of future regret is young age at the time of sterilization. Marital instability is another important factor. Royal College of Obstetricians and Gynaecologists guidelines require a specific interval between obtaining consent and surgical sterilization.

Female sterilization (opposite)

Can be performed at caesarean delivery, immediately postpartum, post-abortion, or as an interval procedure unrelated to pregnancy. Women undergoing sterilization are 4–5 times more likely to eventually undergo hysterectomy (no known biological mechanism).

1 Minilaparotomy

Location of the incision depends on the size of the uterus.
- Interval procedure is performed through a 2–3 cm midline *suprapubic* incision. The abdomen is entered, the uterus is identified, and a finger is used to elevate the fallopian tube. After the tube has been identified by its fimbriated end, the mid-portion of the fallopian tube is grasped with a Babcock clamp. Tubal ligation is then performed.
- Postpartum sterilization (PPS) is either performed at caesarean section or following vaginal delivery. The latter procedure is ideally performed while the uterine fundus is high in the abdomen (within 48 hours of delivery), using a 2–3 cm *subumbilical* incision. Maternal and neonatal well-being should be confirmed prior to PPS.

2 Laparoscopic tubal ligation (LTL)

The most popular method of interval female sterilization in the industrialized world (Chapter 16).
- Mechanical occlusion devices—such as the spring-loaded clip (Filshie clip, Hulka clip) or a silastic ring (Falope ring)—are most commonly used. Special applicators are necessary and each requires skill for proper application. Clips and rings destroy less oviductal tissue than electrocoagulation. However, tubal adhesions or a thickened or dilated fallopian tube increase the risk of misapplication of the clip.
- Bipolar cautery is a less common technique. It is much safer than unipolar cautery, which can cause thermal bowel injury.

- *Advantages:* abdominal and pelvic organs can be inspected, small incision scars, rapid postoperative recovery.
- *Complications.* The mortality rate (1–2/100,000 procedures) is lower than that for childbirth (10/100,000 births). Anaesthetic complications are the leading cause of death. Other potential complications include haemorrhage, infection, erroneous ligation of the round ligament, and injury to adjacent structures. When the risk of pregnancy from contraceptive failure is taken into account, sterilization is the safest of all contraceptive methods.
- *Reversal.* 1 in 500 sterilized women will undergo microsurgical tubal re-anastomosis. This procedure has excellent results if a small segment of the tube has been damaged. Pregnancy rates following re-anastomosis are low with electrocoagulation and higher (70–80%) with clips, rings, and surgical methods. Such pregnancies are more likely to be ectopic (tubal) pregnancies.

3 Transcervical approaches

Involves gaining access to the fallopian tubes through the cervix. A device or occlusive material (essure) is placed hysteroscopically to block each tube. This technique is currently considered experimental.

Failure rates (opposite)

- Dependent upon the specific operation, the skill of the operator, and characteristics of the patient (age, pelvic adhesions, hydrosalpinx).
- Resultant pregnancies are more likely to be ectopic.

Male sterilization (vasectomy)

When compared with female tubal sterilization, vasectomy is safer, less expensive, and equally effective.

Method

- Permanent surgical interruption of the vas deferens (the duct that transports sperm during ejaculation).
- Can be performed on an outpatient basis within 15 minute under local anaesthesia.
- Unlike tubal occlusion in women, vasectomy is not immediately effective. Spermatozoa normally mature in the vas deferens for around 70 days prior to ejaculation. For this reason, 3 months or 20 ejaculations are needed to completely deplete the vas deferens of viable sperm. Post-vasectomy semen analysis should be performed to determine the effectiveness of the procedure prior to unprotected intercourse.
- *Complications.* Mortality is essentially zero. Wound haematomas, infections, and sperm granulomas are rare (<3%). Long-term side-effects (increased risk of prostate cancer, decreased libido) have never been proven.
- *Reversal.* Fewer than 5% of men request vasectomy reversal. Vas deferens re-anastomosis is a difficult and meticulous procedure that has only a 50% success rate.
- *Failure rates* are <1%.

14 Breast disease

ANATOMY OF THE BREAST

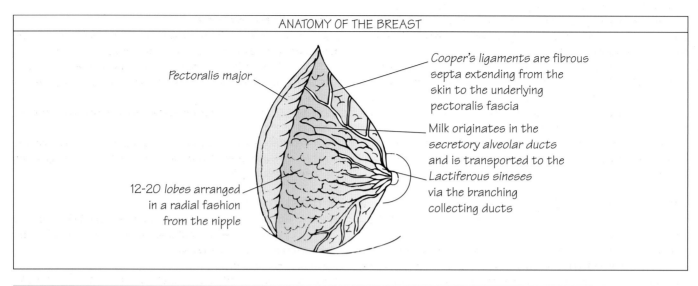

Pectoralis major

Cooper's ligaments are fibrous septa extending from the skin to the underlying pectoralis fascia

Milk originates in the secretory alveolar ducts and is transported to the Lactiferous sineses via the branching collecting ducts

12-20 lobes arranged in a radial fashion from the nipple

Risk factors for breast cancer

Age (risk increases in each decade)	
Previous cancer in the contralateral breast	
Family history of 2 close relatives	>4-fold
BRCA1 or BRCA2 mutation carrier	
Previous biopsy with premalignant histology	
Radiation exposure	2.1-4 fold
Nulliparity	
Residence in North America or Northern Europe	
First birth age 35 or older	
Early menarche	
Late menopause	1.1-2 fold
Obesity	
Urban residence	
Upper socioeconomic status	
Other primary cancer in ovary or endometrium	

Fine needle aspiration

Needle is rotated, moved back and forth, and slightly in and out to aspirate representative specimen

Mammogram

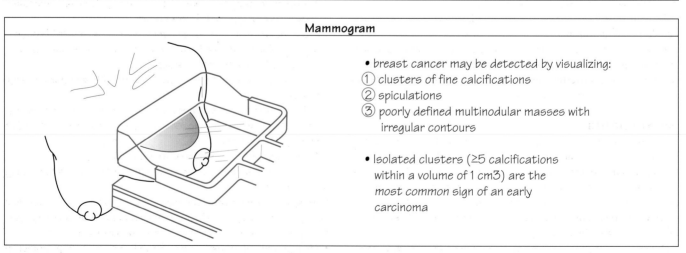

- breast cancer may be detected by visualizing:
  1. clusters of fine calcifications
  2. spiculations
  3. poorly defined multinodular masses with irregular contours

- Isolated clusters (≥5 calcifications within a volume of 1 cm3) are the most common sign of an early carcinoma

Anatomy and development *(opposite)*

• The breasts are large, modified sebaceous glands contained within the superficial fascia of the anterior chest wall.
• The average weight is 200–300 g during the menstruating years
• Composed of 20% glands and 80% fat and connective tissue.
• Breast tissue is sensitive to the cyclic changes in hormonal levels — women often experience breast tenderness and fullness during the luteal phase of the cycle. Premenstrual symptoms are produced by an increase in blood flow, vascular engorgement, and water retention.
• Nearing the onset of puberty, the first change in the breast is the formation of the breast bud (Chapter 19). The areola subsequently enlarges, and then the nipple begins to grow outwards.
• Oestrogen is responsible for the initial stages of breast development, but further development requires adult levels of progesterone.

Physical examination

• Breast examination is particularly important when symptoms are present. Patients should be instructed in the technique of life-long periodic self-examination.
• *Inspection* is the first step. This is usually done with the arms raised overhead, then with tension on the pectoralis muscles (by having the patient place her hands on her hips and press inward) and finally with the patient relaxed and leaning forward. These manoeuvres accentuate skin and contour changes such as retraction, oedema, or erythema, and nipple changes such as retraction, eczema or erosion.
• *Palpation* is best performed with the patient in both sitting and supine positions. The examination is done in concentric circles, starting with the outermost breast tissue. The physician should attempt to elicit nipple discharge and examine the axilla carefully for adenopathy.

Benign breast disease

Fibrocystic changes

• *Definition:* exaggeration of the normal physiological response of breast tissue to the cyclic levels of ovarian hormones.
• *Frequency:* the most common of all benign breast conditions.
• *Symptoms and signs:* cyclic bilateral breast pain, increased engorgement and density of the breasts, excessive nodularity, rapid change and fluctuation in the size of cystic areas, increased tenderness and occasionally spontaneous clear nipple discharge.
• *Physical examination:* marked tenderness of well-delineated, slightly mobile cystic nodules or thickened areas.
• *Diagnosis:* a wide variety of histopathological findings (cysts, adenosis, fibrosis, duct ectasia).
• *Treatment:* well-fitting brassieres and light, loose clothing. Decreased intake of coffee, chocolate, tea and smoking cessation. Oral contraceptives or progestins are helpful in up to 90% of patients. Danazol is effective for severe symptoms.

Fibroadenomas

• *Definition:* firm, rubbery, freely mobile, solid, usually solitary masses.
• *Frequency:* the 2nd most common type of benign breast disease.
• *Symptoms and signs:* typically a young woman in her 20s discovers the painless mass accidentally while bathing. Growth of the mass is usually extremely slow, but occasionally can be quite rapid.
• *Physical examination:* average size is 2.5 cm; multiple lesions are found in 15–20% of women.
• *Diagnosis:* mammography is rarely indicated in a woman under age 30. Ultrasound may be helpful to distinguish a solid from a cystic mass.

• *Treatment:* if the aetiology cannot be established by fine-needle aspiration (FNA), surgical removal is indicated. Any mass that rapidly increases in size should be removed as should any solid mass in a woman over age 30.

Other benign conditions

• *Mastodynia* (breast pain) is a common symptom affecting women. Reduction of dietary fat can result in significant improvement.
• *Galactorrhoea* (Milky discharge) usually results from medication (hormones, phenothiazines) side-effects, but may suggest a prolactin-secreting tumour.
• *Intraductal papilloma* is usually solitary and often causes a serous or bloody discharge.
• *Duct ectasia* results from subareolar dilation and periductal mastitis.
• *Fat necrosis* usually results from trauma and is the only benign lesion that causes skin dimpling.

Breast cancer

• More than 1 million new cases occur each year worldwide—making it the most common malignancy of women. 1 in 8 women will be diagnosed with breast cancer by age 80.
• *Risk factors (opposite)*
• *Inherited* cases (5–10%) are usually due to BRCA1 or BRCA2 germline mutations. Carriers have a 55–85% risk of developing cancer.
• *Prevention* by using tamoxifen or raloxifene in high-risk women is currently being evaluated. Prophylactic mastectomy is chiefly reserved for BRCA1 or BRCA2 mutation carriers.
• *Mammogram (opposite)* is the best technique for early detection, but the false-negative rate is 10%.
• *Screening recommendations*
  UK: Mammogram every 3 years beginning at age 50.
  USA: Mammogram every 1–2 years for women aged 40–49 years and annually beginning at age 50.
• *Histopathology.* The most common type (70–80%) is infiltrating ductal carcinoma, followed by lobular carcinoma (5–8%). The incidence of ductal carcinoma in situ (DCIS) has increased dramatically with the advent of widespread mammography screening.
• *Staging* is based on the TNM system to determine the anatomical extent of malignant disease: primary tumour (T), lymph node involvement (N), and metastasis (M).
• *Surgical procedures:*
  1 *FNA (opposite)* and *core biopsy*: office procedures commonly used to diagnose palpable breast masses.
  2 *Excisional biopsy*: outpatient procedure with complete histology.
  3 *Needle-localized excisional biopsy* or *sterotactic mammography*: performed for non-palpable lesions.
  4 *Lumpectomy*: breast-conserving surgery with superior cosmetic results.
  5 *Modified radical mastectomy*: complete removal of the breast tissue, underlying fascia of the pectoralis major muscle and removal of axillary lymph nodes.
  6 *Reconstruction*: to implant or myocutaneous flap.
• *Postoperative radiation* can benefit high-risk patients by preventing local recurrence.
• *Adjuvant chemotherapy* commonly incorporates doxorubicin and cyclophosphamide. Tamoxifen is often used to prevent relapse in premenopausal women with oestrogen-receptor positive tumours.
• *Management* of breast cancer depends on the histopathological cell type, stage, and other clinical features. Clinicians commonly sequence surgery, radiation and chemotherapy.

15 Miscarriage and termination of pregnancy

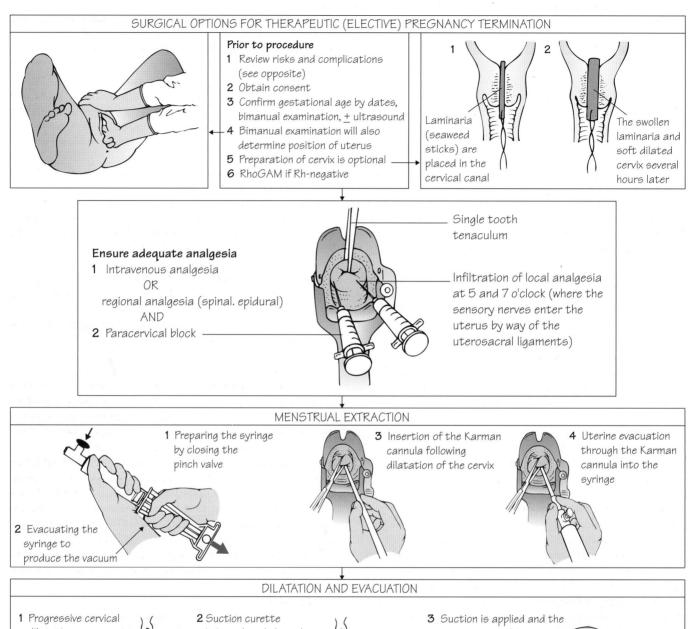

SURGICAL OPTIONS FOR THERAPEUTIC (ELECTIVE) PREGNANCY TERMINATION

Prior to procedure
1 Review risks and complications (see opposite)
2 Obtain consent
3 Confirm gestational age by dates, bimanual examination, ± ultrasound
4 Bimanual examination will also determine position of uterus
5 Preparation of cervix is optional
6 RhoGAM if Rh-negative

1 2
Laminaria (seaweed sticks) are placed in the cervical canal

The swollen laminaria and soft dilated cervix several hours later

Ensure adequate analgesia
1 Intravenous analgesia
   OR
   regional analgesia (spinal. epidural)
   AND
2 Paracervical block

Single tooth tenaculum

Infiltration of local analgesia at 5 and 7 o'clock (where the sensory nerves enter the uterus by way of the uterosacral ligaments)

MENSTRUAL EXTRACTION

1 Preparing the syringe by closing the pinch valve

2 Evacuating the syringe to produce the vacuum

3 Insertion of the Karman cannula following dilatation of the cervix

4 Uterine evacuation through the Karman cannula into the syringe

DILATATION AND EVACUATION

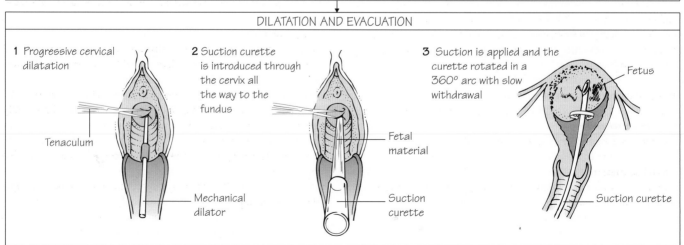

1 Progressive cervical dilatation

Tenaculum

Mechanical dilator

2 Suction curette is introduced through the cervix all the way to the fundus

Fetal material

Suction curette

3 Suction is applied and the curette rotated in a 360° arc with slow withdrawal

Fetus

Suction curette

36 Gynaecology Miscarriage and termination of pregnancy

- *Definition:* expulsion or removal of an embryo or fetus from the uterus before it is capable of independent survival.
- 50–75% of all conceptions abort spontaneously. Most are unrecognized because they occur before or at the time of the next expected menses.

Spontaneous miscarriage

- *Definition:* loss of a clinically recognized pregnancy prior to 20 weeks gestation.
- *Incidence:* 15–20% of clinically diagnosed pregnancies.
- *Risk factors:* advanced maternal age, increasing gravidity, prior miscarriage, smoking.

Diagnosis

- *History.* Vaginal bleeding is the most common presenting complaint. Abdominal pain is also frequent.
- *Physical examination.* Vital signs should be taken to rule out haemodynamic instability. Pelvic examination is useful to estimate gestational age. Speculum examination should be performed to exclude a local cause of vaginal bleeding and to rule out expulsion of products of conception.
- *Laboratory tests.* Quantitative serum human chorionic gonadotropin (hCG), full blood count, and blood typing should be sent.

Aetiology

First trimester miscarriage (<12 weeks gestation)

Most have a chromosomal abnormality. 45,XO (Turner syndrome) is the single most common type. Other common causes include a blighted ovum (gestational sac without embryo or yolk sac) or an endocrine disorder (diabetes). Many cases are idiopathic.

Second trimester miscarriage (12–20 weeks gestation)

Structural abnormalities of the uterus (Müllerian anomalies, fibroids; Chapter 10) or cervix (cervical incompetence; Chapter 55) are the most common causes.

Classification and treatment

Threatened miscarriage

- *Definition*: uterine bleeding before 20 weeks with a closed cervical os and a confirmed viable intrauterine gestation.
- *Treatment:* expectant, unless the pregnancy is undesired or nonviable. Pelvic rest (nothing placed in the vagina) is usually recommended. Virtually all Rh-negative patients having a miscarriage should receive anti-D immunoglobulin prophylaxis (Chapter 50) to prevent sensitization.

Incomplete (or inevitable) miscarriage

- *Definition*: Partial or imminent expulsion of products of conception through a dilated cervix.
- *Treatment:* uterine evacuation or conservative management.

Complete miscarriage

- *Definition:* Complete expulsion of all products of conception prior to 20 weeks of gestation.

- *Treatment:* uterine evacuation is not necessary unless the diagnosis is unclear or there is excessive bleeding.

Missed abortion

- *Definition:* Intrauterine fetal demise before 20 weeks gestation with complete retention of products of conception.
- *Treatment:* expectant observation or uterine evacuation.

Termination of pregnancy

More than 1.5 million terminations are performed annually in the USA (200,000 in the UK). 30% of pregnancies not ending in spontaneous miscarriage or stillbirth are electively terminated.

Surgical options (*opposite*)

95% of therapeutic abortions are performed in an outpatient setting using vacuum aspiration techniques.

1 Menstrual extraction (performed in USA only) can be performed up to 6–7 weeks gestation without regional anaesthesia. A soft, flexible plastic cannula (Karman) is attached to a self-locking syringe. Evacuation is accomplished by repetitive in and out movements and rotation of the cannula.

2 Dilatation and evacuation (D&E) can be safely performed up to 16 weeks gestation. Wider cervical dilatation and specialized (Sopher) forceps may be necessary to evacuate more advanced pregnancies.

- Identification of products of conception is mandatory to confirm that the entire fetus has been evacuated.

Medical termination

1 RU486 (mifepristone) is a progesterone receptor antagonist that interferes at the level of the uterus and leads to detachment of the embryo. A single oral dose of RU486 followed 36–48 hours later by oral misoprostol is a simple, effective, safe, and inexpensive method of elective pregnancy termination up to <7 weeks gestation.

2 Intra-amniotic infusion of hypertonic saline and/or prostaglandin is considered the safest technique between 16 and 24 weeks gestation. Patients undergo laminaria pretreatment of the cervix for 4–12 hours followed by administration of oral misoprostol and intra-amniotic infusion. Once contractions begin, fetal membranes are ruptured and intravenous oxytocin is given until delivery is complete.

3 Prostaglandin vaginal suppositories can be used to initiate abortion up to 28 weeks gestation. Nausea, vomiting, and diarrhoea may be severe.

Complications

- The frequency of complications depends on operator experience and gestational age (increased if <6 wk or >16 wk). Less than 1% of women have a serious complication.
- *Immediate complications:* haemorrhage, cervical injury, anaesthesia complications. The use of osmotic dilators (laminaria) significantly reduces the risk of uterine perforation.
- *Late complications:* retained products of conception, on-going pregnancy (especially if <6 weeks), infection (endometritis) and Rh sensitization.
- *Mortality rate:* 10/100,000 infusion procedures and 5/100,000 surgical D&E procedures.

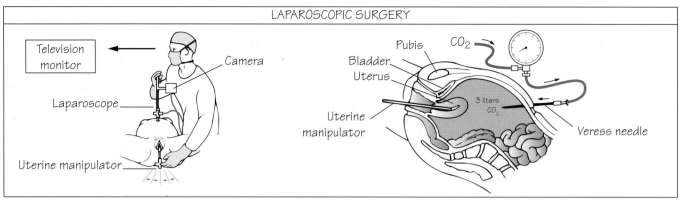

LAPAROSCOPIC SURGERY

Television monitor
Camera
Laparoscope
Uterine manipulator

Pubis
CO_2
Bladder
Uterus
Uterine manipulator
3 liters CO_2
Veress needle

ABDOMINAL SURGERY

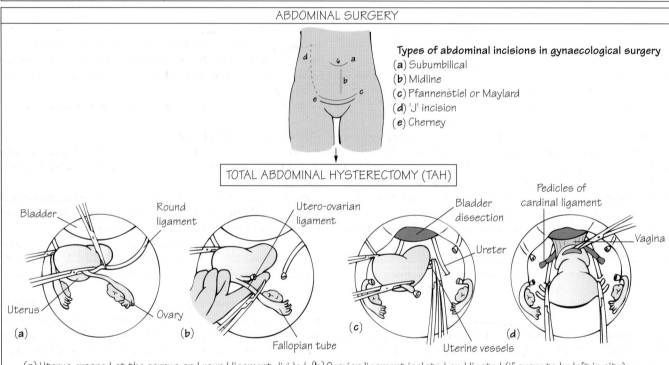

Types of abdominal incisions in gynaecological surgery
(**a**) Subumbilical
(**b**) Midline
(**c**) Pfannenstiel or Maylard
(**d**) 'J' incision
(**e**) Cherney

TOTAL ABDOMINAL HYSTERECTOMY (TAH)

Bladder
Round ligament
Uterus
Ovary
(**a**)

Utero-ovarian ligament
Fallopian tube
(**b**)

Bladder dissection
Ureter
Uterine vessels
(**c**)

Pedicles of cardinal ligament
Vagina
(**d**)

(**a**) Uterus grasped at the cornua and round ligament divided. (**b**) Ovarian ligament isolated and ligated (if ovary to be left in situ).
(**c**) After bladder dissection, uterine vessels are isolated and ligated. (**d**) Cardinal ligaments have been divided and the vagina is entered.
The final step is cuff closure or whip-stitching (not shown).

VAGINAL HYSTERECTOMY

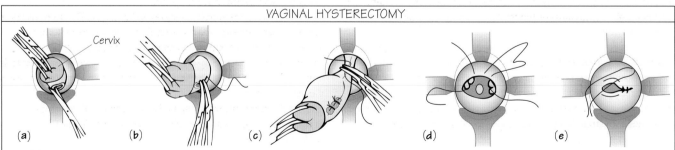

Cervix

(**a**)   (**b**)   (**c**)   (**d**)   (**e**)

(**a**) Traction is placed on cervix. Circumferential incision of cervico-uterine fold has been performed and the posterior
cul-de-sac is entered. (**b**) The cardinal and uterosacral ligaments are ligated. (**c**) Ovarian and round ligaments are ligated.
(**d**) Purse-string closure of peritoneal cavity. (**e**) Reapproximation of the vaginal cuff.

Dilatation and curettage (D & C)
- *Indications:* diagnostic (post-menopausal bleeding) and therapeutic (dysfunctional uterine bleeding; DUB).
- *Surgical technique.* The cervix is placed on traction and the cervical canal is progressively dilated until the internal os is wide enough to admit the curette. The uterine cavity is then circumferentially scraped with a sharp curette.
- *Complications:* bleeding, infection, uterine perforation.

Hysteroscopy (Chapter 4)
- *Indications:* diagnosis of uterine anomalies, resection of submucous fibroids, endometrial ablation, numerous others.
- *Surgical technique.* The hysteroscope is inserted after dilatation of the cervical canal and the uterine cavity is distended with fluid (glycine, saline). A variety of instruments (roller-ball coagulator, scissors, resectoscope) may be passed through the operative sheath to perform the procedure.
- *Complications:* same as D & C, extravasation of pressurized hypotonic fluid into the circulation may cause acute hyponatremia and seizures.

Laparoscopy *(opposite)*
- *Indications:* tubal ligation, unexplained pelvic pain, ectopic pregnancy, adnexectomy, numerous others. This minimally invasive outpatient procedure has many practical applications.
- *Surgical technique.* A Veress needle is inserted at the umbilicus to achieve a pneumoperitoneum (direct trocar insertion is another approach). The surgeon then punctures the abdominal wall with the trocar and inserts the laparoscope. One or more additional operating sites may then be inserted in the lower quadrants for ancillary instruments (probe, forceps, scissors, irrigator, laser). Visualization of the pelvic organs is facilitated by transvaginal placement of an intrauterine manipulator.
- *Complications:* injury to intra-abdominal organs, nerve injury (due to incorrect placement of the legs in surgical stirrups), laceration of large vessels, subcutaneous emphysema.

Abdominal surgery *(opposite)*
The *subumbilical* incision is used for postpartum tubal ligation. The *midline* incision provides excellent exposure to the pelvis and may be extended to the upper abdomen. The *Pfannenstiel* incision is the most common incision in gynaecology. It provides excellent exposure to the pelvis, but can only be extended by making an unsightly 'J' incision. Exposure to the lateral pelvis may be increased by dividing the rectus muscles (Maylard) or the tendon of the rectus muscle from the symphysis pubis (Cherney).

Total abdominal hysterectomy (TAH) *(opposite)*
- The second most common major operation performed in the USA and UK (after caesarean).
- *Indications:* uterine fibroids (most common), endometrial cancer, pelvic pain, dysfunctional uterine bleeding, numerous others.

- *Surgical technique.* (as shown) Supracervical hysterectomy is performed in some circumstances by amputating the cervix after ligation of the uterine vessels and suturing the distal stump.
- *Complications:* bleeding, infection, distal ureteral injury, postoperative ileus.

Salpingo-oophorectomy
- *Indications:* benign ovarian tumours, gynaecological malignancy, pelvic pain, numerous others.
- *Surgical technique.* The retroperitoneal space is entered and the infundibulopelvic ('IP') ligament is clamped proximal to the ovary/tube—above the ureter. The broad ligament attachments are dissected distally and the utero-ovarian ligament divided.
- *Complications:* haematoma, ureteral injury at pelvic brim.

Myomectomy
- *Indications:* symptomatic uterine fibroids, persistent menorrhagia, infertility.
- *Surgical technique.* An incision is made through the uterine musculature overlying the fibroid. The myometrium is bluntly dissected from the fibroid pseudocapsule and the specimen removed. The uterine incisions are then closed to obliterate the dead-space and provide haemostasis.
- *Complications:* bleeding necessitating TAH, postop adhesions.

Radical gynaecological surgery
- *Radical hysterectomy* is used to treat early cervical cancer (Chapter 28). The 'radical' intent is to remove additional soft tissue to achieve widely negative margins for cure.
- *Pelvic and para-aortic lymphadenectomy* is performed for cervical, endometrial (Chapter 30) and ovarian cancer (Chapter 31). It may also be performed laparoscopically or extraperitoneally.
- *Cytoreductive surgery* is performed for advanced ovarian cancer and the aim is to remove all grossly visible disease. The extent of the operation varies, but may include omentectomy, bowel resection +/- splenectomy.
- *Pelvic exenteration* is performed in selected patients with centrally recurrent cervical cancer. This operation involves removal of the bladder (anterior), rectum (posterior), or both organs (total) in addition to the uterus and adjacent soft tissues to achieve a widely negative margin. A urinary conduit is usually part of the surgery.

Vaginal surgery
Vaginal hysterectomy *(opposite)*
- *Indications:* symptomatic uterovaginal prolapse, DUB refractory to medical management, obesity. Morbidity and postoperative recovery time are decreased compared to abdominal surgery.
- *Surgical technique* (as shown) The operative steps are almost in reverse order to TAH. Morcellation of uterine fibroids may allow resection of larger uteri.
- *Complications:* bleeding, vaginal cuff cellulitis, bladder injury.

Other vaginal operations are shown in Chapters 17 and 18.

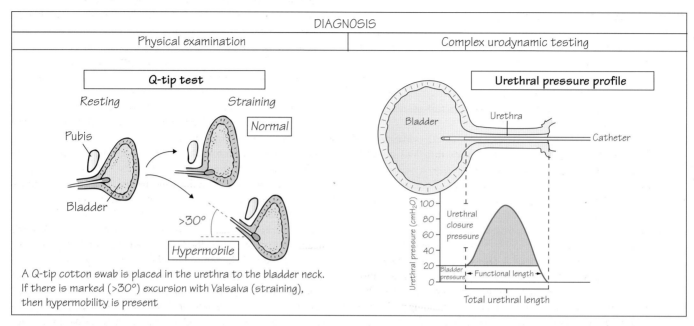

DIAGNOSIS

Physical examination	Complex urodynamic testing

Q-tip test

Resting   Straining

Normal

Pubis

Bladder

>30°

Hypermobile

A Q-tip cotton swab is placed in the urethra to the bladder neck. If there is marked (>30°) excursion with Valsalva (straining), then hypermobility is present

Urethral pressure profile

Bladder   Urethra

Catheter

Urethral pressure (cmH$_2$O)

100, 80, 60, 40, 20, 0

Urethral closure pressure

Bladder pressure

Functional length

Total urethral length

SURGICAL TREATMENT

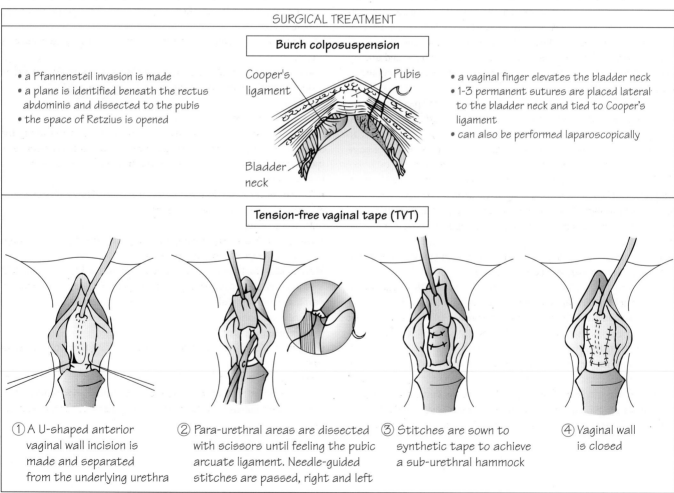

Burch colposuspension

- a Pfannensteil invasion is made
- a plane is identified beneath the rectus abdominis and dissected to the pubis
- the space of Retzius is opened

Cooper's ligament   Pubis

Bladder neck

- a vaginal finger elevates the bladder neck
- 1-3 permanent sutures are placed lateral to the bladder neck and tied to Cooper's ligament
- can also be performed laparoscopically

Tension-free vaginal tape (TVT)

① A U-shaped anterior vaginal wall incision is made and separated from the underlying urethra

② Para-urethral areas are dissected with scissors until feeling the pubic arcuate ligament. Needle-guided stitches are passed, right and left

③ Stitches are sown to synthetic tape to achieve a sub-urethral hammock

④ Vaginal wall is closed

- *Definition:* the involuntary loss of urine that is a social/hygienic problem and that is objectively demonstrable.
- *Incidence:* 4–8% of the population seek medical attention.

Diagnosis (6 basic components)

1 *History.* A detailed history is important to determine the severity of symptoms. Emotional distress often does not correlate well with the amount of urine loss that can be demonstrated.

2 *Physical examination (3 areas):*
- *General examination* to rule out delirium, atrophic urethritis, pharmacological causes, excessive urinary production (diabetes), restricted mobility and stool impaction.
- *Neurological screening examination* (commonly performed in US). Lower extremity reflexes should be evaluated. Lightly stroking the buttocks lateral to the anal sphincter elicits a rapid reflex contraction (ie, anal 'wink') of the external sphincter. Gently tapping the clitoris elicits the bulbocavernosus reflex. Coughing elicits a reflex contraction of the pelvic floor.
- *Urogynaecological examination* Inspection may reveal severe vulvar excoriation from continual dampness and a gaping introitus suggests previous pelvic floor trauma. The vaginal tissue should be inspected for signs of atrophy, stenosis and bladder neck mobility (*Q-tip test: opposite*). The patient is asked to cough or Valsalva repeatedly with a full bladder in the lithotomy or standing position to induce urine leakage. Assessment of pelvic floor strength can be performed during bimanual examination by asking the patient to contract her pelvic muscles. Finally, a rectal examination can evaluate rectal sphincter tone or the presence of faecal impaction.

3 *Urinalysis and urine culture.* Many relevant metabolic and urinary tract disorders can be screened by a simple urinalysis. A culture is essential to rule out infection before proceeding with further evaluation.

4 *Residual urine volume after voiding.* A catheterized post-void residual urine specimen should be obtained to exclude urinary retention or infection.

5 *Frequency-volume bladder chart.* More than 7 voids per day suggest a problem with frequency, but this is highly dependent on habit and fluid intake. Patients are notoriously inaccurate in estimating urinary frequency and should be encouraged to keep a 'urinary diary' for several days as part of their initial evaluation. The volume of each void should be measured and recorded and any episodes of incontinence duly noted.

6 *Urodynamics* are a group of tests designed to aid in determining the aetiology of lower urinary tract dysfunction.
- *Cystometry* involves gradual bladder filling with sterile water. Involuntary 'detrusor' contractions are demonstrated by a rise in water level during filling due to back pressure. Normally, the first sensation to void occurs at 150 mL and bladder capacity is typically 400–600 mL.
- *Uroflowmetry* is used to determine the urinary flow rate and flow time in order to screen for the presence of outflow obstruction and abnormal detrusor contractility. Normally, women achieve a peak flow rate of 15–20 mL/s with a voided volume of 150–200 mL.
- *Complex urodynamic testing (opposite)* requires placement of an intravesical catheter to measure detrusor pressures and a vaginal or rectal catheter to indirectly measure intra-abdominal pressures.

Genuine stress urinary incontinence (GSUI)
- *Definition:* involuntary loss of urine due to weaknesses in urethral supportive structures.
- *Incidence:* the most common form of urinary incontinence.
- *Mechanism.* Increases in intra-abdominal pressure (sneezing, coughing, exercise) cause bladder pressure to exceed urethral sphincter closure pressure, resulting in inadvertent urine loss.
- *Diagnosis.* GSUI is suggested by history, physical examination (positive Q-tip test), and a positive stress test (demonstrable loss of urine while the patient is being examined).
- ***Non-surgical treatment:*** pelvic muscle (Kegel) exercises. Biofeedback is particularly helpful when muscles are extremely weak: a pressure measurement device notifies the patient when correct muscle contraction is performed and reinforces correct technique.
- ***Surgical treatment*** *(opposite):*
  1 *Burch colposuspension* involves suture placement at Cooper's ligament. In the Marshall–Marchetti–Krantz (MMK) procedure, sutures go through the periosteum of the pubic symphysis.
  2 *Tension-free vaginal tape* (TVT) is a newer, minimally invasive procedure that is rapidly becoming the new 'gold standard'. Synthetic tape is placed without tension under the mid-urethra and then fastened to Cooper's ligament. Other needle suspension procedures (Pereyra, Stamey, Raz, Gittes) or pubovaginal slings are less commonly performed.
  3 *Anterior colporrhaphy* (Chapter 18) has a poor long-term success rate.
  4 *Collagen injections* are designed as a treatment for GSUI resulting from intrinsic sphincter deficiency.

Detrusor overactivity
- *Definition:* spontaneous detrusor (bladder) contractions during the filling phase when the patient is attempting to inhibit micturition. The involuntary loss of urine is associated with an abrupt and strong desire to void (urgency).
- *Incidence:* the second most common cause of urinary incontinence, especially prevalent in elderly women.
- *Mechanism:* idiopathic.
- *Diagnosis.* Frequency, nocturia, and urgency are suggestive symptoms. Cystometry may be confirmatory.
- ***Treatment:*** behaviour modification (bladder drills, biofeedback) and/or pharmacological therapy (oxybutynin chloride, imipramine). Surgery is rarely useful.

Overflow incontinence
- *Definition:* any involuntary loss of urine associated with overdistension of the bladder.
- *Mechanism:* dysfunction of either the bladder muscle (multiple sclerosis, spinal cord injury) or the urethral sphincter (severe cystocele).
- ***Treatment:*** catheter drainage, followed by treatment of the underlying condition.

18 Pelvic organ prolapse

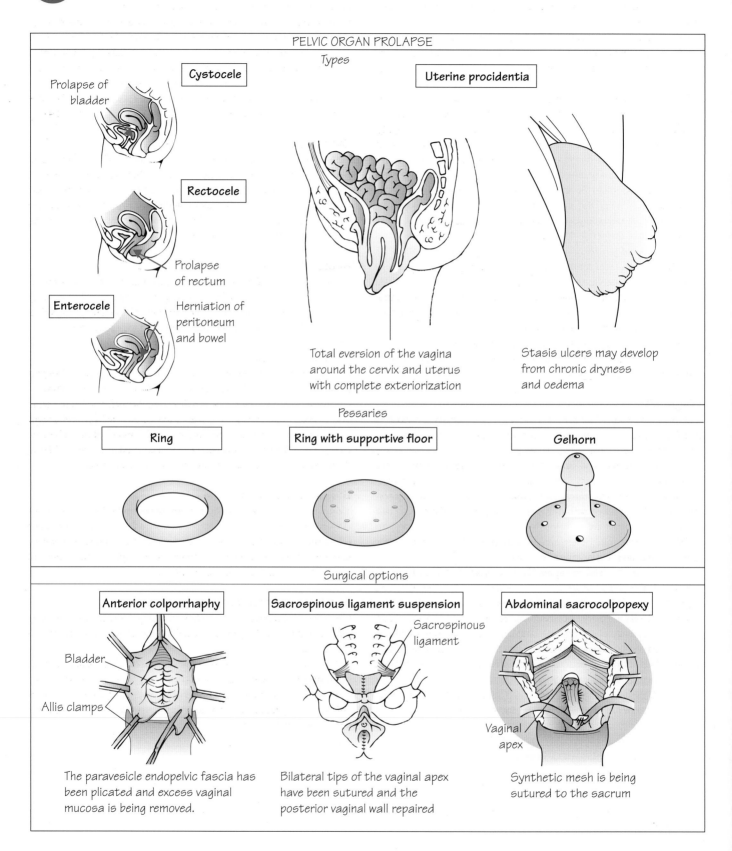

PELVIC ORGAN PROLAPSE

Types

Cystocele

Prolapse of bladder

Rectocele

Prolapse of rectum

Enterocele

Herniation of peritoneum and bowel

Uterine procidentia

Total eversion of the vagina around the cervix and uterus with complete exteriorization

Stasis ulcers may develop from chronic dryness and oedema

Pessaries

Ring

Ring with supportive floor

Gelhorn

Surgical options

Anterior colporrhaphy

Bladder

Allis clamps

The paravesicle endopelvic fascia has been plicated and excess vaginal mucosa is being removed.

Sacrospinous ligament suspension

Sacrospinous ligament

Bilateral tips of the vaginal apex have been sutured and the posterior vaginal wall repaired

Abdominal sacrocolpopexy

Vaginal apex

Synthetic mesh is being sutured to the sacrum

- *Definition:* descent of the pelvic organs through the pelvic floor into the vaginal canal.
- *Incidence:* common in multiparous women, but frequently under-reported.
- *Pelvic support.* The levator ani complex of muscles (Chapter 2) provides the major support for the pelvic organs. Ligaments and endopelvic fascia play a secondary role.
- *Aetiology.*
  1 *Vaginal parity.* Pregnancy, labour and vaginal delivery may result in various degrees of damage to pelvic support structures, including the ligaments, fascia, muscles and their nerve supply. More damage is caused by prolonged labour, large fetal head or shoulders and when difficult forceps operations are required for delivery.
  2 *Race.* Prolapse occurs more frequently among white women than Asians and blacks. Inherited differences in pelvic architecture and the quality of supporting muscles/connective tissue are thought to be responsible.
  3 *Estrogen deficiency.* Pelvic tissues are estrogen sensitive and often prolapse becomes symptomatic during the menopausal years as collagen fibres deteriorate.
  4 *Chronic conditions* that cause repeated increases in intra-abdominal pressure (cough, heavy lifting, constipation) can contribute to significant pelvic relaxation.
  5 *Connective tissue disease.* Chronic steroid use, Ehlers-Danos syndrome and other related conditions can disrupt normal collagen-based pelvic tissue support.

Diagnosis

- *History.* A detailed history is important to identify co-existing medical conditions, prior obstetrical events, past/present medications and to determine the rate of progression.
- *Symptoms.* Mild degrees of genital prolapse are often asymptomatic, but the most common complaint is an annoying protrusion at the vaginal introitus. There may also be a bearing-down sensation that 'everything is falling out', discomfort and aching in the lower back, or difficulties with intercourse.
- *Pelvic examination.* Uterine procidentia *(opposite)* is obvious, but most patients have less pronounced prolapse.
  1 *Lithotomy.* The labia are spread and the protrusion identified. The patient is then asked to strain as though attempting defaecation and also to cough. What appears 1st at the introitus may suggest the location of the major defect. The bony structure of the pelvis, vaginal outlet, anterior and posterior vaginal walls and perineal body should all be evaluated. Rectovaginal examination may indicate an enterocele that bulges into the space between the rectum and upper posterior vaginal wall.
  2 *Standing.* The most reliable information can be obtained by repeating the examination when the patient is standing and straining maximally.

Classification and management

- Women without symptoms or whose symptoms are minimally bothersome may wish to defer any form of therapy.
- *Pessaries (opposite)* can be used to avoid surgery or improve symptoms while awaiting surgical correction. The goal of fitting is to provide satisfactory reduction of the protrusion, without causing discomfort or adversely affecting bladder function. Pessaries are commonly inadequate for posterior defects, procidentia and vault prolapse.
- *Vaginal hysterectomy* (Chapter 16) is usually performed at the same time as primary surgical treatment for pelvic organ prolapse.

Cystocele *(opposite)*
- *Surgical options. Anterior colporrhaphy (opposite)* involves vaginally plicating the endopelvic fascia in the midline to provide support. Variations of this technique have been used for over a century. *Paravaginal repair* replaces the anterolateral vaginal wall to its anatomic position. *McCall's culdoplasty* shortens the uterosacral ligaments and re-attaches them to the vaginal apex.

Rectocele *(opposite)*
- *Surgical options. Posterior colporrhaphy* mimics the anterior procedure with a midline placation of endopelvic fascia. *Perineorrhaphy* is commonly required due to a reduced anovaginal distance (less than 3 cm) or when there is insufficient strength to the perineal body.

Enterocele *(opposite)*
A true herniation of the peritoneal cavity at the pouch of Douglas between the uterosacral ligaments and into the rectovaginal septum.
- *Surgical options. Enterocele repair* is usually performed at the same time as posterior colporrhaphy. The hernia sac is visualized as the vagina is separated from the rectum and it must be dissected free of underlying tissue. The neck of the hernia is then isolated and sutured. Fixing the uterosacral ligaments to the sac will prevent recurrence.

Uterine procidentia *(opposite)*
- *Surgical options.* Vaginal hysterectomy with anterior and posterior colporrhaphy is most commonly performed. *Partial colpocleisis (Lefort procedure)* may be indicated in older women who are no longer sexually active: a strip of anterior and posterior vaginal wall is removed and the underlying tissue sutured together.

Posthysterectomy vaginal vault prolapse
Occurs at some time remote from hysterectomy due to failure of the cardinal and uterosacral ligaments to maintain their tone or attachment to the vagina.
- *Surgical options. Sacrospinous ligament suspension (SSLS) (opposite)* is a vaginal procedure that suspends the fascia of the vaginal apex to one, or both, sacrospinous ligaments. *Abdominal sacrocolpopexy (opposite)* involves attaching a suspensory mesh from the vaginal apex to the sacrum.

19 Puberty and precocious puberty

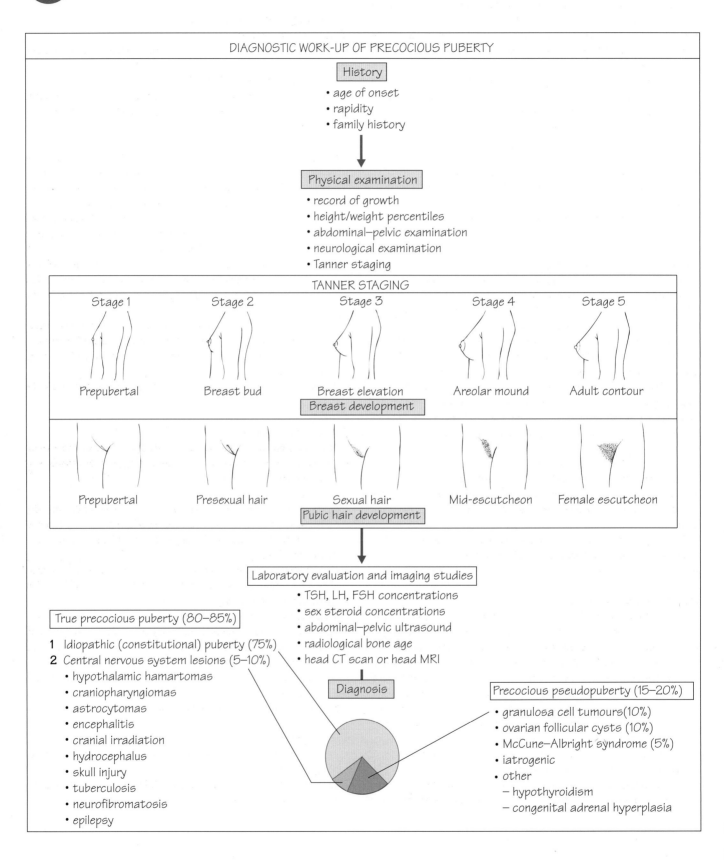

DIAGNOSTIC WORK-UP OF PRECOCIOUS PUBERTY

History
- age of onset
- rapidity
- family history

Physical examination
- record of growth
- height/weight percentiles
- abdominal–pelvic examination
- neurological examination
- Tanner staging

TANNER STAGING

Stage 1	Stage 2	Stage 3	Stage 4	Stage 5
Prepubertal	Breast bud	Breast elevation	Areolar mound	Adult contour

Breast development

Prepubertal	Presexual hair	Sexual hair	Mid-escutcheon	Female escutcheon

Pubic hair development

Laboratory evaluation and imaging studies
- TSH, LH, FSH concentrations
- sex steroid concentrations
- abdominal–pelvic ultrasound
- radiological bone age
- head CT scan or head MRI

Diagnosis

True precocious puberty (80–85%)

1 Idiopathic (constitutional) puberty (75%)
2 Central nervous system lesions (5–10%)
- hypothalamic hamartomas
- craniopharyngiomas
- astrocytomas
- encephalitis
- cranial irradiation
- hydrocephalus
- skull injury
- tuberculosis
- neurofibromatosis
- epilepsy

Precocious pseudopuberty (15–20%)
- granulosa cell tumours(10%)
- ovarian follicular cysts (10%)
- McCune–Albright syndrome (5%)
- iatrogenic
- other
  – hypothyroidism
  – congenital adrenal hyperplasia

Puberty

• *Definition:* the series of events leading to sexual maturity. A time of accelerated growth, skeletal maturation, development of secondary sexual characteristics, and achievement of fertility.

• *Thelarche* (breast development) is the first sign of puberty. It usually begins between 8 and 10 years of age and is associated with increased estrogen production.

• *Adrenarche* (development of pubic and axillary hair) is the second stage in maturation and typically occurs between 11 and 12 years of age. Axillary hair usually appears after the growth of pubic hair is complete.

• *Menarche* (onset of menstruation) usually occurs 2–3 years after thelarche at an average age of 11–13 years. Initial cycles are often anovulatory and irregular.

• The major determinant of the timing of puberty is genetic. Environmental factors (general health, nutritional status, geographic location) are also important.

• Thelarche and adrenarche are occurring significantly earlier than previously suggested—especially in black girls.

Biological basis of puberty

• Pubertal changes are triggered by the maturation of the hypothalamic–pituitary–ovarian axis.

• The onset of puberty is heralded by hypothalamic pulsatile release of gonadotropin-releasing hormone (GnRH).

• Increased pituitary gonadotropin (luteinizing hormone [LH], follicle-stimulating hormone [FSH]) production in response to pulsatile GnRH is the endocrinological *hallmark* of puberty.

• The final maturation phase is the development of a cyclic mid-cycle surge of LH in response to the positive feedback of the steroid hormones, primarily estradiol-17β. This mid-cycle LH surge induces ovulation and the normal female menstrual cycle (Chapter 2).

Precocious puberty

• *Definition:* pubertal changes before 8 years of age.

• *Guidelines for evaluation.* Thelarche or adrenarche should be evaluated if this occurs before age 7 in white girls and before age 6 in black girls.

• The two primary concerns of parents of children are the social stigma associated with the child being physically different from her peers and the diminished ultimate height.

Diagnostic work-up *(opposite)*

• *History.* Determining the age of onset, rapidity and family history is crucial. Co-existing illness (hypothyroidism), medications (estrogen ingestion), or a history of head trauma may be important.

• *Physical examination.* Increased growth is often the first observable change. Abdominal-pelvic examination should focus on examination of the external genitalia, ruling out a pelvic mass, and looking for signs of androgenization. A brief neurological examination may suggest the presence of an intracranial mass. Premature thelarche and pubarche can be quantified by assessment of Tanner stage.

• *Laboratory evaluation.* Thyroid function tests, LH/FSH values, and sex steroid levels may support the diagnosis.

• *Imaging studies.* Abdominal–pelvic ultrasound is an accurate way of detecting ovarian tumours. Bone age may be compared with standards for the patient's age. Head CT scan or MRI should be performed if an intracranial mass is suspected.

Types of precocious puberty *(opposite)*

True precocious puberty

• *Definition:* premature maturation of the hypothalamic–pituitary–ovarian axis.

• *Age of onset:* between the age of 6 and 8.

• *Sequelae.* The most serious adverse effect is short adult stature. Children are transiently tall for their age, but undergo premature epiphyseal fusion.

• *Aetiology.*

(i) *Idiopathic (constitutional) puberty* is most common in girls >4 years. This is a benign process and fundamentally a diagnosis of exclusion. The cause is unknown. Follow-up is necessary to rule out slow growing lesions of the brain, ovary, or adrenal gland.

Treatment: GnRH agonists in girls with menarche <8 years or those with unusually rapid progression of puberty having bone age >2 years ahead of chronologic age. The goals of therapy are to reduce gonadotrophin secretions, decrease the growth rate to normal and slow skeletal maturation to allow development of maximal adult height. Continuous chronic administration is maintained until the median age of puberty.

(ii) *Central nervous system lesions* are often present in girls <4 years Neurological symptoms (visual disturbance, headaches) commonly precede sexual development. Most lesions are located near the hypothalamus.

Treatment: surgery, chemotherapy, and/or irradiation may be indicated.

Precocious pseudopuberty

• *Definition:* premature female sexual maturation that is independent of hypothalamic pituitary control. The underlying process initiates activation of pubertal development.

• *Aetiology.*

(i) *Oestrogen-producing ovarian tumours* account for the majority of cases. Granulosa cell tumours are most common, but follicular cysts, thecomas, and Sertoli–Leydig tumours may also occur.

Treatment: Surgery.

(ii) *McCune–Albright syndrome (polyostotic fibrous dysplasia)* consists of multiple disseminated cystic bone lesions, café-au-lait spots, and sexual precocity.

Treatment: Testolactone (an aromatase inhibitor) prevents the conversion of estrogen precursors to biologically active estrogens and leads to a decreased rate of growth and skeletal maturation. The underlying disease is incurable.

(iii) *Iatrogenic causes* result from excessive exogenous hormonal administration.

Treatment: discontinuation of the medication.

Isolated precocity

• *Definition.* The premature development of a single pubertal event (usually thelarche).

• *Treatment:* reassurance, since this condition is usually self-limiting and resolves spontaneously.

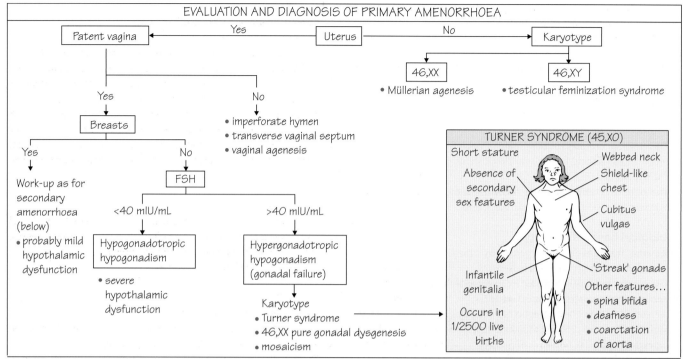

EVALUATION AND DIAGNOSIS OF PRIMARY AMENORRHOEA

Patent vagina ←—Yes— Uterus —No→ Karyotype

Karyotype:
- 46,XX
  - Müllerian agenesis
- 46,XY
  - testicular feminization syndrome

Patent vagina:
- Yes → Breasts
- No →
  - imperforate hymen
  - transverse vaginal septum
  - vaginal agenesis

Breasts:
- Yes → Work-up as for secondary amenorrhoea (below)
  - probably mild hypothalamic dysfunction
- No → FSH

FSH:
- <40 mIU/mL → Hypogonadotropic hypogonadism
  - severe hypothalamic dysfunction
- >40 mIU/mL → Hypergonadotropic hypogonadism (gonadal failure)
  - Karyotype
    - Turner syndrome
    - 46,XX pure gonadal dysgenesis
    - mosaicism

TURNER SYNDROME (45,XO)
- Short stature
- Absence of secondary sex features
- Infantile genitalia
- Occurs in 1/2500 live births
- Webbed neck
- Shield-like chest
- Cubitus vulgas
- 'Streak' gonads
- Other features...
  - spina bifida
  - deafness
  - coarctation of aorta

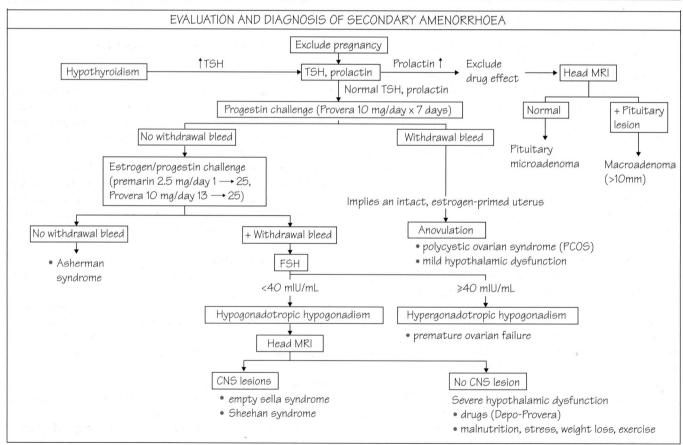

EVALUATION AND DIAGNOSIS OF SECONDARY AMENORRHOEA

Exclude pregnancy → TSH, prolactin

Hypothyroidism ←↑TSH— TSH, prolactin —Prolactin↑→ Exclude drug effect → Head MRI

Head MRI:
- Normal → Pituitary microadenoma
- + Pituitary lesion → Macroadenoma (>10mm)

TSH, prolactin —Normal TSH, prolactin→ Progestin challenge (Provera 10 mg/day x 7 days)

Progestin challenge:
- No withdrawal bleed → Estrogen/progestin challenge (premarin 2.5 mg/day 1 → 25, Provera 10 mg/day 13 → 25)
- Withdrawal bleed → Implies an intact, estrogen-primed uterus → Anovulation
  - polycystic ovarian syndrome (PCOS)
  - mild hypothalamic dysfunction

Estrogen/progestin challenge:
- No withdrawal bleed
  - Asherman syndrome
- + Withdrawal bleed → FSH

FSH:
- <40 mIU/mL → Hypogonadotropic hypogonadism → Head MRI
- ≥40 mIU/mL → Hypergonadotropic hypogonadism
  - premature ovarian failure

Head MRI:
- CNS lesions
  - empty sella syndrome
  - Sheehan syndrome
- No CNS lesion
  - Severe hypothalamic dysfunction
    - drugs (Depo-Provera)
    - malnutrition, stress, weight loss, exercise

- *Definition:* the absence or cessation of menstruation.
- Physiological in prepubertal girls, during pregnancy and lactation, and after menopause.
- Non-physiological (pathological) amenorrhoea occurs in 5% of reproductive-age women and affected patients should be investigated to determine the underlying aetiology.
- It is traditional to categorize amenorrhoea as primary or secondary, but there is often significant overlap.
- There has been a gradual but progressive fall in the mean age of menarche over the past century, largely as a result of improved nutrition and living conditions.

Primary amenorrhoea
- *Definition:* the absence of menstruation by age 16.
- *Prevalence:* 1–2% of girls.
- *Evaluation and diagnosis (opposite).* Clinical evaluation focuses on the presence or absence of the uterus, vaginal patency, and breast development.

Aetiology
Gonadal failure (35%)
- *Description. Hypergonadotropic hypogonadism* is characterized by streak gonads (bands of fibrous tissue in place of the ovary). Synthesis of ovarian steroids does not occur due to the absence of ovarian follicles. Breast development does not occur because of the very low circulating estradiol levels. Since estrogen is not necessary for Mullerian duct development or Wolffian duct regression, the internal and external genitalia are phenotypically normal female.
- *Causes. Turner syndrome* (45,XO) is the single most common cause of primary amenorrhoea *(opposite)*, accounting for >50% of patients with gonadal failure. The remaining causes are commonly due to other non-inherited chromosomal disorders or deletions.
- *Treatment:* oral contraceptives develop breast tissue and prevent osteoporosis. The presence of a Y chromosome on karyotype requires excision of gonadal tissue to prevent the 25% incidence of malignancy.

Hypothalamic dysfunction (20–30%)
- *Description. Hypogonadotropic hypogonadism* results in very low estrogen levels and the aetiology can be morphological or endocrinological.
- *Causes.* Most girls have aetiologies similar to those with secondary amenorrhea (see below). Central nervous system (CNS) lesions (pituitary or hypothalamic tumours) may have elevated prolactin levels. Inadequate GnRH release is due to either insufficient hypothalamic GnRH synthesis or a CNS neurotransmitter defect.
- *Treatment:* oral contraceptives. All patients should have imaging of the hypothalamic-pituitary region to rule out the presence of CNS lesion.

Vaginal agenesis and outflow tract obstruction (15–20%)
- *Description.* Dysmenorrhoea or pelvic pain suggest the possible existence of functional endometrium with obstruction to flow. Conversely, the absence of any symptoms despite normal secondary sexual characteristics would favour a diagnosis involving lack of endometrial tissue.
- *Causes. Vaginal agenesis* (Mayer–Rokitansky–Küster–Hauser syndrome) occurs in 1–2.5/10,000 female births and involves the congenital absence of all or part of the uterus and vagina. Renal abnormalities occur in about one-third of patients and skeletal abnormalities in 12%. These patients can be differentiated from those with testicular feminization syndrome by the presence of normal pubic hair. Imperforate hymen (1/1000 women) or transverse vaginal septum (1/80,000 women) are other variants.
- *Treatment:* creation of a neovagina by progressive dilation or surgery (McIndoe operation).

Testicular feminization syndrome (10%)
- *Description:* androgen insensitivity.
- *Cause.* Pseudohermaphrodites have external genitalia that are opposite of the gonads (testes, 46,XY genotype but female phenotype). Transmission is through an X-linked recessive gene, resulting in absent or markedly diminished androgen receptor activity.
- *Treatment:* This is the only exception to the rule that gonads with a Y chromosome should be removed as soon as the diagnosis is made. The testes should be left in place until after puberty is completed because peripheral conversion of androgen to estrogen promotes breast development and growth.

Secondary amenorrhoea
- *Definition:* the absence of menstruation for >6 months or for ≥3 menstrual cycles in a woman with p47reviously regular cyclic menses.
- *Prevalence:* 3–5% of women (excluding pregnancy).
- *Evaluation and diagnosis (opposite).*

Aetiology
Hypothalamic dysfunction (35%)
- *Causes.* Stress, weight loss, exercise, or drugs can result in a sustained decrease in GnRH pulse frequency and amplitude.
- *Treatment:* oral contraceptives are appropriate for severely affected patients with hypoestrogenism.

Polycystic ovarian syndrome (30%) (Chapter 21)

Pituitary disease (20%)
- *Causes. Prolactin-secreting pituitary adenomas* are the most common lesion. Empty sella syndrome and Sheehan syndrome (pituitary apoplexy, postpartum pituitary necrosis) are rare. Iatrogenic hyperprolactinemic amenorrhoea caused by drugs (especially phenothiazines) should be excluded.
- *Treatment:* surgical resection is usually indicated for patients with pituitary macroadenomas. Other hyperprolactinemic patients should be followed with serial prolactin levels and head imaging to exclude development of a macroadenoma. Therapy of empty sella syndrome and Sheehan syndrome involves hormone replacement.

Premature ovarian failure (10%)
- *Description:* loss of all ovarian follicles with cessation of menstruation prior to age 40.
- *Causes:* intrinsic ovarian defect, genetic mosaicism, autoimmune processes (myasthenia gravis), chemotherapy, radiation, infection.
- *Treatment:* none. Estrogen replacement therapy should be offered. A karyotype should be done if diagnosis occurs before age 30.

Asherman syndrome (5%)
- *Description:* intrauterine synechiae (adhesions) that interfere with normal endometrial growth and shedding.
- *Causes:* vigorous uterine curettage in early pregnancy; pelvic tuberculosis in developing countries.
- *Treatment:* hysteroscopic lysis of intrauterine adhesions and stimulation of the endometrium with oestrogen.

21 Polycystic ovarian syndrome (PCOS)

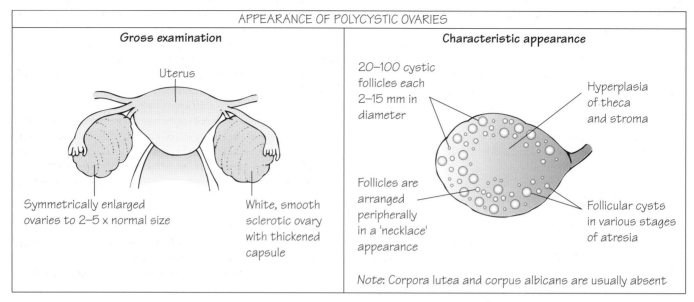

APPEARANCE OF POLYCYSTIC OVARIES

Gross examination

Uterus

Symmetrically enlarged ovaries to 2–5 x normal size

White, smooth sclerotic ovary with thickened capsule

Characteristic appearance

20–100 cystic follicles each 2–15 mm in diameter

Hyperplasia of theca and stroma

Follicles are arranged peripherally in a 'necklace' appearance

Follicular cysts in various stages of atresia

Note: Corpora lutea and corpus albicans are usually absent

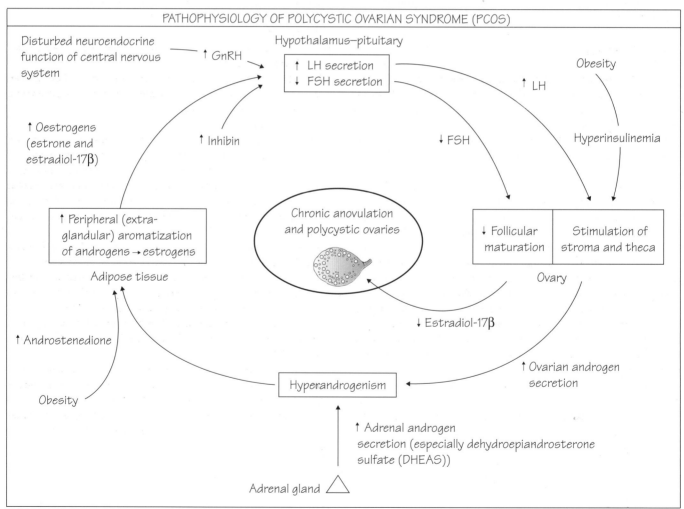

PATHOPHYSIOLOGY OF POLYCYSTIC OVARIAN SYNDROME (PCOS)

Disturbed neuroendocrine function of central nervous system

↑ GnRH

Hypothalamus–pituitary

↑ LH secretion
↓ FSH secretion

Obesity

↑ LH

↑ Oestrogens (estrone and estradiol-17β)

↑ Inhibin

↓ FSH

Hyperinsulinemia

↑ Peripheral (extra-glandular) aromatization of androgens → estrogens

Chronic anovulation and polycystic ovaries

↓ Follicular maturation

Stimulation of stroma and theca

Adipose tissue

Ovary

↓ Estradiol-17β

↑ Androstenedione

↑ Ovarian androgen secretion

Obesity

Hyperandrogenism

↑ Adrenal androgen secretion (especially dehydroepiandrosterone sulfate (DHEAS))

Adrenal gland △

- *Definition:* a heterogeneous disorder of unexplained hyperandrogenic chronic anovulation in which secondary causes (androgen-secreting neoplasms) have been excluded.
- *Prevalence:* 4–6% of reproductive-age women.
- *Aetiology.* Unknown: no gene or specific environmental substance has been identified.

Diagnostic evaluation

- *History.* The history should focus on the menstrual pattern, previous pregnancies (if any), concomitant medications, smoking, alcohol consumption, diet and identification of family members with diabetes and cardiovascular disease.
- *Physical examination* should look for balding, acne, clitoromegaly, body hair distribution and signs of insulin resistance (obesity, centripetal fat distribution, acanthosis nigricans). Bimanual examination may suggest enlarged ovaries *(opposite)*.
- *Laboratory tests* such as testosterone or dehydroepiandrosterone sulfate (DHEAS) are useful for documenting ovarian hyperandrogenism. Androgen-secreting tumours of the ovary or adrenal gland are also invariably accompanied by elevated circulating androgen levels, but there is no absolute level that is pathognomonic for a tumour or minimum level that excludes a tumour.
- *Imaging studies* such as a pelvic sonogram can exclude a solid ovarian tumour and may demonstrate the characteristic 'polycystic' appearance of the ovaries *(opposite)*.

Pathophysiology *(opposite)*

- PCOS represents the end-stage of a 'vicious cycle' of endocrinological events which can be initiated at many different entry points.
- It remains unclear whether the primary pathology resides in the ovary or in the hypothalamus, but the fundamental defect appears to be 'inappropriate' signaling to the hypothalamus and pituitary.
- Elevated LH levels (the hallmark of PCOS) result from increased peripheral strogen production (positive feedback) and increased GnRH secretion.
- Suppressed FSH levels result from increased peripheral estrogen production (negative feedback) and increased secretion of inhibin.
- PCOS is characterized by a 'steady state' of chronically elevated LH and chronically suppressed FSH levels, instead of their cyclic rise and fall in a normal menstrual cycle (Chapter 3).
- Increased LH stimulates ovarian stroma and theca cells to increase production of androgens. Androgens are converted peripherally by aromatization to estrogens, which perpetuate chronic anovulation.
- As a result of suppressed FSH, new follicular growth is continuously stimulated but not to the point of full maturation and ovulation (corpus lutea and corpus albicans are rarely detected). Elevated androgens contribute to the prevention of normal follicular development and induction of premature atresia.
- The *ovary* is the major site of androgen overproduction; the adrenal gland has a minor role.
- Increased adipose tissue in obese patients contributes to the extraglandular aromatization of androgens to estrogens.

- Circulating testosterone is increased (causing hirsutism), because sex hormone-binding globulin (SHBG) levels are decreased in PCOS.

Clinical manifestations

- *Menstrual irregularities* (80%) begin soon after menarche, including secondary amenorrhoea and/or oligomenorrhoea.
- *Hirsutism* (70%) refers to the presence of excessive male pattern (upper lip, chin, chest, back) hair growth in women.
- *Obesity* (50%) contributes substantially to the metabolic abnormalities of PCOS.
- *Infertility* (75%) is due to chronic anovulation.
- *Acanthosis nigricans* is a dermatological marker of insulin resistance and hyperinsulinemia that is marked by grey-brown, velvety, sometimes verrucous, discoloration of the skin at the neck, groin, and axillae.
- *HAIR–AN syndrome* (*H*yper*A*ndrogenism, *I*nsulin *R*esistance, and *A*canthosis *N*igricans) represents the extreme effects of hyperandrogenic chronic anovulation.

Long-term sequelae

- *Endometrial hyperplasia or adenocarcinoma* (Chapter 30) can develop from chronic estrogenic uterine exposure.
- *Glucose intolerance or non-insulin-dependent diabetes mellitus* is increased 2–5 fold.
- *Cardiovascular disease and dyslipidemia* are common.

Management

Directed toward interrupting the self-perpetuating cycle of hyperandrogenic chronic anovulation.
- Weight reduction can reduce androgen secretion in obese women with hirsutism by (i) decreasing peripheral oestrogen aromatization and (ii) decreasing hyperinsulinemia.
- *Medical therapy*
  1 *Oral contraceptives* have been the mainstay of long-term management of PCOS by: decreasing LH and FSH secretion and ovarian production of androgens, increasing hepatic production of SHBG, decreasing levels of DHEA and preventing endometrial neoplasia. Cyproterone acetate (UK standard), spironolactone or topical eflornithine may be helpful in patients with excessive hirsutism.
  2 *Progestins* have been shown to suppress pituitary LH and FSH and circulating androgens, but break-through bleeding is common.
  3 *Insulin-sensitizing agents* (metformin) decrease circulating androgen levels, improve the ovulation rate and improve glucose tolerance, but these drugs are not currently approved for use in PCOS.
  4 *Clomiphene citrate* (Chapter 24) has traditionally been the first-line treatment for women desiring pregnancy.
- *Surgical therapy*
  1 *Ovarian drilling* with laser or diathermy has few advantages over medical therapy for infertility and does not appear to have significant long-term benefits in improving metabolic abnormalities.
  2 *Mechanical hair removal* (laser vaporization, electrolysis, depilatory creams) often is the front line of treatment for hirsutism.

Recurrent pregnancy loss

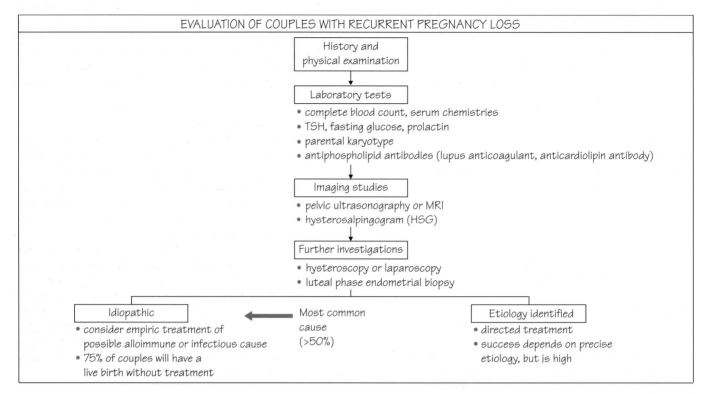

EVALUATION OF COUPLES WITH RECURRENT PREGNANCY LOSS

History and physical examination
↓
Laboratory tests
- complete blood count, serum chemistries
- TSH, fasting glucose, prolactin
- parental karyotype
- antiphospholipid antibodies (lupus anticoagulant, anticardiolipin antibody)
↓
Imaging studies
- pelvic ultrasonography or MRI
- hysterosalpingogram (HSG)
↓
Further investigations
- hysteroscopy or laparoscopy
- luteal phase endometrial biopsy

Idiopathic ← Most common cause (>50%) → Etiology identified

Idiopathic
- consider empiric treatment of possible alloimmune or infectious cause
- 75% of couples will have a live birth without treatment

Etiology identified
- directed treatment
- success depends on precise etiology, but is high

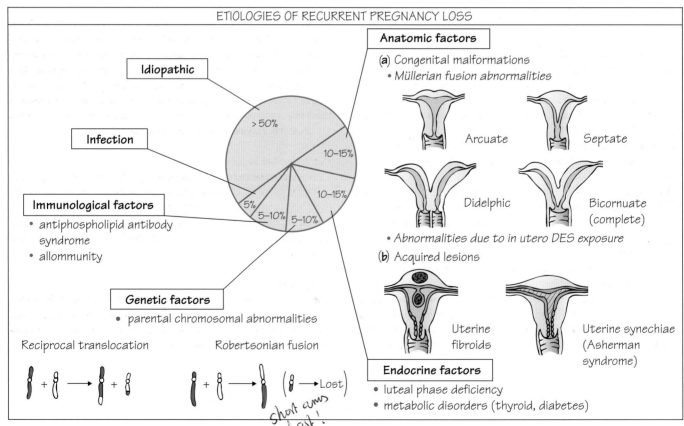

ETIOLOGIES OF RECURRENT PREGNANCY LOSS

Idiopathic

Infection

Immunological factors
- antiphospholipid antibody syndrome
- allommunity

Genetic factors
- parental chromosomal abnormalities

Reciprocal translocation   Robertsonian fusion

short arms lost!

> 50%
10–15%
10–15%
5%
5–10%
5–10%

Anatomic factors

(a) Congenital malformations
- Müllerian fusion abnormalities

Arcuate   Septate

Didelphic   Bicornuate (complete)

- Abnormalities due to in utero DES exposure

(b) Acquired lesions

Uterine fibroids   Uterine synechiae (Asherman syndrome)

Endocrine factors
- luteal phase deficiency
- metabolic disorders (thyroid, diabetes)

- *Definition:* Two or more consecutive pregnancy losses.
- *Prevalence:* 1% of reproductive-age women.

Diagnostic evaluation of couples *(opposite)*

- *History.* The pattern, trimester and characteristics of prior pregnancy losses should be reviewed. Exposure to environmental toxins and drugs, prior gynaecological or obstetric infections and excluding the possibility of consanguinity are important.
- *Physical examination* may reveal evidence of maternal systemic disease or uterine anomalies.
- *Laboratory tests and imaging studies* should be individually utilized.

Aetiology *(opposite–clockwise)*

Most couples will have no clear explanation for their recurrent pregnancy loss. Several alleged causes are controversial and anxious patients/physicians often explore empirical or alternative treatments having dubious benefit.

Idiopathic (>50%)

- Informative and supportive counselling serves an important role because 60–70% of women with at least one previous live birth will have a successful next pregnancy.

Anatomic factors (10–15%)

- *Uterine anomalies* are most often associated with 2nd trimester loss. Congenital malformations (Chapter 10) result from Mullerian fusion abnormalities and acquired lesions have a more controversial impact. Surgical revision may be helpful in some circumstances.
- *Incompetent cervix* (Chapter 55) also accounts for mainly 2nd trimester losses. Cerclage placement may be beneficial in selected patients.

Endocrine factors (10–15%)

- *Luteal phase deficiency* is purported to result from insufficient progesterone secretion by the corpus luteum, resulting in inadequate preparation of the endometrium for implantation and/or an inability to maintain early pregnancy. Two 'out-of-phase' endometrial biopsies (in which histological dating lags behind menstrual dating by ≤ 2 days) in consecutive cycles are required for the diagnosis. Progesterone supplementation is commonly prescribed, but therapeutic benefit is speculative.
- *Metabolic disorders* (hypothyroidism, poorly controlled diabetes, PCOS [Chapter 21]) require diagnosis and treatment of the underlying disease. Mild or sub-clinical endocrine diseases are not causative.

Genetic factors (5–10%)

- *Parental chromosomal abnormalities* are the *only proven cause* of recurrent pregnancy loss. The most frequent karyotypic abnormality is a balanced translocation–found most often in the female partner. 2/3 are reciprocal (exchange of chromatin between any two non-homologous chromosomes without loss of genetic material). 1/3 are Robertsonian (fusion of chromosomes that have the centromere very near one end of a chromosome (typically 13, 14, 15, 21, or 22) with loss of one centromere and two short arms). The overall risk of spontaneous miscarriage in couples with a balanced translocation is >25%. The only treatment option may be in vitro fertilization (Chapter 25) with donor sperm or ova.

- *Recurrent embryonic aneuploidy* may represent non-random events in some predisposed couples. Most aneuploid losses are the result of advanced maternal age. Prenatal diagnosis via amniocentesis or chorionic villus sampling may be useful in some situations—but no treatment is available.

Immunological factors (5–10%)

- *Antiphospholipid antibody syndrome* is an autoimmune disorder characterized by circulating antibodies against membrane phospholipids and at least one specific clinical syndrome (recurrent pregnancy loss, unexplained thrombosis, fetal death). The diagnosis requires at least one confirmatory serological test (lupus anticoagulant, anticardiolipin antibody). The treatment of choice is aspirin plus heparin (or prednisone in some circumstances).
- *Alloimmunity* (immunological differences between individuals) has been proposed as a factor between reproductive partners that causes otherwise unexplained recurrent pregnancy loss. During normal pregnancy, the mother's immune system is thought to recognize semiallogeneic (50% 'non-self') fetal antigens and to produce 'blocking' factors to protect the fetus. Failure to produce these blocking factors may play a role, but there is no direct scientific evidence to support this theory and there is no specific diagnostic test. Immunotherapy has been used in an attempt to promote immune tolerance to paternal antigen.

Infection (5%)

- *Listeria monocytogenes, mycoplasma hominis, Ureaplasma urealyticum, Toxoplasma gondii* and *viruses* (herpes simplex, cytomegalovirus, rubella) have been variously associated with spontaneous abortion, but none have been proven to cause recurrent pregnancy loss. Diagnosis can be made using cervical cultures, viral titres, or serum antibodies. Directed antibiotic therapy may be useful if a causative agent is identified. However, empirical treatment with doxycycline or erythromycin may be more cost effective and efficient.

Other possible factors

- *Environmental toxins* such as smoking, alcohol, and heavy coffee consumption have been associated with an increased risk of spontaneous miscarriage, but not recurrent pregnancy loss.
- *Drugs* such as folic acid antagonists, valproic acid, warfarin, anaesthetic gases, tetrachloroethylene, and Isotretinoin (Accutane) are also not proven causes.

Prognosis

Couples with recurrent pregnancy losses are often anxious, frustrated, and on the verge of despair. Fortunately, the possibility of achieving a live birth is high. Success depends chiefly on maternal age and the number of previous losses, but also on the precise aetiology.

23 The infertile couple

CAUSES OF INFERTILITY

FEMALE FACTOR

1 Ovarian factors
- polycystic ovarian syndrome (chronic anovulation)
- premature ovarian failure
- hypothalamic amenorrhoea

2 Tubal and peritoneal factors
- pelvic adhesions
- endometriosis
- prior ruptured ectopic pregnancy

Note: tubal obstruction can be demonstrated by either hysterosalpingogram (HSG) or during laparoscopy

3 Cervical factors
- cervical stenosis
- cervicitis

Basal body temperature chart

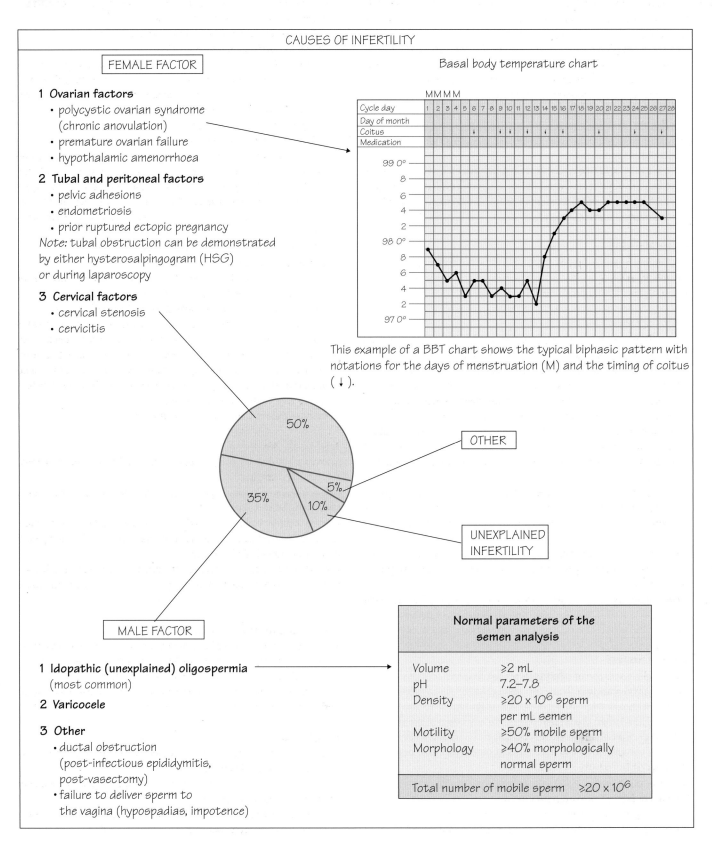

This example of a BBT chart shows the typical biphasic pattern with notations for the days of menstruation (M) and the timing of coitus (↓).

OTHER

UNEXPLAINED INFERTILITY

MALE FACTOR

1 Idopathic (unexplained) oligospermia (most common)

2 Varicocele

3 Other
- ductal obstruction (post-infectious epididymitis, post-vasectomy)
- failure to deliver sperm to the vagina (hypospadias, impotence)

Normal parameters of the semen analysis	
Volume	≥2 mL
pH	7.2–7.8
Density	≥20 × 10^6 sperm per mL semen
Motility	≥50% mobile sperm
Morphology	≥40% morphologically normal sperm
Total number of mobile sperm	≥20 × 10^6

Definitions
- *Fertility:* the capacity to conceive and produce offspring.
- *Fecundity:* the probability of conceiving during a single monthly cycle. The fecundity of 'normal' couples is 20–25%, with a cumulative 85–90% chance of pregnancy in 12 months.
- *Infertility:* the inability to conceive after 12 months of frequent intercourse without contraception. Primary infertility refers to couples who have never achieved a pregnancy. Secondary infertility implies that at least one previous conception has taken place.

Incidence
- 10–15% of reproductive-age married couples are considered infertile.
- The prevalence of infertility has remained constant, but the number of office visits to physicians by 'infertile' couples has tripled over the past 20 years. This 'infertility epidemic' has been attributed primarily to elective postponement of childbearing.

Risk factors
- Fecundity in women peaks at age 25 and declines thereafter.
- Cigarette smoking, illicit drug use and occupational and environmental exposures decrease the fecundity rate.

Initial assessment
- A basic infertility investigation is indicated if a couple has been trying to conceive for ≤1 year. In some cases, it may be appropriate to initiate an evaluation sooner (for example, in women >35 years).
- Infertility is a condition with a unique and profound psychological and emotional impact. Most couples view their 'failure' to achieve pregnancy as a life crisis in which they feel powerless.
- The primary goals of an infertility evaluation are to provide a rational approach to diagnosis, to present an accurate assessment of ongoing progress and prognosis and to educate the couple about reproductive physiology.
- *History.* Relevant details include the couples' age, previous pregnancies, and length of time attempting conception. A sexual history is particularly important, focusing on the frequency and timing of intercourse, lubricant use and impotence.
- *Physical examination.* Features of an endocrine disorder (hirsutism, galactorrhoea, thyromegaly) or gynaecological pathology (fibroids) may be evident.
- *Laboratory tests.* A complete blood count, urinalysis, Papanicolaou smear, and fasting blood glucose may indicate an underlying illness.

Basic work-up
- The common causes of infertility are evaluated by:
    - (i) documentation of ovulation
    - (ii) semen analysis
    - (iii) evaluation of tubal patency
    - (iv) diagnostic laparoscopy (if indicated).

Causes of infertility *(opposite)*
Female factor (50%)
1 Ovarian factor (anovulation) (20%)
- *History:* secondary amenorrhoea, irregular menses.
- *Physical examination:* obesity, hirsutism, galactorrhoea.

- *Screening tests. Urinary kits* are available to accurately detect the mid-cycle LH surge—indicating ovulation. Other methods include recording daily basal body temperature recordings or measuring the luteal phase progesterone concentration.
- *Treatment:* ovulation induction (Chapter 24).

2 Tubal and peritoneal factors (20%)
- *History.* Prior pelvic infection or ectopic pregnancy may suggest pelvic adhesions. Secondary dysmenorrhoea or cyclic pelvic pain should prompt consideration of endometriosis. However, there are no identifiable risk factors in 50% of patients.
- *Physical examination:* stigmata of endometriosis.
- *Screening tests. Hysterosalpingogram* involves injection of a radio-opaque dye through the cervix into the uterus with spillage into the peritoneal cavity. It assesses tubal patency as well as outlining the uterine cavity. Hysterosalpingo contrast sonography (HyCoSy) is another less commonly used method. Laparoscopy with tubal lavage is the 'gold standard' diagnostic test because it can exclude adhesions and endometriosis.
- *Treatment:* surgery or *in vitro* fertilization (Chapter 25).

3 Cervical factor (10%)
- *History:* prior cervical surgery (cone biopsy, cautery), infection, or *in utero* diethylstilbestrol (DES) exposure.
- *Physical examination:* cervical abnormalities, lesions.
- *Screening tests.* None are reliable. However, the post-coital test is a historical method to evaluate sperm–cervical mucus interaction. Mucus from the endocervical canal is examined after intercourse. The finding of 5–10 progressively motile sperm per high-power field in clear, acellular mucus with a spinnbarkeit (stretchability) of >8 cm generally excludes a cervical factor.
- *Treatment:* intrauterine insemination (IUI).

Male factor (35%)
- *History:* testicular injury, genito-urinary infection, chemotherapy, post-pubertal mumps.
- *Physical examination:* hypospadias, varicocele, cryptorchism (small testes), penile anomalies.
- *Screening test. Semen analysis* is the primary screening test for male infertility. Several samples should be analysed over a 1–3 month period because of individual fluctuations.
- *Treatment:* surgical correction of varicocele; *in vitro* fertilization with or without intracytoplasmic sperm injection (ICSI) or donor insemination.

Unexplained infertility (10–15%)
- *History:* female member is ovulatory and has patent oviducts; male member has at least 20 million motile sperm in the ejaculate.
- *Physical examination and screening tests:* normal.
- *Treatment:* ovulation induction and IUI with a washed sample of freshly prepared, recently ejaculated sperm.

Prognosis
- 50% of couples will successfully achieve pregnancy among the couples with an identifiable cause.
- 60% of couples with unexplained infertility who receive no treatment will conceive within 3–5 years.
- The most difficult decision for a couple is deciding when to cease intervention and consider adoption.

WORLD HEALTH ORGANIZATION (WHO) CLASSIFICATION OF OVULATORY DISORDERS			
	Group 1	**Group 2**	**Group 3**
Mechanism	Hypothalamic–pituitary failure	Hypothalamic–pituitary dysfunction	Ovarian (end-organ) failure
Effect on: 1 LH+FSH	(GnRH→) $\downarrow\downarrow\downarrow$	Normal	(GnRH→) $\uparrow\uparrow\uparrow$
2 Estradiol-17β	$\downarrow\downarrow\downarrow$	Normal	−ve feedback $\downarrow\downarrow\downarrow$
Frequency	Common	Most common	Least common
Main diagnosis	Hypothalamic amenorrhoea	Polycystic ovarian syndrome (PCOS) ⊕LH	Ovarian failure
Treatment	Gonadotropin (hMG) or GnRH therapy	Clomiphene citrate	Ovum donation

OVARIAN HYPERSTIMULATION SYNDROME (OHSS)			
	Mild	**Moderate**	**Severe**
Frequency	Common	Uncommon	<2%
Symptoms/signs (usually occur 5–7 days after ovulation)	Mild pelvic discomfort	Nausea/vomiting Abdominal distension Weight gain	Rare events include ovarian rupture with haemorrhage and adult respiratory distress syndrome (ARDS) • Pleural effusions • Ascites • Ovarian enlargement >12 cm • Thrombo-embolism • Oliguria, electrolyte imbalance
Ovarian enlargement	<6 cm	6–12 cm	>12 cm
Estradiol-17β level	2000–4000 pg/mL	4000–6000 pg/mL	>6000 pg/mL
Treatment	Observation	Close monitoring, avoid pelvic or abdominal examinations	Hospitalization with supportive care Note: potentially life threatening

Note: • if no pregnancy occurs, symptoms usually resolve within 7 days
• if pregnancy occurs, symptoms may persist for weeks

Classification of ovulatory disorders
• Ovarian factor infertility (anovulation) is the primary abnormality in 20% of infertile couples.
• Patients are classified into three groups *(opposite)*.
• Ovulation induction is one of the most successful means of treating infertility, but careful patient selection is essential.

Methods of ovulation induction
Clomiphene citrate
• *Indications.* The most common medication used to induce ovulation and the treatment of choice for women with unexplained infertility or chronic anovulation but adequate levels of estrogen and gonadotropins (WHO group 2).
• *Advantages/disadvantages:* safe, effective, cheap, orally administered.
• *Mode of action.* Clomiphene is a non-steroidal estrogen receptor antagonist (a weak estrogen) that is structurally related to tamoxifen and DES. It reduces the negative feedback effect of circulating estrogen, thereby triggering hypothalamic GnRH secretion. Enhanced release of pituitary gonadotropins (FSH, LH) leads to follicular recruitment, selection, and ovulation 5–10 days after the last dose.
• *Dosage.* Initial dose (Clomid®) is 50 mg daily for 5 days beginning on the fifth day of the menstrual cycle. The dose is increased in each cycle in 50 mg increments until ovulation is observed. If there is no response to 150 mg daily dosage, further evaluation is warranted.
• *Monitoring response to therapy.* Follicular development can be monitored ultrasonographically or by measuring serum estradiol-17β concentrations 6–7 days after the last dose of clomiphene. An increased progesterone level 14–15 days after the last clomiphene dose is the hallmark of the luteal phase and implies that ovulation has occurred. At the conclusion of a cycle, either the patient is pregnant or menses occurs and a further cycle is initiated. Once ovulation has been documented at a given dose of clomiphene, there is no advantage to increasing the dose in subsequent cycles.
• *Adjunctive therapy.* The addition of hCG may be necessary in women who exhibit complete ovarian follicular development but not ovulation.
• *Prognosis:* 80% of selected women will ovulate on clomiphene, although only 40% will become pregnant. Success is highest in the first few months of therapy. Failure to conceive within 6 ovulatory clomiphene cycles should prompt re-evaluation.
• *Side-effects:* vasomotor flushes, breast tenderness, visual symptoms, and nausea are common, but not dose-related.
• *Contraindications:* liver disease, pregnancy.
• *Complications:* multiple pregnancies (5–10%).

Human menopausal gonadotropins (hMG)
• *Indications.* The treatment of choice for ovulation induction in women with ovulatory dysfunction and low levels of estrogen and gonadotropins (WHO group 1). It is also used in women who fail to ovulate on clomiphene.
• *Advantages/disadvantages:* expensive.
• *Mode of action.* hMG is a purified preparation of gonadotropins extracted from the urine of post-menopausal women. Administration promotes follicular growth and maturation by increasing estradiol-17β secretion.
• *Dosage.* The recommended initial daily dose is 75–150 IU intramuscularly, but should be individualized.
• *Monitoring response to therapy.* Ultrasonography and serial estradiol-17β measurements are required during each cycle to monitor ovarian response to therapy. In general, hMG is administered daily until the serum estradiol-17β level is >100 pg/mL (usually 7–12 d). hMG is then continued at the same dose and ultrasound examinations are initiated to document the number of follicles and their size. The subsequent rise in serum estradiol-17β levels during this active phase is rapid and follicles typically enlarge by 2–3 mm/d.
• *Adjunctive therapy.* When the leading follicle(s) is 16–20 mm in diameter, a single dose of 5000–10,000 IU of hCG is administered intramuscularly to substitute for the endogenous LH surge. This triggers ovulation.
• *Prognosis.* 90% of selected women ≤35 years will conceive within 6 treatment cycles (lower success rates for older individuals).
• *Complications:* multiple pregnancy (10–30%), ectopic pregnancy, ovarian hyperstimulation syndrome *(opposite)*.

Bromocriptine mesylate (Parlodel®)
• *Indications.* Bromocriptine is only indicated for women with hyperprolactinemic ovulatory dysfunction due to prolactin-secreting pituitary adenomas or idiopathic hyperprolactinemia.
• *Advantages/disadvantages:* reduces the size of prolactin-secreting tumours.
• *Mode of action.* Elevated prolactin levels interfere with the normal menstrual cycle by suppressing pulsatile secretion of GnRH by the hypothalamus. Bromocriptine is a dopamine agonist that inhibits the pituitary secretion of prolactin.
• *Dosage.* The initial dose of 1.25 mg daily may be increased weekly in 1.25 mg increments until normal menstruation is achieved.
• *Prognosis.* Bromocriptine will restore menstruation in 90% of hyperprolactinemic women and 80% will get pregnant.
• *Side-effects:* nausea, vomiting, headaches, postural hypotension (may be minimized by bedtime administration).

Gonadotropin-releasing hormone
• *Indications.* Pulsatile GnRH therapy is used in patients with WHO group 1 or hyperprolactinemic ovulatory dysfunction.
• *Advantages/disadvantages.* GnRH is less expensive than hMG and does not require intensive monitoring. However, a portable pump with a catheter must be worn continuously.
• *Mode of action:* exogenous pulsatile GnRH serves as an artificial hypothalamus to stimulate pituitary gonadotropin release and thus ovulation.
• *Dosage.* GnRH is administered via intravenous (5–10 μg per pulse) or subcutaneous (10–20 μg per pulse) injection.
• *Prognosis:* 80% of selected patients conceive within 6 cycles.
• *Complications.* Ovarian hyperstimulation and multiple gestation are rare, because only 'physiological' levels of FSH are generated by the GnRH pump. Local, mild catheter-related complications are common.

25 Assisted reproductive technology (ART)

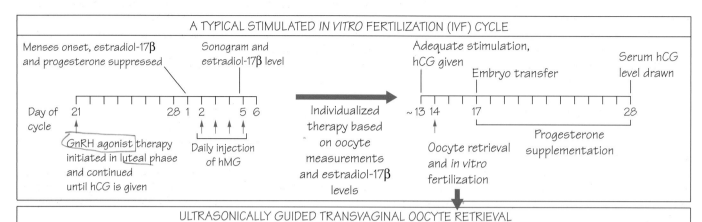

A TYPICAL STIMULATED *IN VITRO* FERTILIZATION (IVF) CYCLE

Menses onset, estradiol-17β and progesterone suppressed

Sonogram and estradiol-17β level

Adequate stimulation, hCG given

Embryo transfer

Serum hCG level drawn

Day of cycle: 21 ... 28 1 2 ... 5 6

GnRH agonist therapy initiated in luteal phase and continued until hCG is given

Daily injection of hMG

Individualized therapy based on oocyte measurements and estradiol-17β levels

~13 14 ... 17 ... 28

Oocyte retrieval and in vitro fertilization

Progesterone supplementation

ULTRASONICALLY GUIDED TRANSVAGINAL OOCYTE RETRIEVAL

Individual follicles are serially punctured and follicular fluid is aspirated and transferred to an embryology laboratory for oocyte identification

Aspiration needle can be seen evacuating follicles (care must be taken to avoid major blood vessels)

Ovary

Transducer

Inspiration needle

TRANSCERVICAL EMBRYO TRANSFER

Embryos are injected at the fundus

OR

Ultrasonographic localization

One tube is selectively cannulated and gametes (GIFT) or zygotes (ZIFT) are injected

IVF

GIFT/ZIFT

(may also be achieved by laparoscopic embryo transfer)

EFFECT OF ASSISTED REPRODUCTIVE TECHNOLOGY ON MULTIFETAL PREGNANCY

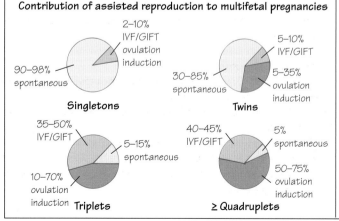

Contribution of assisted reproduction to multifetal pregnancies

2–10% IVF/GIFT ovulation induction
90–98% spontaneous
Singletons

5–10% IVF/GIFT
5–35% ovulation induction
30–85% spontaneous
Twins

35–50% IVF/GIFT
5–15% spontaneous
10–70% ovulation induction
Triplets

40–45% IVF/GIFT
5% spontaneous
50–75% ovulation induction
≥ Quadruplets

Multifetal pregnancy rates with different infertility treatment strategies

Percentage of multifetal pregnancies

Infertility treatment	Twins	Triplets (%)	Higher order (%)
None	1–2	<0.05	<0.001
Ovulation induction			
Clomiphene	5–10	0.5	<0.5
hMG	15–30	5–8	0.5–4
Pulsatile GnRH	5–10	2–5	<0.1
Assisted reproduction			
IVF	10–50	4–8	05–6
GIFT/ZIFT	20–25	2–8	0.1–2

- *Definition:* direct handling and manipulation of oocytes and sperm to enhance the probability of achieving a pregnancy.
- *Classification.* In vitro fertilization (IVF) is the prototype ART procedure. Other techniques include gamete or zygote intrafallopian tube transfer (GIFT, ZIFT), intracytoplasmic sperm injection (ICSI) and cryo-embryo transfer.
- *Frequency.* The first 'test tube' baby conceived by IVF was delivered in 1978. Since that historic birth, ART has undergone rapid growth and is very commonly performed.
- *Goal:* to maximize the chance of a successful pregnancy while minimizing the risk of multiple gestation.

In vitro fertilization
Patient selection
- Since IVF bypasses the fallopian tubes, it was originally developed for tubal factor infertility. However, it is now also used for all infertility conditions that have not been successfully treated with other modalities.
- Maternal age is strongly predictive of IVF success. Most IVF programs limit treatment to women ≤42 years.
- A serum FSH level of >15 mIU/mL on day 3 of the menstrual cycle is suggestive of diminished ovarian responsiveness and poor outcome.
- IVF with donor ovum may be recommended for women over 42 years, those with a day-3 FSH >15 mIU/mL and those who have traditionally been considered sterile (Turner syndrome).

Ovarian stimulation
- Although unstimulated ('natural cycle') or clomiphene-stimulated IVF cycles are less costly, few oocytes are harvested and success rates are low. These techniques are rarely used. Controlled ovarian hyperstimulation maximizes the retrieval of multiple healthy oocytes.
- A typical stimulated IVF cycle *(opposite)* is initiated by the administration of a GnRH agonist (leuprolide acetate, nafarelin) in the late luteal phase of the cycle. GnRH prevents premature (natural cycle) ovulation, decreases cycle cancellation, and increases the number of successful pregnancies per cycle. *human menopausal gonadotrophin*
- Follicular growth and development is achieved with daily intramuscular administration of hMG (Chapter 24). Once 'adequate' ovarian stimulation is achieved (lead follicle >16 mm diameter, at least 3 or 4 other follicles >13 mm diameter, and a serum estradiol level ≥200 pg/mL per large follicle), hCG is given as a substitute for the LH surge to promote maturation of the oocytes in preparation for ovulation.
- 10–30% of IVF cycles are cancelled due to inadequate follicular response.

Oocyte retrieval
- Ultrasound-guided transvaginal oocyte retrieval *(opposite)* is performed 24–36 hours after hCG administration.
- The number of harvested oocytes depends on the number of follicles >12 mm. Retrieved oocytes are scored for maturity.

Fertilization
- Semen is collected the day of oocyte retrieval. The sperm are 'washed' and incubated in supplemented medium.

- 4–5 hours after oocyte retrieval, 50,000–150,000 motile sperm are added to each dish containing a single mature oocyte.
- 18 hours after insemination, the ova are examined microscopically for evidence of fertilization (the presence of two pronuclei). Mature oocytes have a fertilization rate of 50–70%.
- 4–5 embryos are then selected for further development. Extra embryos can be cryopreserved.
- To demonstrate complete failure of fertilization, at least 3 cycles are necessary.

Embryo culture and transfer
- The fertilized oocytes are placed in growth medium and usually not examined until the day of transfer (typically 3 days after oocyte retrieval).
- Transcervical embryo transfer *(opposite)* consists of loading the embryos into a flexible catheter, which is then placed through the cervix, and the contents injected. Patients are discharged home 30–60 minutes later.

Luteal phase support
- Progesterone supplementation is started on the day of embryo transfer and continued until the placenta takes over progesterone production or implantation fails. Progesterone supplementation improves pregnancy outcome.
- A quantitative β-subunit of hCG measurement can be obtained 11–12 days after transfer to check for successful implantation.

Gamete/zygote intrafallopian transfer
- GIFT is a modification of IVF in which oocytes and sperm are placed into the fallopian tube instead of the uterus *(opposite)*. It is an alternative approach for infertile women with functional fallopian tubes.
- ZIFT is similar to GIFT but with placement of fertilized oocytes (zygotes) into the fallopian tube.

Intracytoplasmic sperm injection (ICSI)
- Direct injection of a single sperm into the cytoplasm of the oocyte and the treatment of choice for refractory male factor infertility.
- Success rates approach 30%.
- May cause an increase in the rate of congenital abnormalities.

Cryo-embryo transfer
- Transfer of thawed embryos into the uterus.
- Two-thirds of cryopreserved embryos survive.
- The major advantage is the ability to avoid repeated ovarian stimulation and oocyte retrieval.

Pregnancy outcome
- The field of ART is often criticized for a lack of randomized clinical trials demonstrating superior fecundity.
- The live birth rate per cycle initiated ranges from 15 to 35% for all ART procedures.
- Ectopic pregnancies occur in 3–5% of cycles.
- *Effect of ART on multifetal pregnancy (opposite).* Transfer of several embryos increases the pregnancy rate, but also increases the number of multiple pregnancies.

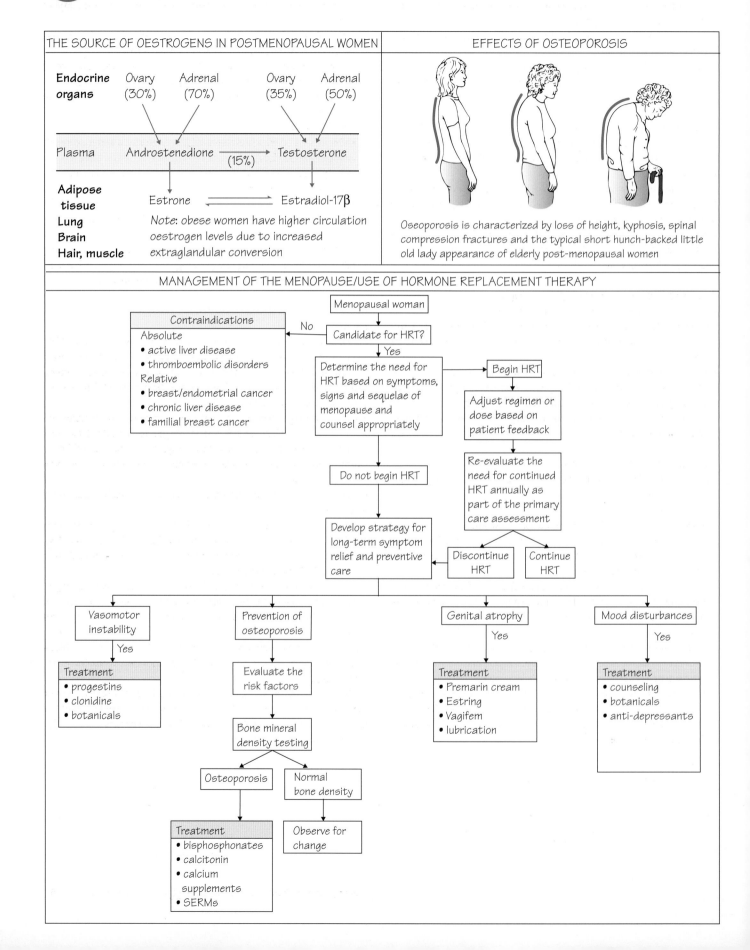

THE SOURCE OF OESTROGENS IN POSTMENOPAUSAL WOMEN

| Endocrine organs | Ovary (30%) | Adrenal (70%) | Ovary (35%) | Adrenal (50%) |

Plasma   Androstenedione ⟷(15%)⟷ Testosterone

Adipose tissue
Lung
Brain
Hair, muscle

Estrone ⟷ Estradiol-17β

Note: obese women have higher circulation oestrogen levels due to increased extraglandular conversion

EFFECTS OF OSTEOPOROSIS

Oseoporosis is characterized by loss of height, kyphosis, spinal compression fractures and the typical short hunch-backed little old lady appearance of elderly post-menopausal women

MANAGEMENT OF THE MENOPAUSE/USE OF HORMONE REPLACEMENT THERAPY

Menopausal woman

Candidate for HRT? — No → Contraindications

Contraindications
Absolute
• active liver disease
• thromboembolic disorders
Relative
• breast/endometrial cancer
• chronic liver disease
• familial breast cancer

Yes → Determine the need for HRT based on symptoms, signs and sequelae of menopause and counsel appropriately → Begin HRT → Adjust regimen or dose based on patient feedback → Re-evaluate the need for continued HRT annually as part of the primary care assessment → Discontinue HRT / Continue HRT

Do not begin HRT

Develop strategy for long-term symptom relief and preventive care

Vasomotor instability
Yes
Treatment
• progestins
• clonidine
• botanicals

Prevention of osteoporosis
Evaluate the risk factors → Bone mineral density testing → Osteoporosis / Normal bone density

Osteoporosis →
Treatment
• bisphosphonates
• calcitonin
• calcium supplements
• SERMs

Normal bone density → Observe for change

Genital atrophy
Yes
Treatment
• Premarin cream
• Estring
• Vagifem
• lubrication

Mood disturbances
Yes
Treatment
• counseling
• botanicals
• anti-depressants

Menopause

• *Definition:* the permanent cessation of menstruation caused by failure of ovarian follicular development in the presence of elevated gonadotrophin (FSH, LH) levels.

• *Age:* 51 years (mean; range, 45–55 years). The timing is genetically predetermined.

• *Risk factors* for early menopause include cigarette smoking and surgery (hysterectomy without oophorectomy hastens menopause by 2–3 years).

Climacteric (perimenopause)

• *Definition:* the period of time leading up to the menopause when a woman passes from the reproductive stage of life to the post-menopausal years.

• *Menstrual irregularities.* 10% of women cease menstruating abruptly, but the vast majority experience 4–5 years of varying cycle length due to progressive ovarian failure.

• *Hormone production:* characterized by elevated FSH, decreased inhibin, but normal levels of estradiol-17β and LH. However, there is wide individual variation.

Post-menopausal ovarian physiology

• *Oestrogens.* The ovary produces almost no oestrogen after menopause due to the absence of ovarian follicles. The source of oestrogens *(opposite)* is derived primarily from peripheral conversion of androgens.

• *Gonadotropins.* There is a 10- to 20-fold increase in FSH and a three-fold increase in LH that peaks 1–3 years after menopause. Thereafter, there is a gradual decline in both gonadotropins over time.

• *Androgens.* Elevated gonadotropins drive the ovarian stroma to increase production of androgens.

Hypooestrogenic changes

Oestrogen deficiency causes the majority of symptoms, signs, and sequelae of menopause.

1 *Vasomotor instability*

• Hot flushes affect 70% of perimenopausal women.

• Characterized by the sensation of intense warmth of the upper body, and generally last for 1–5 minutes. Ascending flushing and profuse perspiration may also occur.

• Result from acute oestrogen withdrawal and not from hypooestrogenism *per se.* As such, hot flushes lessen in frequency and intensity with advancing age. Obese women are less symptomatic.

2 *Osteoporosis*

• Oestrogens inhibit bone resorption. Post-menopausal women experience increased bone resorption, diminished formation and resultant bone fragility that often leads to fracture.

• Defined as a bone mineral density 2.5 standard deviations or more below the young adult peak mean on the basis of axial skeleton measurements. Osteopenia refers to a bone density 1.0–2.5 standard deviations below the mean.

• Effects of osteoporosis *(opposite)* are profound: 50% of women >75 years have vertebral fractures and 25% will develop hip fractures by age 80 with devastating health consequences of disability or death.

• Risk factors include Caucasian or Asian descent, low body-mass index, smoking and a family history of osteoporosis.

• Bone mineral density testing (dual energy X-ray absorptiometry) should be performed on the basis of a patient's risk profile and is not indicated unless the results will influence a treatment or management decision.

3 *Genital atrophy*

• The tissues of the lower vagina, labia, urethra, and trigone are all oestrogen-dependent.

• Dyspareunia, vaginismus, dysuria, urgency and urinary incontinence are common symptoms.

4 *Mood disturbances*

• Menopause does not have a measurable affect on mental health.

• Fatigue, nervousness, headaches, insomnia, depression and irritability are seen more frequently during the perimenopause, but their causal relationship with oestrogen withdrawal is uncertain.

Hormone replacement therapy (HRT)
(opposite)

• *Benefits.* Oestrogen given to post-menopausal women will effectively treat hot flushes, osteoporosis, genital atrophy and perhaps mood disturbances. The risk of Alzheimer's disease, osteoarthritis, colon cancer, tooth loss and skin aging may also be decreased. There is no reduction in cardiovascular disease.

• *Risks.* Oestrogen increases the risk of endometrial hyperplasia and adenocarcinoma (Chapter 30), unless progestins are added (women with prior hysterectomy do not need progestins). The risk of breast cancer is moderately increased, depending on the length of use and pre-existing family history.

• *Side-effects:* nausea, erratic vaginal bleeding, headaches and breast tenderness.

• *Regimens:* cyclic oestrogen (Premarin® 0.625 mg, estradiol 0.1 mg) on days 1–25 of the calendar month and Provera®(10 mg on days 13–25); continuous daily oestrogen (Premarin, estradiol, transdermal oestrogen 0.05 mg) and Provera 2.5 mg.

• *New medications.* Raloxifene (Evista®) is a selective oestrogen receptor modulator (SERM) that has oestrogen-agonist effects on bone and cholesterol, but oestrogen-antagonist effects on breast and endometrium.

• *Botanicals.* Soy products, isoflavones, St. John's wort and black cohosh may be helpful in the short-term treatment of vasomotor symptoms or depression.

• *Compliance* remains a significant problem with HRT because most of the benefits are long-term and no immediate results (except relief of hot flushes) are evident. Recently, the fear of breast cancer has been a major cause of HRT discontinuation.

27 Dysplasia and colposcopy

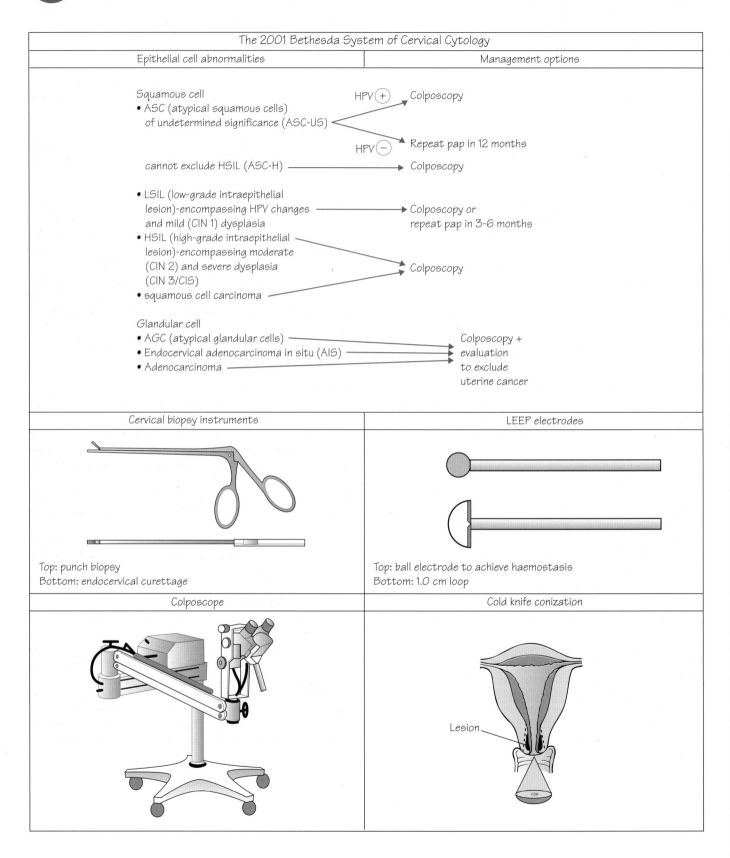

The 2001 Bethesda System of Cervical Cytology	
Epithelial cell abnormalities	Management options

Squamous cell
• ASC (atypical squamous cells) of undetermined significance (ASC-US)

HPV (+) → Colposcopy

HPV (−) → Repeat pap in 12 months

cannot exclude HSIL (ASC-H) → Colposcopy

• LSIL (low-grade intraepithelial lesion)-encompassing HPV changes and mild (CIN 1) dysplasia → Colposcopy or repeat pap in 3-6 months
• HSIL (high-grade intraepithelial lesion)-encompassing moderate (CIN 2) and severe dysplasia (CIN 3/CIS) → Colposcopy
• squamous cell carcinoma

Glandular cell
• AGC (atypical glandular cells)
• Endocervical adenocarcinoma in situ (AIS)
• Adenocarcinoma
→ Colposcopy + evaluation to exclude uterine cancer

Cervical biopsy instruments	LEEP electrodes
Top: punch biopsy Bottom: endocervical curettage	Top: ball electrode to achieve haemostasis Bottom: 1.0 cm loop
Colposcope	Cold knife conization
	Lesion

Cervical intraepithelial neoplasia (CIN)

Papanicolaou (Pap) smear

• *Purpose.* Pap smear screening has substantially decreased the incidence and mortality from cervical cancer because precursor lesions (dysplasia) can be identified and treated. Progression of CIN to invasive cancer usually occurs over many years.

• *Natural history.* CIN usually originates at the transformation zone (TZ), a circumferential ring of metaplasia at the squamo-columnar junction of the cervix.

• *Abnormal smears.* 9/10 smear results are normal. 1/20 shows equivocal or mild cell changes, 1/100 smears shows moderate cell changes, 1/200 shows severe changes and <1/1000 shows an invasive cancer.

• *Technique.* Performing a Pap smear is simple to perform and painless (Chapter 1).

• *Sensitivity.* 10–25% of lesions will be missed on a single Pap smear due to errors in sampling or interpretation.

• *Types.* Conventional Pap smears are prepared by manually smearing the cervical cells onto a glass slide and spraying fixative. Liquid-based cytology (LBC) is an increasingly popular preparation that requires collection of the cells into a vial where cells are better preserved and sensitivity is increased.

• *Frequency*

USA: Pap smear screening should begin 3 years after initiation of sexual intercourse, but no later than age 21. Women <30 years should undergo annual cervical cytology screening. Those ≥30 years who have had 3 consecutive negative Pap smears and no high risk features may extend the interval to every 2–3 years. Screening may be discontinued at age 70 in low-risk women.

UK: Screening should begin at age 25. The interval is every 3 years for women age 25–49 and every 5 years for women age 50–64. Screening may be discontinued at 64 years if the last 3 smears were normal.

• *Classification*

USA: The 2001 Bethesda System *(opposite)* was developed to standardize Pap smear interpretation. Atypical squamous cell diagnoses are now further designated as 'undetermined significance' (ASC-US) or cannot exclude a 'high-grade' lesion (ASC-H). The LSIL and HSIL categories are unchanged. Glandular lesions now consist of 'atypical glandular cells' (AGC) or a more targeted diagnosis of endocervical AIS or adenocarcinoma to help guide management.

UK: Pap smears are reported as CIN 1, CIN 2, CIN 3 or cervical glandular intraepithelial lesion (CGIN). This classification is not strictly accurate as CIN can only really be diagnosed with a biopsy *(opposite)*.

Human papillomavirus (HPV) testing

• *Method.* Hybrid Capture II detects the presence of 1 or more of 13 high- and intermediate-risk HPV types (i.e., 16, 18, 31).

• *Utility:* primary triage of cervical cytology tests read as ASC-US in the USA. >80% of LSIL and HSIL Pap smears are HPV-positive, making the test less useful.

• *Requirement:* residual LBC sample or a separate conventional Pap slide.

Colposcopy

• *Indications*

USA: ASC-US (HPV-positive or repeated smears), ASC-H, LSIL (1st or repeated smear), HSIL and AGC.

UK: CIN 1 (1st or repeated smear), CIN 2, CIN 3 and CGIN.

• *Purpose.* The Pap smear is a screening test to detect cervical abnormalities. Colposcopy is a microscopic evaluation of the TZ to identify the most worrisome areas (aceto-white epithelium, mosaicism, punctation, and/or atypical vessels) for directed, diagnostic cervical biopsies. This is a more accurate method than biopsies performed by gross visualization alone.

• *Colposcope: (opposite)* a binocular instrument allowing stereoscopic inspection of the cervix at 5–40 × magnification. A green filter is helpful to emphasize vascular patterns by giving red vessels a black color against a pale green background.

• *Procedure.* The cervix is cleaned and 3–5% acetic acid is liberally applied with cotton swabs. Dysplastic epithelium turns white 1–2 minutes after application and the degree of whiteness correlates with the histological grade of the lesion. If the TZ and the extent of the lesion cannot be fully visualized, the examination is called 'unsatisfactory'.

• *Biopsies* should be performed at the areas appearing most abnormal. Sedation or local anaesthesia is rarely needed and bleeding can be quickly controlled with cauterization using silver nitrate or ferrous subsulfate (Monsel's solution). An endocervical curettage (ECC) can also be performed if endocervical disease or extension is a possibility.

Management of CIN

• *Treatment* of CIN is indicated for biopsy-proven CIN 2, CIN 3 and persistent CIN 1 (does not resolve after 1 year).

• *Loop electrosurgical excision procedure (LEEP)* is the most common method *(opposite)*. The procedure is done under local anaesthesia and removes, rather than destroys, the affected tissue—allowing for diagnosis and treatment during a single visit.

• *Cold knife conization (opposite)* is indicated for glandular disease (adenocarcinoma in situ) or squamous lesions that may extend up the canal.

• *Ablative options.* Laser vaporization and cryotherapy destroy the dysplastic cells, but do not provide tissue for diagnosis and to rule out invasive disease.

Vaginal intraepithelial neoplasia (VAIN)

• Most patients have an antecedent or coexistent neoplasia of the lower genital tract (i.e., CIN).

• The diagnosis should be suspected in patients with persistently abnormal Pap smears and negative cervical colposcopy. It arises most commonly at the vaginal apex and is often multifocal.

• **Treatment.** Local excision is the treatment of choice and the only modality to rule out invasive disease. Intravaginal 5-fluorouracil cream is particularly useful in multifocal lesions or in patients with immunosuppression. Laser therapy has rapid healing and few side-effects.

STAGING OF CERVICAL CARCINOMA

Cancer is confined to the cervix and identified only microscopically with invasion up to 5.0 mm and width up to 7.0 mm • Stage Ia-1: up to 3.0 mm depth and 7.0 mm width • Stage Ia-2: 3.1–5.0 mm depth and up to 7.0 mm width	Cancer is confined to the cervix and larger than stage Ia-2 OR associated with a visible lesion • Stage Ib-1: up to 4.0 cm cervical tumour diameter • Stage Ib-2: >4.0 cm cervical tumour diameter
Stage Ia	**Stage Ib**
Involvement of the upper two-thirds of the vagina, but no evidence of parametrial involvement	Infiltration of the parametria, but not out to the sidewall
Stage IIa	**Stage IIb**
Involvement of the lower third of the vagina, but not out to the pelvic sidewall if the parametria are involved	Ureter Ureteral obstruction by tumour Extension to the pelvic sidewall and/or hydronephrosis or non-functional kidney (unless known to be attributable to other causes)
Stage IIIa	**Stage IIIb**
Extension outside the reproductive tract with involvement of the mucosa of the bladder OR rectum	Distant metastases, including supraclavicular, brain, subcutaneous, or pulmonary sites
Stage IVa	**Stage IVb**

Brachytherapy

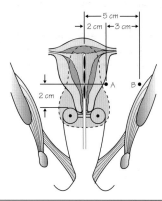	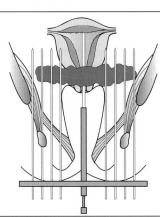
Tandem and ovoid	**Interstitial implant**
• Pear-shaped distribution of radiation delivered	• Used for advanced disease with anatomical distortion

Cervical cancer

Epidemiology and risk factors

• *Incidence (annual)*. USA: 10370 new cases and 3710 deaths; UK: 2991 new cases and 1123 deaths. Cervical cancer is the most frequent cause of cancer death in third-world nations because of a lack of effective screening.

• *Median age:* 52 years.

• *Risk.* Cervical cancer is a disease of sexually active women. It is more prevalent in women of lower socioeconomic status and is correlated with early age at first coitus and having multiple sexual partners.

• *Human papillomavirus (HPV)* is the primary causative agent in cervical cancer. HPV serotypes 6 and 11 predispose to benign condylomas. HPV serotypes 16, 18, 31, and 45 account for 80% of all invasive cervical cancers.

Prevention and diagnosis

• *Screening.* Regular Pap smear screening reduces a woman's chance of dying of cervical cancer by 90%.

• *Symptoms and physical findings.* Postcoital bleeding is the most common early symptom. Late symptoms include menorrhagia and flank or leg pain. The cervical lesion may appear exophytic, barrel-shaped, or ulcerative.

Pathology

• *Squamous cell carcinoma* (75–80%) is the most common type of cervical cancer, but the incidence is decreasing in countries with widespread Pap smear screening.

• *Adenocarcinomas* (20–25%) are more difficult to detect and appear to be increasing in incidence, especially among younger women.

• Cancer of the cervix spreads primarily by direct local extension. Lymphatic and haematogenous spread occurs more frequently in larger tumours.

Staging *(opposite)*

• *NOTE:* cervical cancer is *clinically* staged.

• Stage Ia cancer is most commonly diagnosed by cone biopsy. Stage Ib-1 cancer is usually diagnosed by visualizing a small gross lesion. Stage Ib-2 to stage IV cases require formal staging with an examination under anaesthesia, chest X-ray, cystoscopy, proctoscopy, and in some cases, an intravenous pyelogram or barium enema.

Treatment

• *Primary therapy by stage:*

  Ia-1 disease is treated by cone biopsy or simple hysterectomy in the absence of high-risk features.

  Ia-2/Ib-1 disease is usually treated by radical hysterectomy. This procedure differs from simple hysterectomy by removal of parametrial tissue to the pelvic sidewall, resection of the uterine artery at its origin, removal of the upper third of the vagina and resection of one-half of the uterosacral ligaments to achieve negative margins. Pelvic +/-paraaortic lymphadenectomy is also routinely performed.

  Ib2/IIa disease is usually treated by primary chemoradiation therapy: weekly cisplatin and external beam radiation (teletherapy) followed by local radiation implants (brachytherapy: *opposite*). Radical hysterectomy may also be appropriate, but most patients will require postoperative chemoradiation for high-risk features (lymph node metastases, deep cervical invasion).

  IIb/IIIa/IIIb/IVa disease is treated by primary chemoradiation because there is minimal likelihood of safely performing an operation that will achieve negative margins.

  IVb cervical cancer is treated with palliative intent using chemotherapy +/– directed radiation.

• *Adjuvant therapy.* Patients with high-risk early stage disease (positive lymph nodes, deep invasion) benefit from postoperative chemoradiation. Postradiation hysterectomy is not generally advocated.

• *Recurrent disease.* Patients who develop recurrence after surgery alone are candidates for radiation therapy. Pelvic exenteration (removal of bladder, uterus, rectum, and other involved structures) is the only curable option for postradiation recurrence with central pelvic disease.

• *Palliation.* Most patients with recurrent cervical cancer are not candidates for exenteration due to sidewall disease or distant metastases. The combination of cisplatin and topotecan is the most effective palliative chemotherapy regimen. Regional radiotherapy may be effective in reducing pain symptoms from lesions outside the original radiation field.

Prognostic factors

Excluding clinical stage, lymph node metastases are the most significant pathologic variable. Other prognostic factors include tumour size, depth of invasion, lymph-vascular space invasion and positive surgical margins.

Vaginal cancer

One of the *rarest* malignancies of the human body. Extension of cervical cancer and secondary metastases from other gynaecological malignancies are far more common.

• *Staging:* similar to cervical cancer.

• *Pathology:* squamous cell carcinoma (85–90%) is the most common histological type, followed by adenocarcinoma (5%).

• **Treatment:** radiation therapy is the treatment of choice because anatomical distortion makes primary surgical management more difficult.

• *Clear cell adenocarcinoma.* Maternal use of DES in the 1960s was followed by a dramatic increase in the incidence of this disease among exposed female fetuses. However, the risk is still only 1/1000.

STAGING OF VULVAR CANCER

Ia Lesions 2 cm or less in size confined to the vulva or perineum and with stromal invasion no greater than 1.0 mm (no nodal metastasis)

Ib Lesions 2 cm or less in size confined to the vulva or perineum and with stromal invasion greater than 1.0 mm (no nodal metastasis)

II Tumour confined to the vulva and/or perineum—more than 2 cm in greatest dimension (no nodal metastasis)

III Tumour any size with
    (a) adjacent spread to the lower urethra and/or the anus, and/or
    (b) unilateral regional lymph node metastasis

IVa Tumour invades any of the following: upper urethra, bladder, mucosa, rectal mucosa, bone, and/or bilateral regional node metastasis

IVb Any distant metastasis including pelvic lymph nodes

MANAGEMENT OF VULVAR CANCER

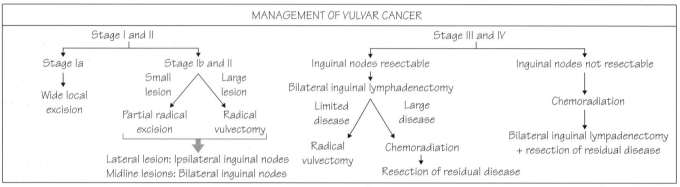

Stage I and II
- Stage Ia → Wide local excision
- Stage Ib and II
  - Small lesion → Partial radical excision
  - Large lesion → Radical vulvectomy

Lateral lesion: Ipsilateral inguinal nodes
Midline lesions: Bilateral inguinal nodes

Stage III and IV
- Inguinal nodes resectable → Bilateral inguinal lymphadenectomy
  - Limited disease → Radical vulvectomy
  - Large disease → Chemoradiation → Resection of residual disease
- Inguinal nodes not resectable → Chemoradiation → Bilateral inguinal lymphadenectomy + resection of residual disease

SURGERY FOR VULVAR CANCER

Radical vulvectomy and bilateral inguinal lymphadenectomy

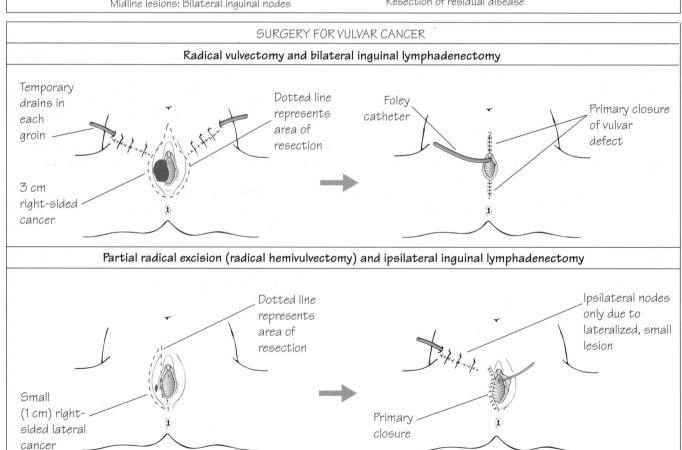

Temporary drains in each groin

Dotted line represents area of resection

3 cm right-sided cancer

Foley catheter

Primary closure of vulvar defect

Partial radical excision (radical hemivulvectomy) and ipsilateral inguinal lymphadenectomy

Dotted line represents area of resection

Small (1 cm) right-sided lateral cancer

Ipsilateral nodes only due to lateralized, small lesion

Primary closure

Vulvar intraepithelial neoplasia (VIN)

- Vulvar pruritis is the most common symptom but 50% of patients are asymptomatic.
- 20% have a coexistent invasive vulvar cancer.
- *Mean age:* 40 years. Pre-menopausal women are more likely to have HPV-related, multifocal lesions.
- *Diagnosis.* Careful inspection of the vulva during routine gynaecological examinations remains the most productive diagnostic technique. Application of acetic acid using soaked cotton balls for at least 5 minutes is necessary before many lesions are colposcopically apparent. Keyes dermatological punch biopsies should be performed liberally under local anaesthesia.
- *Treatment.* Wide local excision with negative margins is the treatment of choice. 'Skinning' vulvectomy is indicated for large, confluent lesions. Laser therapy is particularly useful for scattered, multifocal lesions.

Vulvar cancer

Epidemiology and risk factors
- *Incidence.* 5% of all gynaecological cancers.
- *Median age:* 65 years.
- *Risk factors.* Inadequate personal hygiene and inadequate medical care.

Prevention and diagnosis
- *Screening.* Annual vulvar examination is the most effective way to prevent vulvar cancer. However, many women do not seek medical evaluation for months or years despite noticing an abnormal 'lump'.
- *Symptoms and signs.* Vulvar pruritis or a vulvar mass is present in >50% of patients. All suspicious lesions should be biopsied, even if patients are asymptomatic.

Pathology
- *Squamous cell carcinoma* (90%) is the most common histological type, followed by melanoma (5%).
- Primary disease can occur anywhere on the vulva. 70% of lesions arise on the labia, most commonly the labia majora.
- Vulvar cancer spreads primarily via the lymphatics to the superficial inguinal lymph nodes. Metastases to the intra-abdominal pelvic nodes almost never occur if the inguinal nodes are negative. Direct extension to the vagina, urethra, and anus is another common method of disease growth.

Staging (opposite)
- *NOTE:* vulvar cancer is *surgically* staged.
- 30–40% of patients present with stage III or IV disease.

Management of vulvar cancer (opposite)

- *Surgery* for vulvar cancer (opposite) depends primarily on the size of the lesion and ideally achieves negative margins. Radical procedures are designed to encompass the entire tumour with ≥2 cm gross lateral margins and the dissection is taken down to the underlying pelvic fascia. Drains are placed after inguinal lymphadenectomy until lymphatic drainage ceases. Advanced (stage III and IV) disease usually requires a combination of surgery, chemotherapy and radiotherapy. Skin grafts, myocutaneous flaps or other reconstructive procedures may be required to close the surgical defect in some cases.
- *Operative morbidity.* The incidence of surgical wound breakdown is high (>50%) following radical vulvectomy due to the difficulty in keeping the postoperative area clean and dry. Chronic lower extremity lymphedema may also occur—especially if postoperative radiation is performed.
- *Adjuvant therapy.* Metastasis to the inguinal lymph nodes is the primary indication for adjuvant external beam radiation (teletherapy). The utility of concomitant weekly cisplatin (as in cervical cancer [Chapter 28]) is currently being investigated.
- *Recurrent disease.* Most recurrences occur near the site of the primary lesion and can be surgically resected. Distant metastases usually respond poorly to palliative chemotherapy.

Prognostic factors
The *number of positive inguinal lymph nodes* is the single most important prognostic variable.

Vulvar melanoma
- The second most common vulvar malignancy occurring predominantly in post-menopausal white women.
- Most are located on the labia minora or clitoris.
- The FIGO staging system is not applicable: prognosis is primarily related to the depth of invasion. Clark's or Breslow's classification is used and the prognosis decreases considerably with level of extension.
- *Treatment:* radical excision with ≥2 cm gross lateral margins. Inguinal lymphadenectomy is more prognostic than therapeutic.

Paget's disease of the vulva
- A rare intraepithelial neoplasm that predominantly affects post-menopausal white women.
- 20% have a co-existing adenocarcinoma.
- *Treatment:* wide local excision is the treatment of choice, but positive margins and recurrent disease are very common. The clinical course may be prolonged and indolent.

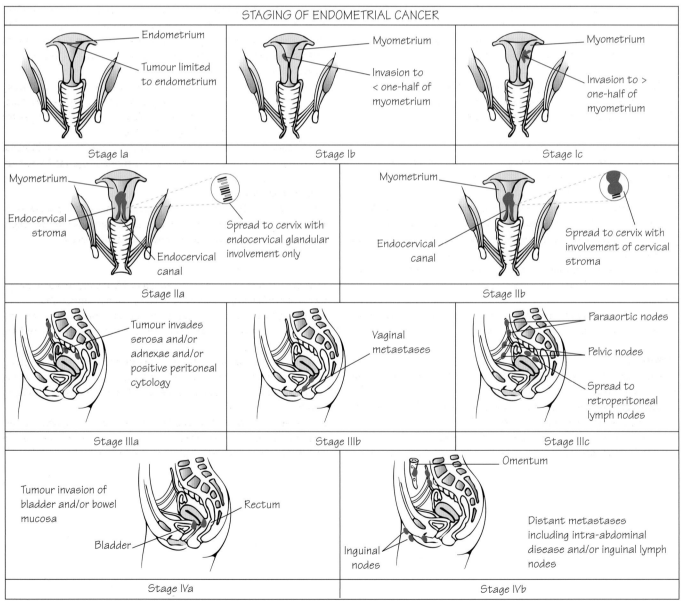

UNOPPOSED OESTROGEN

1 Obesity
  • Increased adipose tissue causes aromatization of androgens → oestrogens
2 Tamoxifen
  • Oestrogenic effect on uterus
  • Anti-oestrogen effect on breast tissue
3 Polycystic ovarian syndrome
  • Chapter 21
4 Exogenous oestrogen
  • Postmenopausal oestrogen without progestin
  • alternative medications (ie, St. Johns Wort) with 'natural' hormones

STAGING OF ENDOMETRIAL CANCER

Endometrium
Tumour limited to endometrium

Stage Ia

Myometrium
Invasion to < one-half of myometrium

Stage Ib

Myometrium
Invasion to > one-half of myometrium

Stage Ic

Myometrium
Endocervical stroma
Endocervical canal
Spread to cervix with endocervical glandular involvement only

Stage IIa

Myometrium
Endocervical canal
Spread to cervix with involvement of cervical stroma

Stage IIb

Tumour invades serosa and/or adnexae and/or positive peritoneal cytology

Stage IIIa

Vaginal metastases

Stage IIIb

Paraaortic nodes
Pelvic nodes
Spread to retroperitoneal lymph nodes

Stage IIIc

Tumour invasion of bladder and/or bowel mucosa
Rectum
Bladder

Stage IVa

Omentum
Distant metastases including intra-abdominal disease and/or inguinal lymph nodes
Inguinal nodes

Stage IVb

Endometrial hyperplasia

• *Definition:* abnormal endometrial glandular proliferation.
• *Aetiology:* prolonged unopposed estrogenic stimulation.
• *Classification.*
  (i) *Hyperplasia with cytological atypia* exhibits an increased nuclear/cytoplasmic ratio, hyperchromasia and loss of cell polarity. More than 20% will progress to endometrial adenocarcinoma without treatment.
  (ii) *Hyperplasia without cytologic atypia* is clinically benign.
• *Diagnosis.* Patients typically present with abnormal uterine bleeding or a Pap smear having atypical glandular cells. An office endometrial biopsy (Chapter 4) makes the diagnosis.
• *Treatment.* Fertility sparing treatment involves oral contraceptives or progestins followed by a repeat endometrial biopsy in 3–6 months to confirm resolution. Hysterectomy is recommended for most women with cytologic atypia.

Endometrial cancer (95%)

Epidemiology and risk factors
• *Incidence (annual).* USA: 40,880 new cases and 7310 deaths; UK: 5624 new cases and 1073 deaths. The lifetime risk is 2%.
• *Median age:* 60 years.
• *Aetiology (opposite).* Exposure to unopposed estrogen increases the risk of endometrial cancer. Protective factors include high parity, pregnancy and smoking.
• *Hereditary factors.* Women with a hereditary non-polyposis colorectal cancer (HNPCC) gene mutation (MLH1, MSH2) have a 40–60% lifetime risk of developing endometrial cancer.

Prevention and diagnosis
• *Screening.* Endometrial biopsy is NOT recommended for routine screening, even in patients on tamoxifen. Pap smear screening is not a sensitive means of detection.
• *Chemoprevention.* Oral contraceptive use decreases the risk of developing endometrial cancer. Hormonal treatment of endometrial hyperplasia will usually prevent progression to cancer.
• *Symptoms and physical findings.* Abnormal uterine bleeding occurs frequently. Intermenstrual or heavy, prolonged bleeding in premenopausal women and any post-menopausal bleeding should be evaluated.
• *Diagnostic work-up.* Initial evaluation should include a pelvic examination, Pap smear and endometrial biopsy.

Pathology
• Adenocarcinoma (80%) is by far the most common and most curable histological type.
• Adenosquamous and clear cell adenocarcinoma are infrequent, but have a more aggressive clinical course.
• Uterine papillary serous carcinoma often presents with extensive intra-abdominal disease despite minimal or absent myometrial inva-

sion. Advanced disease is usually treated like epithelial ovarian cancer (Chapter 31), but survival is very poor.
• Many 'high-risk' tumours will have mixed cell types.
• The histological grade is based on tumour architecture and reflects the amount of non-gland-forming (solid) tumour. Grades 1, 2, and 3 indicate solid growth patterns in ≤5%, 6–50%, and >50% of the tumour, respectively.
• Endometrial carcinoma spreads by lymphatic or haematological dissemination, direct extension and transtubal passage.

Staging (opposite)
• Endometrial cancer is *surgically* staged.
• 75% of patients present with stage I disease.

Treatment
• *Primary therapy.* Exploratory laparotomy, peritoneal washings, total abdominal hysterectomy (TAH) and bilateral salpingo-oophorectomy (BSO) is standard treatment. Pelvic and paraaortic node dissection may be performed, depending on the tumour grade and depth of myometrial invasion. Primary radiation therapy is primarily used in women with unacceptable surgical risks but the cure rate is diminished by 10–15%.
• *Adjuvant therapy.* External beam radiation and/or vaginal brachytherapy can reduce the incidence of pelvic recurrence in women with grade 3 tumours +/- deep invasion. Chemotherapy may be beneficial in selected patients.
• *Recurrent disease.* Radiation or pelvic exenteration (Chapter 28) may be curative options for locally recurrent endometrial cancer. Combination chemotherapy (paclitaxel, doxorubicin, cisplatin; 'TAP') has the highest response rate for more systemic disease.
• *Palliation.* Hormonal therapy (progestin, tamoxifen) has minimal toxicity and reasonable response rates—especially in grade 1 tumours.

Prognostic factors
Patient age, histological type, histological grade, surgical stage, peritoneal cytology, tumour size, lymph-vascular space invasion and depth of myometrial invasion are independent prognostic factors.

Uterine sarcomas (5%)
Uterine sarcomas are aggressive tumours with a poor prognosis. Surgical resection is the only treatment of any proven curative value.
1 Leiomyosarcomas are uterine smooth muscle tumours that are distinguished from benign fibroids by the increased number of cellular mitoses.
2 Mixed Müllerian mesodermal tumours are a combination of carcinoma and sarcoma. Malignant elements are usually inherent to the uterus (homologous), but may include bone, cartilage or skeletal muscle (heterologous).
3 Endometrial stromal sarcomas are soft, fleshy, polypoid masses that protrude into the endometrial cavity. Low-grade and high-grade tumours are distinguished by the number of mitoses.

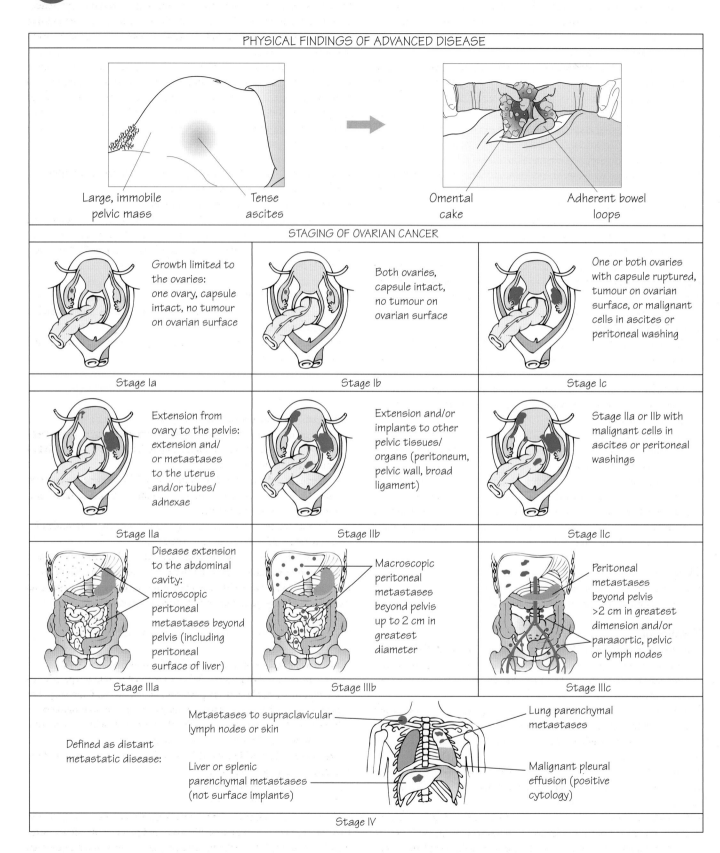

PHYSICAL FINDINGS OF ADVANCED DISEASE

Large, immobile pelvic mass — Tense ascites

Omental cake — Adherent bowel loops

STAGING OF OVARIAN CANCER

Growth limited to the ovaries: one ovary, capsule intact, no tumour on ovarian surface

Stage Ia

Both ovaries, capsule intact, no tumour on ovarian surface

Stage Ib

One or both ovaries with capsule ruptured, tumour on ovarian surface, or malignant cells in ascites or peritoneal washing

Stage Ic

Extension from ovary to the pelvis: extension and/or metastases to the uterus and/or tubes/adnexae

Stage IIa

Extension and/or implants to other pelvic tissues/organs (peritoneum, pelvic wall, broad ligament)

Stage IIb

Stage IIa or IIb with malignant cells in ascites or peritoneal washings

Stage IIc

Disease extension to the abdominal cavity: microscopic peritoneal metastases beyond pelvis (including peritoneal surface of liver)

Stage IIIa

Macroscopic peritoneal metastases beyond pelvis up to 2 cm in greatest diameter

Stage IIIb

Peritoneal metastases beyond pelvis >2 cm in greatest dimension and/or paraaortic, pelvic or lymph nodes

Stage IIIc

Defined as distant metastatic disease:

Metastases to supraclavicular lymph nodes or skin

Liver or splenic parenchymal metastases (not surface implants)

Lung parenchymal metastases

Malignant pleural effusion (positive cytology)

Stage IV

Epithelial ovarian cancer (85–90%)

• *Incidence (annual).* USA: 22,220 new cases and 16,210 deaths; UK: 6734 new cases and 4687 deaths. More patients die from this malignancy in industrialized Western countries than all other gynaecological cancers combined.

• *Median age:* 60 years.

• *Risk factors* include low parity, family history of breast or ovarian cancer and living in industrialized Western countries. Protective factors include multiparity, breast-feeding and chronic anovulation.

• *Hereditary factors* account for 5–10% of all cases. Women with two 1st or 2nd-degree relatives having pre-menopausal breast or ovarian cancer (any age) should be referred to genetic counselling. Testing can identify BRCA1 or BRCA2 mutation carriers.

• *Screening.* There is no known precursor lesion. No combination of CA125, transvaginal sonography and pelvic examination has been shown to reliably detect early disease or decrease mortality. CA125 should not be used routinely as a screening test.

• *Chemoprevention.* Oral contraceptive use decreases the incidence of ovarian cancer by up to 50%.

• *Surgical prophylaxis.* High-risk women (BRCA1 mutation carriers) may be offered prophylactic bilateral salpingo-oophorectomy (BSO) at age 35 or at completion of childbearing. This reduces their ovarian cancer risk by 90% and their breast cancer risk by 50%. Primary peritoneal carcinoma can still occur rarely.

• *Signs and symptoms.* Women with ovarian cancer frequently report symptoms such as bloating, increased abdominal size and urinary symptoms. Most often these are vague symptoms that are overlooked by the doctor or patient. Early satiety, recent bowel changes or 'indigestion' are common complaints of advanced disease. Significant weight loss is unusual.

• *Physical findings.* Early ovarian cancer may be suspected by detection of an adnexal mass on pelvic examination. Advanced disease *(opposite)* is more clinically obvious.

• *Diagnostic work-up.* Transvaginal sonography is the most sensitive method to evaluate an adnexal mass. Computed tomography (CT) of the abdomen-pelvis and a chest x-ray are most helpful for treatment planning in advanced disease. Diagnostic paracentesis in the presence of a pelvic mass is not indicated.

Staging *(opposite)*

• Ovarian cancer is *surgically* staged.

• 75% of patients present with stage III–IV disease.

Treatment

• *Primary therapy* includes exploratory laparotomy, TAH, BSO, appropriate staging (peritoneal cytology, peritoneal biopsies, infracolic omentectomy, pelvic and para-aortic node dissection) and removal of all gross disease.

• *Adjuvant therapy.* Patients with stage IA–IB grade 1–2 disease do not benefit from postoperative chemotherapy. Carboplatin with or without paclitaxel is recommended for at least 6 cycles in women with more advanced disease.

• *Prognostic factors* include surgical stage (most important), extent of residual disease, volume of ascites, patient age and clinical performance status.

• *Surveillance.* Response to therapy is monitored by regular physical examination and serum CA125 levels. CT scans are often helpful when an abnormality is detected. 'Second-look laparotomy' at the completion of primary chemotherapy to look for residual cancer does not improve survival.

• *Relapse* eventually occurs in 80% of patients with advanced disease. Patients with a prolonged clinical response to initial carboplatin-based therapy should be re-evaluated for 'secondary' tumour cytoreduction and/or re-treatment with carboplatin. Otherwise, second-line chemotherapy using paclitaxel, Doxil®, topotecan or another agent should be considered.

• *Palliation.* Most patients eventually develop several areas of small bowel obstruction and subsequent malnutrition from intraperitoneal tumour spread. Palliative therapy aimed at temporary relief of symptoms is critical to maximize patient comfort. Gastrostomy tube placement and IV hydration may be appropriate in selected cases of terminal care.

Borderline (low malignant potential) ovarian tumours

• 10–15% of epithelial ovarian cancers.

• Younger age at diagnosis (mean: 35 years).

• Treatment includes TAH, BSO (or fertility sparing unilateral salpingo-oophorectomy [USO]) and surgical staging. Postoperative chemotherapy is rarely indicated. Prognosis is excellent: 95% will survive at least 10 years.

Primary peritoneal cancer

• Accounts for fewer than 10% of epithelial 'ovarian' cancers and is histologically identical.

• Clinical features, staging, treatment and prognosis are virtually the same as ovarian cancer.

Malignant germ cell ovarian tumours (5–7%)

• Younger age at diagnosis (mean: 20 years).

  1 Dysgerminomas (50%) are most common. Lactate dehydrogenase may be a useful tumour marker, up to 20% of tumours are bilateral and two-thirds are stage I.

  2 Endodermal sinus (yolk-sac) tumours (20%) have characteristic microscopic Schiller–Duval bodies. Alpha-fetoprotein (AFP) is a highly accurate tumour marker.

  3 Immature teratomas (15–20%) are distinct from dermoids by the presence of immature neural elements.

• *Treatment:* fertility-sparing USO and surgical staging is usually indicated due to patient age (otherwise TAH and BSO). Bleomycin, etoposide and cisplatin (BEP) chemotherapy is indicated for all patients except stage IA dysgerminomas or immature teratomas.

Malignant sex cord-stromal tumours (5–7%)

• Mean age at diagnosis is 50 years, but the range is very broad.

  1 Granulosa cell tumours (70%) are the most common type. Microscopic Call-Exner bodies are pathognomonic. 80–90% are stage I at diagnosis. Inhibin A/B or estradiol may be useful tumour markers.

  2 Sertoli–Leydig tumours (10–20%) present with progressive virilization and >95% are stage I at diagnosis.

• *Treatment:* TAH, BSO (or fertility-sparing USO) and staging. Postoperative BEP is not usually needed.

Fallopian tube cancer

• Very rare. The classic clinical triad of a watery vaginal discharge (*hydrops tubae profluens*), a pelvic mass and pelvic pain occurs infrequently. The staging, treatment and prognosis are similar to ovarian cancer.

Gestational trophoblastic disease (GTD)

CHROMOSOMAL ORIGIN OF HYDATIDIFORM MOLE

Partial hydatidiform mole	Complete hydatidiform mole

Partial hydatidiform mole: Disispermy. Normal ovum → Triploid karyotype with an extra (haploid) set of paternal chromosomes.

Complete hydatidiform mole: Single (haploid) sperm fertilizes empty ovum and then duplicates. Empty ovum (90%). Two sperms fertilize an empty ovum OR (10%). Diploid karyotype all of paternal origin.

FEATURES OF HYDATIDIFORM MOLES

Features	Partial moles	Complete mole
Karyotype	69,XXX or 69,XXY	46,XX or 46,XY
Pathology		
Fetus	Present	Absent
Chorionic villi	Focal, variable oedema	Diffusely hydropic
Trophoblastic hyperplasia	Focal, minimal	Diffuse, severe
Clinical presentation		
Symptoms/signs	Missed abortion	Molar gestation
Uterine size	Appropriate	28% large for dates
GTN		
Non-metastatic	3–4%	15%
Metastatic	0	4%

FIGO STAGING OF GESTATIONAL TROPHOBLASTIC NEOPLASIA (GTN)

Stage I	Disease confined to the uterus	Stage II	GTN extends outside the uterus but is limited to the genital structures (adnexa, vagina, broad ligament)

Stage III	GTN extends to the lungs with or without known genital tract involvement	Stage IV	All other metastatic sites

Stage III: Lung metastases.
Stage IV: Liver, Spleen, Kidney, Bowel, Brain.

Modified WHO prognostic scoring system

Scores	0	1	2	4
Age	<40	≥40	–	–
Antecedent pregnancy	Mole	Abortion	Term	–
Interval months from index pregnancy	<4	4–<7	7–<13	≥13
Pretreatment serum hCG (IU/mL)	$<10^3$	$10^3–<10^4$	$10^4–<10^5$	$\geq 10^5$
Largest tumour size (including uterus)	–	3–<5 cm	≥5 cm	–
Site of metastases	Lung	Spleen, kidney	Gastrointestinal	Liver Brain
Number of metastases	–	1–4	5–8	>8
Previous failed chemotherapy	–	–	Single Drug	2 or more drugs

- *Definition.* A spectrum of histologically distinct diseases originating from the placenta: *partial* and *complete hydatidiform mole, choriocarcinoma,* and *placental-site trophoblastic tumour (PSTT).*
- *Tumour marker.* Serum levels of the β-subunit of hCG are extremely accurate.

Hydatidiform moles

- *Incidence.* Japan has the highest incidence of molar pregnancy (2.0 per 1000 pregnancies vs. 0.6–1.1 for Europe and North America). Variations in the worldwide incidence rates result in part from discrepancies between population-based data and hospital-based data.
- *Risk factors* include maternal age >35 years (>2 × increase), prior molar pregnancy (10 × increase), long-term use of oral contraceptives (2 × increase) and dietary deficiency (β-carotene, vitamin A).
- *Chromosomal origin (opposite)*
- *Clinical presentation.* Partial moles usually present as a missed abortion during the 1st or early 2nd trimester. Normal or marginally elevated β-hCG levels are common. Complete moles typically have abnormal vaginal bleeding (85%) that prompts a health care visit. Fewer than 10% of women will have anaemia, hyperemesis gravidarum or pre-eclampsia. Markedly elevated β-hCG levels (>>100,000 mIU/mL) are characteristic.
- *Sonographic findings.* Partial moles may be suspected by visualizing a fetus with focal cystic spaces in the placenta and an increase in the transverse diameter of the gestational sac. Complete moles classically have a 'snowstorm' appearance of diffuse hydropic swelling without a fetus. However, 1st trimester sonograms may be too early to distinguish small molar villi from degenerating chorionic villi.
- *Diagnosis* of hydatidiform moles is made by histopathological analysis. Partial moles have a non-viable fetus with malformations (syndactyly, hydrocephalus, growth restriction), variably hydropic (swollen) villi and minimal trophoblastic hyperplasia. Complete moles have no fetal tissue and consist of diffusely hydropic villi (grape-like vesicles) with widespread trophoblastic hyperplasia. Immunostaining with p57 or ploidy analysis may be indicated in some equivocal cases.
- **Treatment.** Dilatation and evacuation (D & E) is the most common initial treatment for molar pregnancy. Hysterectomy is an alternative in selected patients who desire surgical sterilization.
- *Prophylaxis.* Anti-D immunoglobulin should be administered to appropriate Rh-negative patients.
- *Surveillance.* β-hCG levels should be monitored until they are undetectable.
- *Hormonal contraception* should be encouraged to prevent pregnancy and reduce the potential for complicating β-hCG interpretation.
- *Future pregnancies.* Patients may expect normal reproductive outcome of subsequent conceptions. The risk of developing another hydatidiform mole is approximately 1%.

Gestational trophoblastic neoplasia (GTN)

- *Antecedent gestation:* most commonly occurs following a molar pregnancy, but may occur after any gestational event (termination or spontaneous miscarriage [Chapter 15], ectopic pregnancy [Chapter 5], term pregnancy).
- *Diagnosis* is not uniform worldwide, but includes one of these criteria:
    1 β-hCG plateau of 4 measurements over a period of at least 3 weeks
    2 β-hCG rise of 3 measurements over a period of at least 2 weeks
    3 β-hCG level remains elevated for more than 6 months
    4 Histological diagnosis of choriocarcinoma.
- *Choriocarcinoma* consists of sheets of anaplastic cytotrophoblast and syncytiotrophoblast cells without chorionic villi. Invasive moles may have the histological features of either choriocarcinoma or hydatidiform mole, but metastases are always choriocarcinoma.
- *PSTT* is a rare variant of choriocarcinoma that is insensitive to chemotherapy and usually requires hysterectomy.

Staging (opposite)

- GTN is *anatomically staged.*
- The combination of a chest X-ray, abdominal-pelvic CT scan and pelvic examination is an effective strategy to determine the extent of disease. Chest and head CT are indicated if the chest X-ray is abnormal.
- Biopsy of suspected metastatic lesions is not recommended and may cause haemorrhage.
- The modified World Health Organization (WHO) prognostic scoring system *(opposite)* is used to categorize patients with GTN into low-risk (score: 0–6) or high-risk (score: 7 or higher) groups.

Treatment

- Low-risk GTN is most frequently treated by methotrexate. If the tumour is resistant, the patient may be switched to dactinomycin.
- High-risk GTN is usually best managed by combination chemotherapy (etoposide, methotrexate, dactinomycin, cytoxan, vincristine [EMA/CO]) due to the increased risk of tumour resistance to a single agent.
- *Surveillance.* β-hCG levels are measured until undetectable and therapy is completed. Follow-up should continue for 12 (stage I–III) to 24 months (stage IV).
- *Prognosis.* 98–100% of stage I–III patients and 75–80% of stage IV patients will be cured.

Phantom hCG

- *Definition:* persistent mild elevations of hCG leading physicians to treat patients for GTN when in reality no true hCG or trophoblast disease is present.
- *Cause:* some individuals have circulating factors in their serum (heterophilic antibodies) that interact with the hCG antibody and cause false-positive results.
- *Diagnosis:* negative urine test or serial dilutions of the serum hCG.
- **Treatment:** recognition of the false-positive test. No treatment is needed.

33 Embryology and early fetal development

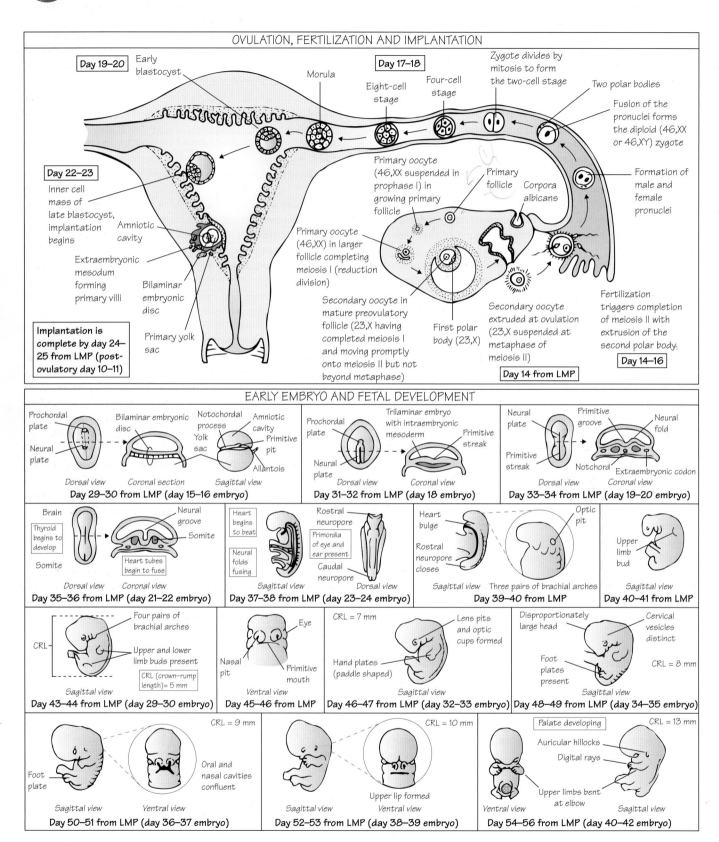

OVULATION, FERTILIZATION AND IMPLANTATION

Day 19–20 — Early blastocyst

Morula

Day 17–18 — Eight-cell stage

Four-cell stage

Zygote divides by mitosis to form the two-cell stage

Two polar bodies

Fusion of the pronuclei forms the diploid (46,XX or 46,XY) zygote

Formation of male and female pronuclei

Day 22–23 — Inner cell mass of late blastocyst, implantation begins

Extraembryonic mesodum forming primary villi

Amniotic cavity

Bilaminar embryonic disc

Primary yolk sac

Primary oocyte (46,XX suspended in prophase I) in growing primary follicle

Primary follicle

Corpora albicans

Primary oocyte (46,XX) in larger follicle completing meiosis I (reduction division)

Secondary oocyte in mature preovulatory follicle (23,X having completed meiosis I and moving promptly onto meiosis II but not beyond metaphase)

First polar body (23,X)

Secondary oocyte extruded at ovulation (23,X suspended at metaphase of meiosis II)

Fertilization triggers completion of meiosis II with extrusion of the second polar body

Day 14–16

Implantation is complete by day 24–25 from LMP (post-ovulatory day 10–11)

Day 14 from LMP

EARLY EMBRYO AND FETAL DEVELOPMENT

Prochordal plate / Neural plate — Bilaminar embryonic disc — Notochordal process / Yolk sac — Amniotic cavity / Primitive pit / Allantois

Dorsal view | Coronal section | Sagittal view
Day 29–30 from LMP (day 15–16 embryo)

Prochordal plate / Neural plate — Trilaminar embryo with intraembryonic mesoderm — Primitive streak

Dorsal view | Coronal view
Day 31–32 from LMP (day 18 embryo)

Neural plate / Primitive streak — Primitive groove — Neural fold — Notchord — Extraembryonic codon

Dorsal view | Coronal view
Day 33–34 from LMP (day 19–20 embryo)

Brain / Thyroid begins to develop / Somite — Neural groove — Somite / Heart tubes begin to fuse

Dorsal view | Coronal view
Day 35–36 from LMP (day 21–22 embryo)

Heart begins to beat / Neural folds fusing — Rostral neuropore / Primordia of eye and ear present / Caudal neuropore

Sagittal view | Dorsal view
Day 37–38 from LMP (day 23–24 embryo)

Heart bulge / Rostral neuropore closes — Optic pit

Sagittal view | Three pairs of brachial arches
Day 39–40 from LMP

Upper limb bud

Sagittal view
Day 40–41 from LMP

Four pairs of brachial arches / Upper and lower limb buds present / CRL (crown–rump length) = 5 mm

CRL

Sagittal view
Day 43–44 from LMP (day 29–30 embryo)

Nasal pit — Eye / Primitive mouth

Ventral view
Day 45–46 from LMP

CRL = 7 mm — Lens pits and optic cups formed / Hand plates (paddle shaped)

Sagittal view
Day 46–47 from LMP (day 32–33 embryo)

Disproportionately large head — Cervical vesicles distinct / Foot plates present / CRL = 8 mm

Sagittal view
Day 48–49 from LMP (day 34–35 embryo)

CRL = 9 mm / Foot plate — Oral and nasal cavities confluent

Sagittal view | Ventral view
Day 50–51 from LMP (day 36–37 embryo)

CRL = 10 mm / Upper lip formed

Sagittal view | Ventral view
Day 52–53 from LMP (day 38–39 embryo)

Palate developing / CRL = 13 mm / Auricular hillocks / Digital rays / Upper limbs bent at elbow

Ventral view | Sagittal view
Day 54–56 from LMP (day 40–42 embryo)

Ovulation, fertilization and implantation
(opposite)

Definitions
• *Gestational age* refers to the duration of pregnancy dated from the first day of the last menstrual period (LMP) which precedes ovulation and fertilization by around 2 weeks.
• From fertilization to 10 weeks of gestation (8 weeks post-conception), the conceptus is called an *embryo*. From 10 weeks to birth, it is a *fetus*.

Follicular development and ovulation
• Primitive germ cells are present in the female embryo by the end of the third week of intrauterine life. The number of germ cells in the fetal ovary peak at around 7 million at 5 months. Degeneration occurs thereafter, with only 2 million primary oocytes surviving in the ovary at birth and as few as 300,000–400,000 in the ovary of pre-pubertal women.
• Primary oocytes have a diploid number of chromosomes (46,XX) which are suspended in prophase of meiosis I. During the follicular phase of the menstrual cycle, several primary oocytes mature under the influence of follicle-stimulating hormone (FSH) with completion of meiosis I. This results in formation of the secondary oocyte with a haploid number of chromosomes (23,X) and extrusion of the first polar body. The mature follicle is known as a Graafian follicle (described by de Graaf in 1677). Secondary oocytes enter meiosis II but become suspended in metaphase. Selection of a single dominant follicle occurs at this time.
• The mid-cycle surge of luteinizing hormone (LH) results in ovulation and extrusion of the secondary oocyte into the abdominal cavity.

Fertilization
• Fertilization of a mature ovum by a single spermatozoon (23,X or 23,Y) occurs in the fallopian tube within the first few hours after ovulation. The genetic composition of the spermatozoon thus determines the gender of the conceptus.
• Fertilization serves as a trigger for the secondary oocyte to complete meiosis II. The male and female pronuclei (each haploid) fuse to form the zygote which has a diploid number of chromosomes (46,XX or 46,XY).

Preimplantation embryo development
• Mitotic division of the zygote (known as segmentation or cleavage) gives rise to daughter cells called *blastomeres*. The initial division results in a 'two-cell' stage followed by a 'four-cell' stage and an 'eight-cell' stage. Such divisions continue while the embryo is still in the fallopian tube. As the blastomeres continue to divide, a solid ball of cells is produced known as the *morula*.
• The morula enters the uterine cavity around 3–4 days after fertilization. The accumulation of fluid between blastomeres results in formation of a fluid-filled cavity, converting the morula to a *blastocyst*.
• A compact mass of cells (the *inner cell mass*) collect at one pole of the blastocyst. These cells are destined to produce the embryo. The outer rim of trophectoderm cells are destined to become the trophoblast (placenta).

Implantation
• Implantation usually occurs in the upper part of the uterus and more often on the posterior uterine wall.
• Prior to implantation, the collection of cells surrounding the blastocyst (known as the zona pellucida) disappears and the blastocyst adheres to the endometrium. This is known as *apposition*.
• The blastocyst then proceeds to invade the endometrium. Implantation is usually completed by day 24–25 of gestation (day 10–11 post-conception).

Early embryo and fetal development
(opposite)

Embryonic development after implantation
• By day 24–26 of gestation, the embryonic disc is bilaminar, consisting of embryonic ectoderm and endoderm.
• Cellular proliferation in the embryonic disc results in midline thickening known as the *primitive streak*. Cells then spread out laterally from the primitive streak between the endoderm and ectoderm to form the mesoderm. This results in a trilaminar embryonic disc *(opposite)*.
• These three germ layers give rise to all the organs of the embryo. The nervous system and epidermis along with its derivatives (lens of the eye, hair) are derived from *ectoderm*. The gastrointestinal tract and derivatives (pancreas, liver, thyroid) arise from *endoderm*. The skeleton, dermis, muscles, vascular and urogenital systems are derived from *mesoderm*.

Early fetal development
The embryonic period ends after 10 weeks of gestation (8 weeks post-conception). The crown–rump (CR) length of the embryo is now 4 mm. The fetal period is characterized by growth and maturation of structures formed during the embryonic period *(below)*.

Gestational age (weeks)		CR length	Fetal weight	
Menstrual	Fertilization	(mm)	(g)	Main external features
12	10	8	14	Fingers, toes visible; intestines in umbilical cord
16	14	12	110	Sex is distinguishable; well defined neck; head erect.
20	18	16	320	Vernix caseosa present.
24	22	21	630	Skin red and wrinkled; lanugo (body hair) present; limit of fetal survival.
28	26	25	1100	Eyes partly open; eyebrows, eyelashes present.
32	30	28	1800	Body filling out; intact fetal survival >95%.
36	34	32	2500	Skin pink and smooth; body plump; testes descending.
40	38	36	3400	Prominent chest; testes in scrotum; breasts protrude.

34 Fetal physiology

TERM PLACENTAL PHYSIOLOGY

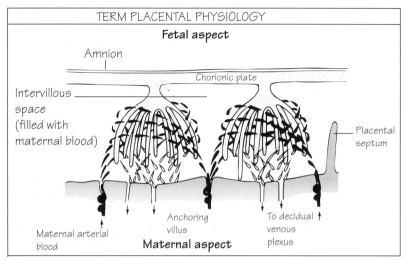

SITES OF HAEMATOPOIESIS AND TYPES OF HAEMOGLOBIN SYNTHESIZED THROUGHOUT GESTATION

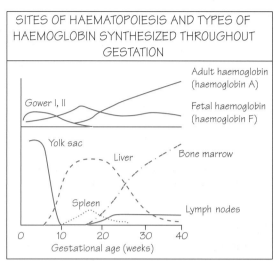

THE FETAL CIRCULATION AND ITS ADAPTATION TO EXTRAUTERINE LIFE

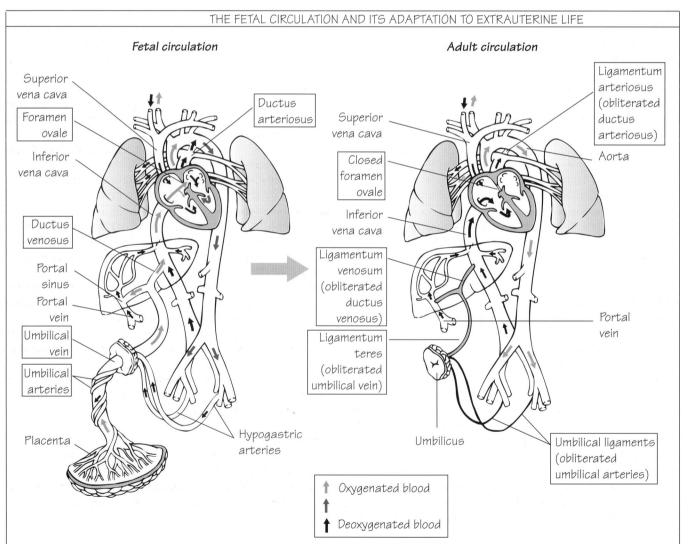

Placental physiology

- The placenta has several functions, including the maternal–fetal transfer of nutrients and oxygen, the clearance of fetal waste, and the synthesis of proteins and hormones.
- The human placenta is classified as *haemochorioendothelial*, because only three cell layers separate the maternal and fetal circulations: fetal trophoblast, fetal villous stroma, and fetal capillary endothelium. Fetal villi are suspended in intervillous spaces bathed with maternal blood (*opposite*).
- Placental villi create a high surface area/volume ratio with a total surface area at term of around $10\,m^2$.
- Transfer across the placenta occurs by passive diffusion (oxygen, CO_2, electrolytes, simple sugars), active transport (iron, vitamin C), or carrier-mediated facilitated diffusion (glucose, immunoglobulins).
- There is a large placental reserve; 30–40% of placental villi can be lost without evidence of placental insufficiency.

Fetal physiology

Nutrition

- The embryo consists almost entirely of water. After 10 weeks, however, the fetus is dependent on nutrients from the maternal circulation via the developing placenta.
- The average term fetus weighs 3400 g. Birthweight is influenced by race, socioeconomic status, parity, genetic factors, diabetes, smoking, and fetal gender. At term, the fetus grows around 30 g/day.

Cardiovascular system

- The fetal heart starts beating at 4–5 weeks of gestation.
- The fetoplacental blood volume at term is 120 mL/kg (or a total of approximately 420 mL).
- After birth, the fetal circulation undergoes profound haemodynamic changes (*opposite*). The umbilical vessels, ductus arteriosus, foramen ovale, and ductus venosus constrict. This is thought to be due to a change in oxygen tension within minutes of birth. The distal portions of the umbilical arteries atrophy within 3–4 days to become the *umbilical ligaments*, and the umbilical vein becomes the *ligamentum teres*. The ductus venosus is functionally closed within 10–90 hours of birth, but anatomic closure and formation of the *ligamentum venosum* is only achieved by 2–3 weeks of life.

Respiratory system

- Within minutes of birth, the fetal lungs must be able to provide oxygen and eliminate CO_2 if the fetus is to survive.
- Movements of the fetal chest can be detected at 11 weeks. The ability of the fetus to 'breathe' amniotic fluid into the lungs at 16–22 weeks appears to be important for normal lung development. Pulmonary hypoplasia may result if this does not occur.
- Surfactant is a heterogeneous detergent-like substance which lowers alveoli surface tension and prevents alveoli collapse after birth. It is made in the lungs by type II pneumocytes.
- Functional maturation results in an increase in surfactant in the lungs. Respiratory compromise due to surfactant deficiency is known as *hyaline membrane disease* (*HMD*) or *respiratory distress syndrome* (*RDS*), and is seen primarily in premature infants. Antenatal *corticosteroid therapy* promotes surfactant production and decreases the risk of RDS by 50%.

Fetal blood

- Sites of haematopoiesis change with gestational age (*opposite*).
- The haemoglobin of fetal blood rises to the adult level of 15 g/dL by mid-pregnancy, and increases to 18 g/dL at term.
- Haemoglobin F (fetal haemoglobin) has a higher affinity for oxygen than haemoglobin A (adult haemoglobin). Haemoglobin A is present in the fetus from 11 weeks and increases linearly with increasing gestational age (*opposite*). A switch from haemoglobin F to haemoglobin A begins at around 32–34 weeks. By term, 75% of total haemoglobin is haemoglobin A.
- The average fetal haematocrit is 50%.

Gastrointestinal system

- The small intestine is capable of peristalsis by 11 weeks. By 16 weeks, the fetus is able to swallow.
- The fetal liver absorbs drugs rapidly but metabolizes them slowly because the hepatic pathways for drug detoxification and inactivation are poorly developed until late in fetal life.
- During the last trimester, the liver stores large amounts of glycogen and the enzyme pathways responsible for glucose synthesis mature.

Genito-urinary system

- Fetal urination starts early in pregnancy, and fetal urine is a major component of amniotic fluid, especially after 16 weeks.
- Renal function improves slowly as pregnancy progresses.

Nervous system

- Neuronal development continues throughout gestation and at least into the second year of extrauterine life. Development of the central nervous system requires normal thyroid activity.
- The fetus is able to perceive sounds at 24–26 weeks. By 28 weeks, the fetal eye is sensitive to light.
- Gonadal steroids are the major determinant of sexual behaviour.

Immune system

- Fetal IgG (immunoglobulin G) is derived almost exclusively from the mother. Receptor-mediated transport of IgG from mother to fetus begins at 16 weeks' gestation, but the bulk of IgG is acquired in the last 4 weeks of pregnancy. As such, preterm infants have very low circulating IgG levels. IgM (immunoglobulin M) is not actively transported across the placenta. As such, IgM levels in the fetus accurately reflect the response of the fetal immune system to infection.
- B lymphocytes appear in the fetal liver by 9 weeks, and in the blood and spleen by 12 weeks. T cells leave the fetal thymus at around 14 weeks.
- The fetus does not acquire much IgG (passive immunity) from colostrum, although IgA (immunoglobulin A) in breast milk may protect against some enteric infections.

Endocrine system (Chapter 35)

- Both oxytocin and vasopressin are secreted by the fetal neurohypophysis by 10–12 weeks.
- The fetal thyroid begins functioning at 12 weeks. Very little fetal thyroid hormone is derived from the mother (Chapter 44).

Endocrinology of pregnancy and parturition

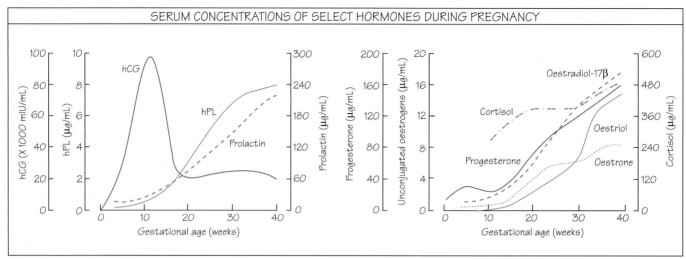

SERUM CONCENTRATIONS OF SELECT HORMONES DURING PREGNANCY

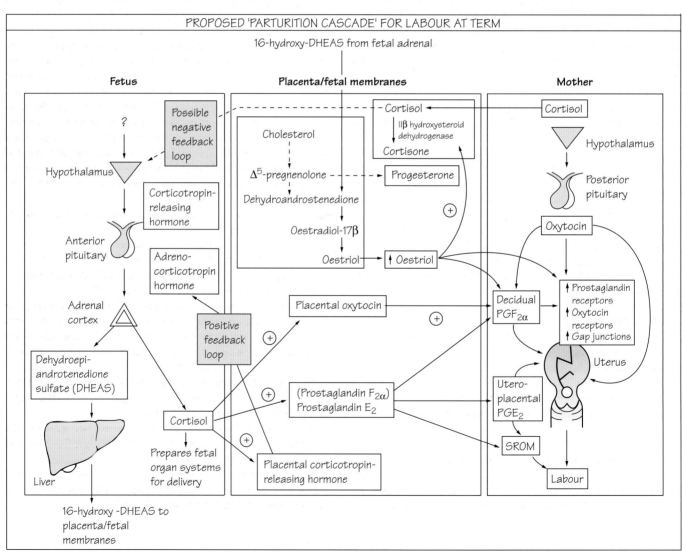

PROPOSED 'PARTURITION CASCADE' FOR LABOUR AT TERM

Endocrinology of pregnancy

The placenta is a rich source of hormones, including human chorionic gonadotropin, human placental lactogen, steroid hormones, oxytocin, growth hormone, corticotropin-releasing hormone, proopiomelanocortin, prolactin, and gonadotropin-releasing hormone. A few are discussed below.

Human chorionic gonadotropin

- Human chorionic gonadotropin (hCG) is a heterodimeric protein hormone that shares a common α-subunit with luteinizing hormone (LH), follicle-stimulating hormone (FSH), and thyroid-stimulating hormone (TSH), but has a unique β-subunit. It is most closely related to LH.
- hCG is produced exclusively by syncytiotrophoblast cells and can be detected in maternal serum 8–9 days post-conception. It is the basis of all standard pregnancy tests.
- hCG levels double every 48 hours in the first several weeks of pregnancy, reaching a peak of 80,000–100,000 mIU/mL at around 8–10 weeks' gestation. Thereafter, hCG concentrations fall to 10,000–20,000 mIU/mL and remain at that level for the remainder of pregnancy (*opposite*).
- The primary function of hCG appears to be maintenance of progesterone production from the corpus luteum of the ovary until the placenta can take over progesterone production at around 6–8 weeks' gestation. Progesterone is essential for early pregnancy success. For example, surgical removal of the corpus luteum or administration of a progesterone receptor antagonist (such as RU 486 (Mifepristone®)) prior to 7 weeks (49 days) of gestation will cause abortion.
- hCG also has thyrotropic activity (0.025% of TSH), which only becomes clinically significant if hCG levels are markedly elevated such as in complete molar pregnancies.

Human placental lactogen

- Human placental lactogen (hPL) is a protein hormone produced exclusively by the placenta that is closely related to both prolactin and growth hormone.
- hPL production is directly proportional to placental mass and levels rise steadily throughout pregnancy (*opposite*).
- The function of hPL is not known, but it has anti-insulin-like activity and may be involved in the development of insulin resistance which characterizes pregnancy.

Steroid hormones

- The placenta is the major source of progesterone and oestrogen production during pregnancy.
- In the placenta, oestrogen is synthesized from androgen precursors and is important for preparing the uterus for labour. Progesterone is derived primarily from maternal substrate (cholesterol) and may be important for maintaining uterine quiescence prior to labour.

Endocrine control of labour

- Reproductive success is critical for survival of the species. Each species has solved the problem of labour in a different way. Such differences may reflect the evolutionary status of the organism in question or may represent solutions to inherent obstacles to reproduction faced by each species (such as differences in placentation, in gestational length, and in the number of offspring per pregnancy).
- The slow progress in our understanding of the mechanisms responsible for the process of labour in humans reflects in large part the difficulty of extrapolating from the endocrine-control mechanisms in many animal species to the paracrine/autocrine mechanisms of parturition in humans.

Initiation of labour

- Considerable evidence suggests that, in most viviparous animals, the fetus is in control of the timing of labour. It is likely that this is achieved through activation of the fetal hypothalamic–pituitary–adrenal (HPA) axis prior to the onset of labour, and that this is common to all species.
- A proposed 'parturition cascade' is outlined opposite.
- The human placenta is an incomplete steroidogenic organ, and oestrogen production by the placenta has an obligate need for androgen precursor. This excess androgen is supplied by the fetus in the form of dehydroepiandrosenedione sulfate (DHEAS).
- Activation of the fetal HPA axis at term results in excess DHEAS release from the intermediate (fetal) zone of the fetal adrenal. DHEAS is 16-hydroxylated in the fetal liver and passes via the fetal circulation to the placenta where it is converted almost exclusively to oestriol (16-hydroxyoestradiol-17β).
- Human pregnancy is characterized by a hyperoestrogenic state of unparalleled magnitude in the entire mammalian kingdom. The placenta is the primary source of oestrogens. The concentration of oestrogens in the maternal circulation increases with gestational age (*opposite*). Placental oestrone and oestradiol-17β are derived primarily from maternal C19 androgens (testosterone and androstenedione), whereas oestriol is derived almost exclusively from fetal DHEAS. Oestrogens do not cause uterine contractions, but do promote a series of myometrial changes (including increasing the number of prostaglandin receptors, oxytocin receptors, and gap junctions) that enhance the capacity of the myometrium to generate contractions.
- In addition to DHEAS, the enlarged fetal adrenal glands also produce cortisol, which has two actions:
  (i) it prepares fetal organ systems for extrauterine life;
  (ii) it promotes expression of a number of placental products, including corticotropin-releasing hormone (CRH), oxytocin, and prostaglandins (especially prostaglandin E_2 (PGE_2)).
- Placental CRH initiates a *positive feedback loop* by stimulating the fetal HPA axis to produce more DHEAS and more cortisol, which then further upregulates placental CRH expression. (This stimulatory effect of cortisol on placental CRH should be contrasted with the feedback inhibition of cortisol on maternal CRH.)
- Placental oxytocin acts directly on the myometrium to cause contractions and indirectly by upregulating prostaglandin production (especially prostaglandin $F_{2\alpha}$ ($PGF_{2\alpha}$)) by the decidua.
- $PGF_{2\alpha}$ is produced primarily by the maternal decidua and acts on the myometrium to upregulate oxytocin receptors and gap junctions and thereby promote uterine contractions.
- $PGE_{2\alpha}$ is primarily of feto-placental origin and is probably more important in promoting cervical 'ripening' (maturation) and spontaneous rupture of the fetal membranes (SROM).

RESPIRATORY SYSTEM

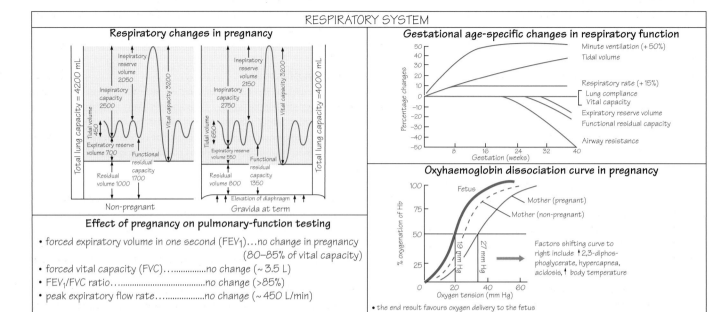

Respiratory changes in pregnancy

Non-pregnant

Gravida at term

Gestational age-specific changes in respiratory function

Minute ventilation (+50%)
Tidal volume
Respiratory rate (+15%)
Lung compliance
Vital capacity
Expiratory reserve volume
Functional residual capacity
Airway resistance

Oxyhaemoglobin dissociation curve in pregnancy

Fetus
Mother (pregnant)
Mother (non-pregnant)

Factors shifting curve to right include ↑2,3-diphos-phoglycerate, hypercapnea, acidosis, ↑ body temperature

• the end result favours oxygen delivery to the fetus

Effect of pregnancy on pulmonary-function testing

• forced expiratory volume in one second (FEV₁)…no change in pregnancy
  (80–85% of vital capacity)
• forced vital capacity (FVC)…..............no change (~3.5 L)
• FEV₁/FVC ratio…...................................no change (>85%)
• peak expiratory flow rate…..................no change (~450 L/min)

WEIGHT GAIN IN PREGNANCY	
Fat	3.5 kg
Breasts	0.4 kg
Uterus	1.0 kg
Blood	1.3 kg
Extracellular fluid	1.5–4.5 kg
Fetus	3.4 kg
Placenta	0.7 kg
Amniotic fluid	0.8 kg
Total weight gain	12.5 kg (range 0–23 kg)
at term	26.5 lls (range 0–50.6lls)

CARDIOVASCULAR SYSTEM

Central haemodynamic changes induced by pregnancy

Measurement	Non-pregnant	Term pregnant	Change
• blood volume (mL)	3500	5000	+40%
• mean arterial BP (mm Hg)	86 ± 8	90 ± 6	no change
• cardiac output (L/min)	4.3 ± 1	6.2 ± 1	+44%
• heart rate (bpm)	71 ± 10	83 ± 10	+17%
• central venous pressure (mm Hg)	4 ± 3	4 ± 3	no change
• pulmonary capillary wedge pressure (mm Hg)	6 ± 2	8 ± 2	no change
• systemic vascular resistance (dyne/sec/cm⁻⁵)	1530 ± 520	1210 ± 266	−21%
• pulmonary vascular resistance (dyne/sec/cm⁻⁵)	119 ± 47	78 ± 22	−35%
• left ventricular stroke work index (g/m/m²)	41 ± 8	48 ± 6	no change

Blood volume changes during pregnancy

Blood volume
Plasma volume
RBC mass
Delivery

Gestational age-specific changes in mean arterial pressure

20% increase in labour
Nadir at 20–24 weeks
Back to baseline at term
Rapid resolution post-partum

First trimester | Second trimester | Third trimester | Labour | Puerperium

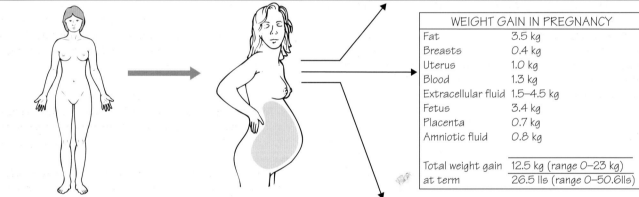

- Physiological adaptations in the mother occur in response to demands created by pregnancy. These include:
  - (i) support of the fetus (volume, nutritional and oxygen support, clearance of fetal waste);
  - (ii) protection of the fetus (from starvation, drugs, toxins);
  - (iii) preparation of the uterus for labour;
  - (iv) protection of the mother from potential cardiovascular injury at delivery.
- Maternal age, ethnicity, and genetic factors affect the ability of the mother to adapt to pregnancy.
- All maternal organ systems are required to adapt to the demands of pregnancy. The quality, degree, and timing of the adaptation varies from one individual to another and from one organ system to another.

Respiratory system (opposite)
- Respiratory adaptations during pregnancy are designed to optimize maternal and fetal oxygenation, and to facilitate transfer of CO_2 waste from the fetus to the mother.
- Many pregnant women complain of a subjective perception of shortness of breath (dyspnoea) in the absence of pathology. The reason for this is unclear.
- The mechanics of respiration change with pregnancy. The ribs flare outward and the level of the diaphragm rises 4 cm.
- During pregnancy, tidal volume increases by 200 mL (40%) resulting in a 100–200 mL (5%) increase in vital capacity and a 200 mL (20%) decrease in the residual volume, thereby leaving less air in the lungs at the end of expiration. The respiratory rate does not change. The end result is an increase in minute ventilation and a drop in arterial P_{CO_2} (below). Arterial P_{O_2} is essentially unchanged. A compensatory decrease in bicarbonate enables the pH to remain unchanged. Pregnancy thus represents a state of **compensated respiratory alkalosis**.

	pH	P_{O_2} (mmHg)	P_{CO_2} (mmHg)
Non-pregnant	7.40	93–100	35–40
Pregnant	7.40	100–105	28–30

Cardiovascular system (opposite)
- Progesterone decreases systemic vascular resistance early in pregnancy leading to a decline in blood pressure. In response, cardiac output increases by 30–50%.
- Activation of the renin–angiotensin system results in increased circulating angiotensin II which encourages sodium and water retention (leading to a 40% increase in blood volume) and directly constricts the peripheral vasculature.

Gastrointestinal tract
- Nausea ('morning sickness') occurs in >70% of pregnancies. Symptoms usually resolve by 17 weeks.
- Progesterone causes relaxation of gastrointestinal smooth muscle resulting in delayed gastric emptying and increased reflux.
- Pregnancy predisposes to cholelithiasis (gallstones). The majority of gallstones in pregnancy are cholesterol stones.
- Pregnancy is a 'diabetogenic state' with evidence of insulin resistance and reduced peripheral uptake of glucose (due to increased levels of placental anti-insulin hormones, primarily human placental lactogen (hPL)). These mechanisms are designed to ensure a continuous supply of glucose to the fetus.

Genitourinary system
- Glomerular filtration rate (GFR) increases by 50% early in pregnancy leading to an increase in creatinine clearance and a 25% decrease in serum creatinine and urea concentrations.
- Increased GFR results in an increase in filtered sodium. Aldosterone levels increase 2- to 3-fold to reabsorb this sodium.
- Increased GFR also results in decreased resorption of glucose. As such, 15% of normal pregnant women exhibit glycosuria.
- Mild hydronephrosis and hydroureter are common sonographic findings that are due to high progesterone levels and partial obstruction from the gravid uterus.
- 5% of pregnant women have bacteria in their urine. Pregnancy does not increase the incidence of asymptomatic bacteriuria, but such women are more likely to develop pyelonephritis (20–30%).

Haematological system
- Increased intravascular volume results in dilutional anaemia. Elevated erythropoetin levels lead to a compensatory increase in total red cell mass, but never fully corrects the anaemia.
- A modest increase in white blood cell count (leukocytosis) can be seen during pregnancy, but the differential count should not change.
- Mild thrombocytopaenia (<150,000 platelets/mL) is seen in 10% of pregnant women. This is probably dilutional and is rarely clinically significant.
- Pregnancy represents a hypercoagulable state with increased circulating levels of factors II (fibrinogen), VII, IX and X. These changes protect the mother from excessive blood loss at delivery, but also predispose to thromboembolism.

Endocrine system (Chapter 35)
- Oestrogen increases hepatic production of thyroid-binding globulin leading to an increase in total thyroid hormone concentration. However, thyroid-stimulating hormone (TSH), free T_3 and free T_4 levels remain unchanged.
- Serum calcium levels decrease in pregnancy leading to an increase in parathyroid hormone, which encourages conversion of cholecalciferol (vitamin D_3) to its active metabolite, 1,25-dihydroxycholecalciferol (DHCC), by 1α-hydroxylase in the placenta. This leads to increased intestinal absorption of calcium.
- Aldosterone and cortisol are increased in pregnancy.
- Prolactin increases in pregnancy, but its function is unknown. It is probably more important for lactation after delivery.

Immune system
Cellular immunity is depressed during pregnancy. As a result, pregnant women may be at increased risk for contracting viral infections and tuberculosis.

Musculoskeletal and dermatological systems
- A shift in posture (exaggerated lumbar lordosis) and lower back strain are common in pregnancy.
- Increased oestrogens and melanocyte-stimulating hormone may cause hyperpigmentation (darkening) of the umbilicus, nipples, abdominal midline (linea nigra), and face (chloasma).
- Increased oestrogen may also lead to skin changes such as spider angioma and palmar erythema.

ROUTINE PRENATAL SCREENING

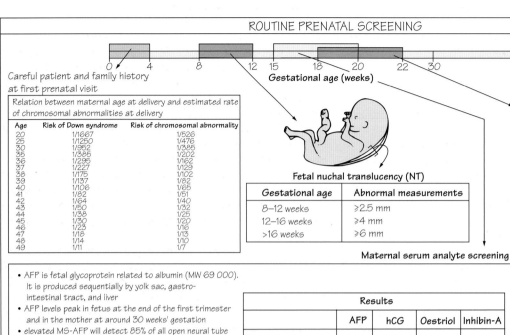

Careful patient and family history at first prenatal visit

Relation between maternal age at delivery and estimated rate of chromosomal abnormalities at delivery

Age	Risk of Down syndrome	Risk of chromosomal abnormality
20	1/1667	1/526
25	1/1250	1/476
30	1/952	1/385
35	1/385	1/202
36	1/295	1/162
37	1/227	1/129
38	1/175	1/102
39	1/137	1/82
40	1/106	1/65
41	1/82	1/51
42	1/64	1/40
43	1/50	1/32
44	1/38	1/25
45	1/30	1/20
46	1/23	1/16
47	1/18	1/13
48	1/14	1/10
49	1/11	1/7

Gestational age (weeks)

Fetal nuchal translucency (NT)

Gestational age	Abnormal measurements
8–12 weeks	≥2.5 mm
12–16 weeks	≥4 mm
>16 weeks	≥6 mm

Maternal serum analyte screening

Routine ultrasound screening
ideally performed 18–22 weeks (see Chapter 39)

Sonographic findings
- trisomy 21 (Down syndrome) thickened nuchal fold, short femur, renal pyelectasis, cardiac defect, duodenal atresia, echogenic bowel, echogenic cardiac focus
- trisomy 13 (Patau syndrome) holoprosencephaly, cardiac defect, omphalocoele, polycystic kidney, IUGR, polydactyly, cleft lip
- trisomy 18 (Edwards syndrome) polyhydramnios, IUGR, micrognathia, clenched hands, choroid plexus cysts, omphalocoele, clubfeet, hyronephrosis

- AFP is fetal glycoprotein related to albumin (MW 69 000). It is produced sequentially by yolk sac, gastro-intestinal tract, and liver
- AFP levels peak in fetus at the end of the first trimester and in the mother at around 30 weeks' gestation
- elevated MS-AFP will detect 85% of all open neural tube defects. Other causes include ventral wall defects, twins, placental abnormalities, congenital nephrosis

Down syndrome — Unaffected (normal) — Spina bifida

MS-AFP ≥2.0 MOM suggestive of NTD

0.2   0.5 0.8   2   3 4 5   10   20
Maternal serum AFP (MoM)

Results

	AFP	hCG	Oestriol	Inhibin-A
Open neural tube defects	↑↑	normal	normal	normal
Trisomy 21 (Down syndrome)	↓	↑	↓	↑
Trisomy 18 (Edwards syndrome)	↓	↓	↓	↓

Down syndrome screening
- 20% of Down syndrome births occur to women ≥35 years of age at delivery
- use of serum analyte screening will increase the detection rate to 60% with a false-positive rate of ~5% (MS-AFP alone will detect 20–25% of Down syndrome conceptions. hCG is the most sensitive maternal marker for Down syndrome)
- ultrasound can increase detection of Down syndrome fetuses to ~85%
- 15% of Down syndrome pregnancies will be missed by maternal age, serum screening, and ultrasound screening
- karyotype provides a definitive diagnosis

INDICATIONS FOR FURTHER PRENATAL SCREENING

Maternal
- maternal age ≥35 years at delivery
- prior child with neural tube defect
- previous child with chromosomal abnormality
- chromosomal abnormality in either parent
- family history of chromosome abnormality

- abnormal maternal serum analyte screening
- teratogen exposure
- maternal medical conditions

Fetal
- abnormal nuchal translucency
- abnormal fetal structural survey

FURTHER PRENATAL TESTING

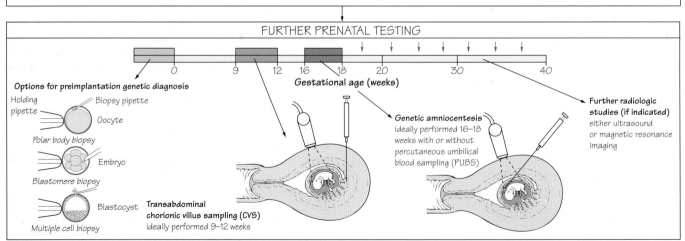

Gestational age (weeks)

Options for preimplantation genetic diagnosis
Holding pipette — Biopsy pipette — Oocyte
Polar body biopsy
Embryo
Blastomere biopsy
Blastocyst
Multiple cell biopsy

Transabdominal chorionic villus sampling (CVS)
ideally performed 9–12 weeks

Genetic amniocentesis
ideally performed 16–18 weeks with or without percutaneous umbilical blood sampling (PUBS)

Further radiologic studies (if indicated)
either ultrasound or magnetic resonance imaging

Congenital disorders and the fetus

- Congenital anomalies refer to structural defects present at birth. Major congenital anomalies (those incompatible with life or requiring major surgery) occur in 2–3% of live births, and 5% have minor malformations.
- 30–40% of congenital anomalies have a known cause, including chromosomal abnormalities (0.5% of live births), single gene defects (1% of births), multifactorial disorders, and teratogenic exposures. 60–70% have no known cause.

Classification of chromosomal abnormalities

Autosomal disorders

- *Trisomy 21 (Down syndrome)*: the most common autosomal disorder. Overall incidence is 1/800 live births, but it is strongly associated with maternal age (*opposite*). Long-term prognosis depends largely on the presence of cardiac anomalies.
- *Trisomy 18 (Edwards syndrome)*: 1/3500 births. It is characterized by intrauterine growth restriction (IUGR), single umbilical artery, overlapping clenched fingers, and 'rocker-bottom' feet. Fewer than 10% of infants survive to age 1.
- *Trisomy 13 (Patau syndrome)*: 1/5000 births. IUGR with facial clefts, ocular anomalies, and polydactyly. Fewer than 3% survive to age 3.
- *5p- (cri du chat syndrome)*: 1/20,000 births. Round facies, epicanthal folds, mental retardation, and a high-pitched, monotonous cry. Variable survival.

Sex chromosomal disorders

- *47,XXY (Klinefelter syndrome)*: the most common sex chromosome disorder. 1/500 births. Male phenotype, but with female adipose distribution and breast development. Normal pubic and axillary hair, scant facial hair. 20-fold increase in breast cancer. Usually infertile.
- *45,X0 (Turner syndrome)*: 1/2500 live births (but accounts for around 25% of early miscarriage). Short female with a webbed neck, primary amenorrhoea, renal anomalies, cardiac defect (aortic coarctation). Affected individuals are infertile.
- *47,XYY*: 1/800 births. Tall male with normal genitalia and testosterone levels, but intellectually limited. Usually fertile.

Classification of genetic disorders

Autosomal dominant (70%)

- Inherited from either parent or a new mutation.
- *Examples:* Huntington's chorea, neurofibromatosis, achondroplasia, Marfan syndrome.

Autosomal recessive (20%)

- Genetic screening is difficult since many different mutations may result in the same clinical disorder.
- *Examples:* sickle cell disease (African carrier rate 1/10), cystic fibrosis (1/20 in Caucasians), Tay–Sachs disease (1/30 in Ashkenazi Jews), β-thalassaemia (1/25 in women of Mediterranean origin).

X-linked recessive (5%)

Examples: Duchenne muscular dystrophy, haemophilia.

X-linked dominant (rare)

Examples: vitamin D-resistant rickets, hereditary haematuria.

Multifactorial inheritance

- May be isolated or part of a clinical syndrome.
- *Examples*: neural tube defect, talipes equinovarus (club feet), hydrocephaly, cleft lip, cardiac anomalies.

Routine prenatal screening (*opposite*)

- *Patient history* may identify a fetus at risk for aneuploidy (genetic anomalies). For example, the risk of recurrent neural tube defect is 1% (as compared with a baseline risk of 0.1%).
- The risk of fetal aneuploidy (primarily Down syndrome) increases with *maternal age* (*opposite*). 'Advanced maternal age' refers to women ≥35 years at delivery. Such women account for 5–8% of deliveries and 20–30% of Down syndrome births.
- *Nuchal translucency (NT)* in early pregnancy correlates with fetal aneuploidy (*opposite*). A measurement of ≤2.5 mm at 8–12 weeks is seen in 2–6% of fetuses of which 50–70% will have a chromosomal anomaly. *First trimester aneuploidy screening* incorporates NT and the serum analyte markers, PAPP-A and free β-human chorionic gonadotropin (β-hCG).
- Second trimester *maternal serum analyte screening* uses a panel of biochemical markers to adjust the maternal age-related risk for fetal aneuploidy (*opposite*). The standard 'quadruple panel' test at 15–20 weeks uses four markers: AFP, β-hCG, inhibin, and oestriol. The most important variable is gestational age which accounts for the majority of false-positive results.

Further prenatal testing

- *Amniocentesis* involves sampling amniotic fluid from around the fetus. The fluid itself or fetal cells can be used for karyotyping, DNA analysis, or enzyme assays. When performed at 16–18 weeks, the procedure-related loss rate is quoted at 1 in 270. US practice favours offering all women ≤35 years of age at delivery elective amniocentesis, because the risk of fetal aneuploidy approximately equals the procedure-related loss rate. Early amniocentesis (≤15 weeks) is associated with a higher rate of pregnancy loss, and should not be performed.
- *Chorionic villus sampling (CVS)* involves sampling of placental tissue at 9–12 weeks. Tissue can be used for DNA analysis, cytogenetic testing, or enzyme assays. Advantages include earlier diagnosis. Disadvantages include high procedure-related loss rate (1–2%), potential for maternal cell contamination, and sampling of cells destined to become placenta rather than fetus. CVS performed ≤9 weeks is associated with a 3-fold increase in limb reduction defects.
- *Percutaneous umbilical blood sampling (PUBS)* involves ultrasound-guided aspiration of fetal blood from the umbilical cord. Advantages include the ability to get a rapid fetal karyotype and to measure several haematological, immunological and acid/base parameters in the fetus. Fetal blood transfusions can also be performed. The procedure-related fetal loss rate is estimated at 1–5%.
- *Other studies* may include magnetic resonance imaging or invasive procedures (fetoscopy, fetal tissue biopsy).
- *Future options.*
  (i) *Preimplantation genetic diagnosis* (*opposite*) involves genetic analysis of a cell(s) removed prior to embryo transfer at *in vitro* fertilization.
  (ii) *Fetal cells* exist in the maternal circulation (~1 fetal cell per 10,000 maternal cells). The ability to isolate such cells (or DNA) may provide an option for fetal genetic analysis.

38 Obstetric ultrasound

INDICATIONS FOR OBSTETRIC ULTRASOUND

Maternal
- pelvic mass
- uterine size > dates
- follow fibroid growth
- cervical length evaluation in women at risk for cervical insufficiency

Fetal
- estimation of gestational age
- evaluation of fetal growth
- determine fetal presentation
- suspected multiple gestation
- suspected fetal death
- follow-up fetal anomaly
- biophysical profile
- suspected ectopic pregnancy

Uteroplacental
- vaginal bleeding of unclear aetiology, suspected abruption
- suspected molar pregnancy
- suspected uterine anomaly
- suspected polyhydramnios or oligohydramnios
- follow-up on placental location in previously identified previa

Other
- amniocentesis
- abnormal MS-AFP
- adjuvant to cervical cerclage placement
- external cephalic version
- adjunct to surgical procedure (embryo transfer, chorionic villus sampling, intrauterine transfusion, fetoscopy)

FIRST TRIMESTER SONOGRAPHY

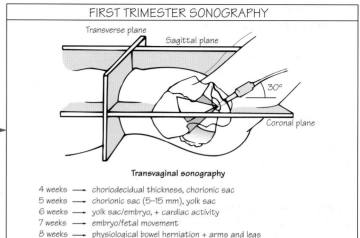

Transverse plane
Sagittal plane
Coronal plane
30°

Transvaginal sonography

4 weeks	→	choriodecidual thickness, chorionic sac
5 weeks	→	chorionic sac (5–15 mm), yolk sac
6 weeks	→	yolk sac/embryo, + cardiac activity
7 weeks	→	embryo/fetal movement
8 weeks	→	physiological bowel herniation + arms and legs

SECOND AND THIRD TRIMESTER SONOGRAPHY

Fetal biometry and estimated fetal weight (EFW)

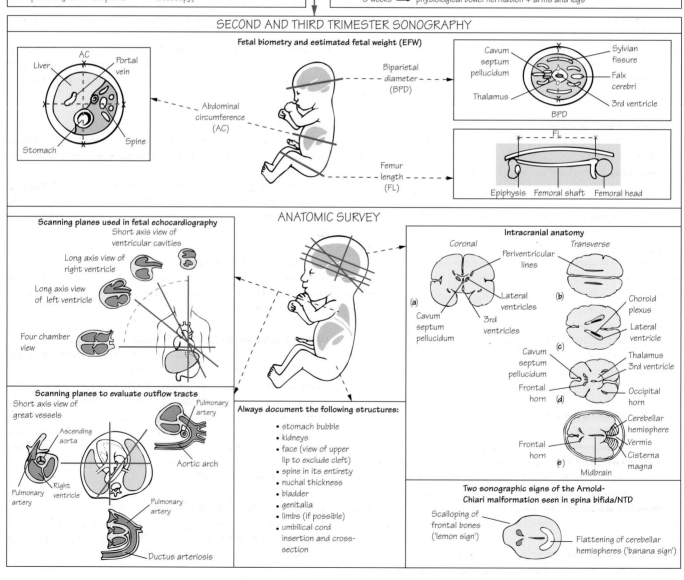

AC
Liver
Portal vein
Stomach
Spine

Abdominal circumference (AC)

Biparietal diameter (BPD)

Femur length (FL)

Cavum septum pellucidum
Thalamus
Sylvian fissure
Falx cerebri
3rd ventricle
BPD

FL
Epiphysis   Femoral shaft   Femoral head

ANATOMIC SURVEY

Scanning planes used in fetal echocardiography

Short axis view of ventricular cavities
Long axis view of right ventricle
Long axis view of left ventricle
Four chamber view

Scanning planes to evaluate outflow tracts

Short axis view of great vessels
Ascending aorta
Pulmonary artery
Right ventricle
Pulmonary artery
Aortic arch
Pulmonary artery
Ductus arteriosis

Always document the following structures:
- stomach bubble
- kidneys
- face (view of upper lip to exclude cleft)
- spine in its entirety
- nuchal thickness
- bladder
- genitalia
- limbs (if possible)
- umbilical cord insertion and cross-section

Intracranial anatomy

Coronal
Transverse

(a)
Cavum septum pellucidum
Periventricular lines
Lateral ventricles
3rd ventricles

(b)
Choroid plexus
Lateral ventricle

(c)
Cavum septum pellucidum
Frontal horn
Thalamus
3rd ventricle
Occipital horn

(d)

(e)
Frontal horn
Cerebellar hemisphere
Vermis
Cisterna magna
Midbrain

Two sonographic signs of the Arnold-Chiari malformation seen in spina bifida/NTD

Scalloping of frontal bones ('lemon sign')
Flattening of cerebellar hemispheres ('banana sign')

Principles of ultrasonography

• Ultrasound uses sound waves delivered at high frequency (3.5–5 MHz for transabdominal and 5–7.5 MHz for transvaginal transducers). The higher the frequency the better the resolution but the less the tissue penetration.
• Interpretation of images requires operator experience.

Indications (opposite)

Routine use of obstetric ultrasound can improve detection of fetal anomalies, accurately determine gestational age, and facilitate early diagnosis of multiple pregnancies. However, it is expensive and has not consistently been shown to improve perinatal outcome.

Complications

There are no confirmed adverse effects of ultrasound on the fetus. The major complication is false-positive and false-negative diagnoses.

Guidelines for obstetric ultrasound

First trimester sonography (opposite)

• Evaluate the uterus for the presence of a *gestational sac*. An intrauterine gestational sac should be seen at a serum β-hCG level of 1000–1200 mIU/mL by transvaginal scan and 6000 mIU/mL by transabdominal ultrasound. If no intrauterine pregnancy is seen, the possibility of an ectopic pregnancy should be entertained.
• If a gestational sac is identified, it should be examined for a *yolk sac* (usually evident at a β-hCG of 7000 mIU/mL) and *embryo* (at 11,000 mIU/mL).
• *Gestational age* should be documented. Crown–rump length (CRL) in the early first trimester is an accurate determinant of gestational age to within 3–5 days (as compared with an error of ± 2 weeks by second trimester measurements and ±3 weeks by third trimester ultrasound).

CRL (in mm) + 6.5 = approximate gestational age in weeks.

In the late first trimester, measurement of the biparietal diameter (BPD) can be used to estimate gestational age.
• Fetal *cardiac activity* is usually evident once the fetal pole is seen. If the CRL is 3–5 mm but no cardiac activity is seen, a follow-up ultrasound is indicated in 3–5 days to evaluate fetal viability. Once fetal cardiac activity has been documented, the fetal loss rate decreases to around 5%.
• Document *fetal number*. If a multiple pregnancy is identified, chorionicity should be determined (Chapter 52).
• Measure *nuchal translucency* (Chapter 37).
• Evaluate the uterus, adnexal structures, and cul-de-sac for anomalies unrelated to pregnancy.

Second trimester sonography (opposite)

• Document fetal cardiac activity and fetal number.
• Estimate *amniotic fluid volume* (Chapter 47).
• Document *placental location*. Overdistention of the maternal bladder or a lower uterine contraction can give a false impression of placenta previa. If placenta previa is identified at 18–22 weeks, serial ultrasound examinations should be performed to follow placental location. Only 5% of placenta previa identified in the second trimester will persist to term.
• The *umbilical cord* should be imaged, and the number of vessels (a single umbilical artery may suggest fetal aneuploidy, especially if associated with other structural anomalies), placental insertion (if possible), and insertion into the fetus (to exclude an anterior abdominal wall defect) should be noted. Extra-abdominal herniation of the midgut into the umbilical cord occurs normally at 8–12 weeks' gestation and should not be misdiagnosed as an abdominal wall defect.
• *Cervical length* should be documented. A shortened cervix is associated with an increased risk for preterm birth.
• Assessment of *gestational age*.
• *Anatomic survey* (opposite) is best done at 18–22 weeks.
• Evaluation of uterus and adnexae.

Third trimester sonography

• As for second trimester sonography.
• Determine *estimated fetal weight* (EFW) using the average of three readings for each of the following three measurements: femur length (FL), abdominal circumference (AC), and BPD. Each of these measurements have been standardized to specific fetal landmarks (opposite). Of the three measurements, the AC is the most important since it is disproportionately weighted in the calculation of EFW. It is also the most difficult to measure. A small difference in AC will result in a large difference in EFW. As a result, sonographic EFW estimations have an error of 15–20%.
• A detailed *anatomic survey* should be performed with each ultrasound even if a prior anatomic survey was reported as normal. Certain fetal anomalies will only become evident later in gestation (such as achondroplastic dwarfism).

Doppler velocimetry

• Doppler velocimetry shows the direction and characteristics of blood flow, and can be used to examine the uteroplacental or fetoplacental circulations.
• Doppler velocimetry should not be performed routinely. Indications include intrauterine growth restriction, cord malformations, unexplained oligohydramnios, preeclampsia, and possibly fetal cardiac anomalies.

Fetal echocardiography (opposite)

Fetal echo is indicated for pregnancies at high risk of a fetal cardiac anomaly (such as pregnancies complicated by maternal diabetes or maternal congenital cardiac disease).

Use of ultrasound to detect fetuses with aneuploidy

• Fetuses with trisomy 13 or trisomy 18 tend to have major structural anomalies that can be detected on ultrasound.
• Fetuses with trisomy 21 (Down syndrome) may have no anomalies, structural malformations that can only reliably be detected late in pregnancy (duodenal atresia), or very subtle biometric or morphologic abnormalities (shortened femurs, renal pyelectasis). Only 30–50% of Down syndrome fetuses will be detected by routine ultrasound (see Chapter 37). A normal anatomic survey decreases the risk of Down syndrome by approximately 50%.

Ultrasound and hydrops fetalis

Hydrops fetalis is a pathologic condition characterized by excessive fluid accumulation in the fetus. It is a sonographic diagnosis (Chapter 50).

BACTERIAL AND PROTOZOAN INFECTIONS IN PREGNANCY

	Diagnosis	Organism	Maternal signs and symptoms	Fetal/neonatal effects
Bacteria	Group B streptococcus	Streptococcus agalactiae	Asymptomatic colonization Urinary tract infection Chorioamnionitis Endomyometritis	Early onset: neonatal sepsis Late onset: meningitis
	Chorioamnionitis	Polymicrobial • bacteroides • Strep agalactiae • E. coli	Presents with fever; tachycardia, uterine tenderness, leukocytosis, and/or malodorous discharge	Neonatal sepsis
	Listeriosis	Listeria monocytogenes	Asymptomatic (most common) Flu-like symptoms Fatigue (similar to infectious mononucleosis) Meningitis (rare)	Early onset: neonatal sepsis Late onset: meningitis
	Tuberculosis	Mycobacterium tuberculosis	Asymptomatic (most common) Active disease: cough, night sweats, weight loss, haemoptysis	Congenital tuberculosis may be fatal (especially tuberculous meningitis)
	Bacterial vaginosis	Overgrowth of normal vaginal bacteria	Preterm labour	Prematurity Low birth weight
	Gonorrhoea	Neisseria gonorrhoeae	Preterm labour Chorioamnionitis Disseminated gonococcal infection	Neonatal sepsis Neonatal gonococcal ophthalmia
	Chlamydia	Chlamydia trachomatis	Preterm labour Chorioamnionitis	Conjunctivitis Pneumonia
Protozoa	Toxoplasmosis	Toxoplasma gondii	Asymptomatic Fatigue Lymphadenopathy, myalgias	Abortion Intracranial calcifications Hepatosplenomegaly Chorioretinitis, convulsions
	Trichomoniasis	Trichomonas vaginalis	Premature rupture of fetal membranes	Low birth weight

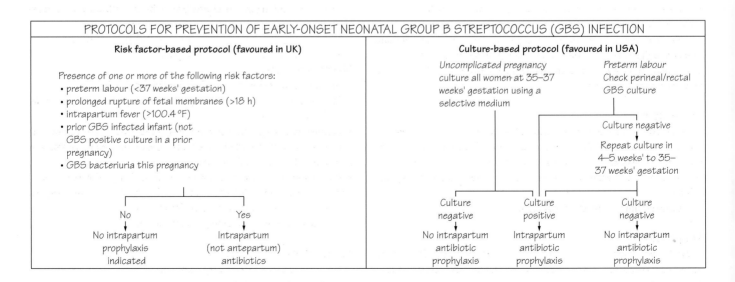

PROTOCOLS FOR PREVENTION OF EARLY-ONSET NEONATAL GROUP B STREPTOCOCCUS (GBS) INFECTION

Risk factor-based protocol (favoured in UK)

Presence of one or more of the following risk factors:
• preterm labour (<37 weeks' gestation)
• prolonged rupture of fetal membranes (>18 h)
• intrapartum fever (>100.4 °F)
• prior GBS infected infant (not GBS positive culture in a prior pregnancy)
• GBS bacteriuria this pregnancy

No → No intrapartum prophylaxis indicated

Yes → Intrapartum (not antepartum) antibiotics

Culture-based protocol (favoured in USA)

Uncomplicated pregnancy culture all women at 35–37 weeks' gestation using a selective medium

Preterm labour Check perineal/rectal GBS culture

Culture negative → Repeat culture in 4–5 weeks' to 35–37 weeks' gestation

Culture negative → No intrapartum antibiotic prophylaxis

Culture positive → Intrapartum antibiotic prophylaxis

Culture negative → No intrapartum antibiotic prophylaxis

Bacterial infection (opposite)
Group B streptococcus
• *Incidence.* In developed countries, neonatal group B streptococcus (GBS) sepsis complicates 1.8/1000 live births.
• *Maternal signs/symptoms.* 20% of all pregnant women are asymptomatically colonized in the vaginal or perianal region.
• *Fetal/neonatal effects.* Two clinically distinct neonatal GBS infections have been identified.

  (i) *Early-onset* neonatal GBS infection (80%) results from transmission during labour or delivery. Signs of serious infection (respiratory distress, septic shock) usually develop within 6–12 hours of birth. The mortality rate is 25% and surviving infants frequently exhibit neurological sequelae.

  (ii) *Late-onset* GBS infection (20%) is a nosocomial or community-acquired infection. It presents more than a week after birth, usually as meningitis. The mortality rate is lower than for early onset disease, but neurological sequelae are equally common.
• *Prevention.* Strategies to prevent early-onset neonatal GBS infection vary. In the UK, a risk-factor based protocol is used. Patients are treated in labour if one of the following risk factors is present: a prior affected infant (not GBS +ve in a prior pregnancy), GBS UTI in index pregnancy, preterm labour, fever, or rupture of membranes ≥18 hours. This protocol results in the treatment of 15–20% of pregnant women and prevents 65–70% of early-onset GBS sepsis. US practice favours a universal screening protocol. All women are screened for GBS carrier status at 35–37 weeks (*opposite*). Women who are GBS carriers receive intrapartum antibiotics. The latter protocol results in the treatment of 25–30% of pregnant women and prevents 85–90% of early-onset GBS sepsis. Patients with unknown GBS carrier status in labour should be treated according to the risk factor-based protocol.
• *Treatment:* intrapartum penicillin (2nd generation cephalosporin, erythromycin, or clindamycin if penicillin allergic).

Chorioamnionitis
• *Incidence.* 1–10% of pregnancies.
• *Maternal signs/symptoms.* Chorioamnionitis is a clinical diagnosis. Definitive diagnosis requires a positive amniotic fluid culture. Maternal complications may include sepsis, adult respiratory distress syndrome (ARDS), pulmonary oedema, and death.
• *Fetal/neonatal effects:* neonatal sepsis, pneumonia, death.
• *Prevention:* avoidance of rupture of membranes >18 hours.
• *Treatment:* prompt administration of broad-spectrum antibiotics and immediate delivery. Chorioamnionitis is not an indication for caesarean delivery; however, the caesarean rate is increased due to dystocia and non-reassuring fetal testing.

Listeriosis
• Listeriosis is an uncommon cause of neonatal sepsis that may be acquired transplacentally. Cervical and blood cultures should be obtained in women with suspicious symptoms. Listeriosis is a common cause of intrauterine fetal demise and neonatal mortality rate is high.
• Treatment: ampicillin and gentamicin.

Tuberculosis
• *Incidence.* Tuberculosis (TB) in pregnant women is rare in developed countires. Cases occur most commonly among recent immigrants.
• *Maternal signs/symptoms.* Most infected women are asymptomatic. Active disease at presentation is rare.
• *Fetal/neonatal effects.* Congenital or neonatal TB is a highly morbid condition that may be fatal if misdiagnosed.
• *Prevention.* Intradermal placement of purified protein derivative (PPD) is an accurate way to screen for TB. Interpretation of the PPD test depends on the risk status of the patient (*below*).
• *Treatment.* A positive PPD necessitates a chest X-ray. If the X-ray is normal, 6 months of isoniazid (INH) is recommended in women less than 35 years of age (can be deferred until after delivery). If the chest X-ray is abnormal, immediate treatment with INH and ethambutol is indicated, and three early morning sputum cultures should be sent to exclude active pulmonary TB.

Interpretation of the PPD screening test for TB

Very high risk	High risk	No risk factors
HIV positive	Foreign-born	↓
Abnormal chest X-ray	Intravenous drug use	↓
Recent contact with	Medical condition	↓
an active case of TB	increasing the risk	↓
↓	of TB	≥15 mm of induration
↓	↓	(not redness)
≥5 mm is positive	≥10 mm is positive	is positive

Bacterial vaginosis (Chapter 7)
Bacterial vaginosis (BV) is the most common cause of vaginal discharge in pregnancy. It is associated with pre-term delivery in high-risk women. However, it remains unclear whether treatment for asymptomatic BV will reduce the risk of pre-term delivery.

Chlamydia and gonorrhoea (Chapters 7 and 8)
• *Incidence:* very prevalent sexually transmitted diseases.
• *Maternal signs/symptoms:* usually asymptomatic.
• *Fetal/neonatal effects.* Untreated maternal chlamydia and gonorrhoea are associated with increased neonatal morbidity.
• *Prevention.* Cervical cultures in early pregnancy in high-risk women reliably detect infection. Instillation of prophylactic antibiotic ointment into the eyes of all newborns prevents eye infection.
• *Treatment:* chlamydia: oral erythromycin or azithromycin; gonorrhoea: intramuscular or oral cefuroxime, ceftriaxone.

Protozoan infections (opposite)
Toxoplasmosis
• *Incidence.* Acute toxoplasmosis during pregnancy is rare.
• *Maternal signs/symptoms.* Most patients are asymptomatic, but some have flu-like symptoms.
• *Fetal/neonatal effects.* Only acute toxoplasmosis in pregnancy is capable of being transmitted to the fetus. 10% of infected newborns will have clinical evidence of disease.
• *Prevention.* Toxoplasmosis is acquired through ingestion of encysted organisms in raw or undercooked meat or through contact with infected cat faeces. Avoid cleaning litter box. Strict hygiene.
• *Treatment:* sulfadiazine with pyrimethamine.

Trichomoniasis (Chapter 7)
• *Vaginal trichomoniasis* is very common.
• *Treatment:* metronidazole .

Infections in pregnancy: viruses and spirochetes

	Organism	Maternal signs and symptoms	Fetal/neonatal effects	Prevention	Management
	VIRAL AND SPIROCHETE INFECTIONS IN PREGNANCY				
Viruses	Rubella	Mild illness (rash, arthralgia, diffuse lymphadenopathy)	*Congenital rubella syndrome* • deafness, eye lesions (cataracts), heart disease (patent ductus arteriosus), mental retardation, IUGR	MMR to children and non-immune (non-pregnant) adults	None
	Cytomegalovirus	• asymptomatic (common) • mild viral illness • infectious mononucleosis-like syndrome • hepatitis (rare)	*CMV inclusion disease* • hepatosplenomegaly, intracranial calcification, chorioretinitis, mental retardation, interstitial pneumonitis • 30% mortality	None	None
	HIV	• asymptomatic • mild viral illness • AIDS	Childhood AIDS	Barrier contraception, abstinence, avoid IV drug use	Zidovudine (ZDV) and possibly elective caesarean delivery to prevent vertical transmission
	Varicella zoster	• "chickenpox" (most common) • pneumonitis (10–20%) • meningitis (rare)	*Congenital varicella syndrome* • chorioretinitis, cerebral cortical atrophy, hydronephrosis, longbone defects • exposure <20 weeks' gestation *Near-term infection* • benign chickenpox • fulminant disseminated infection can be fatal	•VZV vaccine to non-immune (non-pregnant) adults •VZIG within 96 hours of VZV exposure and to neonates, if indicated	Acyclovir
	Herpes simplex virus (HSV)	*First-episode primary* •systemic illness, fever, arthralgias, painful genital lesions, adenopathy *Recurrent infection* •painful genital lesions (blister, ulcer)	• herpetic lesions of the skin and mouth • viral sepsis • herpes encephalitis • disseminated herpes simplex virus infection (long-term neurological sequelae, high mortality rate)	Caesarean delivery if primary HSV lesion is present in labour	Prophylactic acyclovir from 35–36 weeks to decrease incidence of active lesions in labour
	Hepatitis B and C	Mild/moderate viral illness (nausea, vomiting, hepatosplenomegaly, jaundice, right upper quadrant pain)	Chronic hepatitis carrier	• avoid sexual contact with infected partners, IV drug abuse, infected blood • hepatitis B vaccine (no vaccine for HCV)	Hepatitis B immune globulin (HBIG) and hepatitis B vaccine to neonate
Spirochetes	Syphilis (*Treponema pallidum*)	• primary (solitary genital tract lesion or gumma) • secondary (rash, snail-track ulcers in the mouth, adenopathy, condylomata lata) • tertiary neurosyphilis or meningovascular syphilis	• stillbirth *Early congenital syphilis* • maculopapular rash • 'sniffles' • hepatosplenomegaly • chorioretinitis *Late congenital syphilis* • Hutchinson's teeth • mulberry molars • saber shins • cardiovascular anomalies • sensorineural deafness	• avoid sexual contact with infected partners • treat infected women to prevent vertical transmission	Penicillin (in pregnancy, women who are allergic to penicillin should undergo penicillin desensitization and then be treated with penicillin)
	Lyme disease (*Borrelia burgdorferi*)	• local infection (fever, erythema chronicum migrans, adenopathy) • disseminated disease	• prematurity • stillbirth • rash-like neonatal illness	Avoid tick bites (long trousers, sprays, remove all ticks)	Erythromycin

Viral infections (opposite)
Rubella
- *Incidence*: rare in developed countries.
- *Transmission:* airborne.
- *Maternal signs/symptoms*. Rubella ('German measles') is usually a mild viral illness.
- *Diagnosis*. Serological diagnosis requires either the presence of IgM or a significant rise in IgG antibody titer (fourfold rise over 4–6 weeks).
- *Fetal/neonatal effects*. The risk of congenital rubella syndrome is 90% if maternal infection is acquired <11 weeks, 33% if 11–12 weeks, 11% if 13–14 weeks, 4% if 15–16 weeks, 0% if >16 weeks.
- *Prevention*. Measles/mumps/rubella (MMR) immunization. MMR is a live vaccine and is not recommended in pregnancy.
- *Management:* there is no treatment.

Cytomegalovirus
- *Incidence:* 1–2% of all births.
- *Transmission:* contact with body fluids, sexual contact.
- *Maternal signs/symptoms*: 20% of women have a non–specific viral syndrome (fever, pharyngitis, lymphadenopathy).
- *Diagnosis*. The high prevalence of CMV seroreactivity (>50%) and multiple CMV serotypes limits the value of serological screening.
- *Fetal/neonatal effects*. 90% of infected newborns are asymptomatic at birth, but many later demonstrate deafness, mental retardation, and/or delayed psychomotor development.
- *Prevention:* there is no vaccine.
- *Management:* there is no treatment.

Human immunodeficiency virus
- *Incidence*. Rare in developed countries, but very high prevalence in developing countries (e.g., 1 in 3 pregnant women in South Africa is HIV-positive).
- *Transmission:* sexual contact, intravenous drug use, vertical transmission.
- *Maternal signs/symptoms:* variable.
- *Diagnosis:* serum enzyme-linked immunosorbent assay (ELISA) and confirmatory western blot.
- *Fetal/neonatal effects*. HIV-positive infants may develop AIDS with high perinatal mortality rate.
- *Prevention:* safe sexual practices, avoidance of high-risk drug behaviour, serial serum viral load measurements and antiviral therapy, if indicated.
- *Management*. Prenatal HIV testing. Zidovudine (AZT) therapy reduces the risk of vertical transmission from 25–33% to 8%, with a further reduction to 0–2% if the viral load is <1000 copies/mL. Elective caesarean delivery may reduce vertical transmission if viral load is ≥1000 copies/mL.

Varicella zoster virus
- *Incidence:* 1 in 7500 pregnancies.
- *Transmission:* airborne (highly infectious).
- *Maternal signs/symptoms:* 'chickenpox'. The maternal mortality rate approaches 50% for adults with pneumonitis or encephalitis.
- *Diagnosis:* clinical suspicion. Confirmatory serological tests.
- *Fetal/neonatal effects*. First trimester varicella zoster virus (VZV) has a 2–3% risk of congenital varicella syndrome. Near-term infections resemble benign childhood infection.

- *Prevention*. Only 5% of adults are not immune to VZV.
- *Management:* delivery should be avoided at the time of acute maternal infection. At-risk neonates should receive VZIG. Acyclovir may also be helpful.

Herpes simplex virus (Chapter 7)
- *Incidence:* neonatal herpes simplex virus (HSV) infection occurs in 2–4 per 10,000 births
- *Transmission:* direct contact.
- *Maternal signs/symptoms*. First-episode primary genital HSV may be associated with systemic symptoms. Both primary and recurrent HSV are characterized by painful, vesicular lesions.
- *Fetal/neonatal effects*. Neonatal herpes is acquired from passage through an infected birth canal. The risk of vertical transmission is 50% for primary HSV infection and 0–4% in women with recurrent disease.
- *Prevention:* Caesarean delivery is recommended for all pregnancies complicated by primary genital HSV in labour. The management of women with a recurrent genital HSV outbreak (either lesion and/or symptoms) in labour is less clear. In the UK, such women are allowed to deliver vaginally. US practice favours caesarean delivery for such women.
- *Management*. Prophylactic acyclovir from 35–36 weeks may be useful in preventing active lesions in labour in some high-risk women.

Hepatitis B and C
- *Incidence:* 1–2% of pregnancies.
- *Transmission:* sexual contact, intravenous drug use, vertical transmission.
- *Maternal signs/symptoms:* usually mild/moderate viral illness.
- *Diagnosis:* serological testing.
- *Fetal/neonatal effects*. Hepatitis B and C are not teratogenic, but affected infants may become carriers. Vertical transmission rates of hepatitis B range from 15% (in women who are e-antigen negative) to 80% (e-antigen positive), and of hepatitis C from 0 to 5% (HIV-negative women) to 35–50% (HIV-positive women).
- *Prevention:* safe sexual practices, avoidance of high-risk drug behaviour. Avoid breast-feeding. Hepatitis B has an effective vaccine.
- *Management:* infants born to women with detectable hepatitis B surface antigen (HBsAg) should receive hepatitis B immunoglobulin (HBIG) and hepatitis B vaccine within 12 hours of birth. There is no effective treatment for hepatitis C.

Spirochete infections (opposite)
Syphilis (Chapter 7)
- *Incidence:* rare in developed countries.
- *Transmission:* sexual contact.
- *Maternal signs/symptoms*. Patients may exhibit primary, secondary, or tertiary syphilis.
- *Diagnosis:* serum *r*apid *p*lasma *r*eagin (RPR) or *v*enereal *d*isease *r*esearch *l*aboratory (VDRL) test. Confirmatory tests are required before instituting treatment.
- *Fetal/neonatal effects*. Affected infants may be stillborn or exhibit signs of early or late congenital syphilis.
- *Prevention:* safe sexual practices. Congenital syphilis is unusual if the mother is treated.
- *Management*. Penicillin.

41 Hypertensive disorders of pregnancy

RISK FACTORS FOR PREECLAMPSIA

Nulliparity
African-American/African race
Prior history of preeclampsia
Extremes of maternal age (≤15 or ≥35 years)
Family history of preeclampsia
Multiple gestation
Chronic hypertension
Chronic renal disease
Antiphospholipid antibody syndrome
Collagen vascular disease
Angiotensinogen gene T235 mutation

DIAGNOSIS OF PREECLAMPSIA

Hypertension

Clinical triad

Proteinuria   ± Non-dependent oedema

CLASSIFICATION OF PREECLAMPSIA

'Mild' pre-eclampsia

- includes all women with a diagnosis of preeclampsia, but without features of 'severe' pre-eclampsia

'Severe' pre-eclampsia

Note: only one of the features listed below is required for diagnosis

Symptoms	Signs	Laboratory findings
• symptoms of central nervous system dysfunction (severe headache, blurred vision, scotomata) • symptoms of liver capsule distention (right upper quandrant and/or epigastric pain)	• severe elevations in BP (defined as BP ≥160/110 on two occasions at least 6 hours apart) • pulmonary oedema • eclampsia (generalized seizures or unexplained coma) • cerebrovascular accident • IUGR	• proteinuria (>5 g/24 h) • renal failure or oliguria (<500 mL/24 h) • hepatocellular injury (serum transaminase levels >2x normal) • thrombocytopenia (<100 000 platelets/mm^3) • coagulopathy • HELLP (haemolysis, elevated liver enzymes, low platelets)

SHORT-TERM COMPLICATIONS

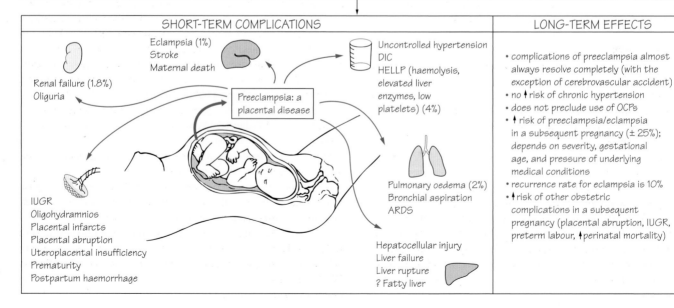

Eclampsia (1%)
Stroke
Maternal death

Renal failure (1.8%)
Oliguria

Preeclampsia: a placental disease

Uncontrolled hypertension
DIC
HELLP (haemolysis, elevated liver enzymes, low platelets) (4%)

IUGR
Oligohydramnios
Placental infarcts
Placental abruption
Uteroplacental insufficiency
Prematurity
Postpartum haemorrhage

Pulmonary oedema (2%)
Bronchial aspiration
ARDS

Hepatocellular injury
Liver failure
Liver rupture
? Fatty liver

LONG-TERM EFFECTS

- complications of preeclampsia almost always resolve completely (with the exception of cerebrovascular accident)
- no ↑ risk of chronic hypertension
- does not preclude use of OCPs
- ↑ risk of preeclampsia/eclampsia in a subsequent pregnancy (± 25%); depends on severity, gestational age, and pressure of underlying medical conditions
- recurrence rate for eclampsia is 10%
- ↑ risk of other obstetric complications in a subsequent pregnancy (placental abruption, IUGR, preterm labour, ↑perinatal mortality)

Hypertensive disorders of pregnancy are the second most common cause of maternal death in developed countries (after embolism) accounting for 15% of all maternal deaths.

Effects of pregnancy on maternal cardiovascular system

- Blood volume increases 1 L by 12 weeks (2 L in twins).
- BP decreases in early pregnancy (due primarily to a decrease in systemic vascular resistance secondary to progesterone), nadirs in mid-pregnancy, and returns to baseline by term.

Classification

1 Chronic hypertension

- *Definition:* hypertension prior to pregnancy. The diagnosis should also be entertained in women with BP ≥140/90 mmHg prior to 20 weeks' gestation.
- *Complications.* Such pregnancies are at increased risk of superimposed preeclampsia, intrauterine fetal growth restriction (IUGR), placental abruption, and stillbirth.
- *Management.* Continue antihypertensive medications with the exception of angiotensin converting enzyme (ACE) inhibitors. These drugs are not teratogenic *per se*, but have been associated with progressive and irreversible renal injury in the fetus. Diuretic therapy is generally discouraged.
- Fetal testing (serial ultrasound examinations for fetal growth with or without fetal non-stress testing) should be initiated after 32 weeks gestation. Delivery should be achieved by 40 weeks.

2 Chronic hypertension with superimposed preeclampsia

3 Pregnancy-induced hypertension (PIH)

- Also known as gestational non-proteinuric hypertension.
- *Diagnosis:* persistent elevation of BP ≥140/90 in the third trimester without evidence of preeclampsia in a previously normotensive woman. It is a diagnosis of exclusion.
- *Aetiology.* It probably represents an exaggerated physiological response of the maternal cardiovascular system to pregnancy.
- Rarely associated with adverse maternal or fetal outcome.

4 Preeclampsia

- Also known as gestational proteinuric hypertension, preeclamptic toxemia (PET).
- *Definition:* a multisystem disorder specific to pregnancy and the puerperium. More precisely, it is a disease of the placenta since it occurs in pregnancies where there is trophoblast but no fetal tissue (complete molar pregnancies).
- *Incidence*: 6–8% of all pregnancies.
- *Risk factors:* (*opposite*).
- *Diagnosis.* A clinical diagnosis with three elements.
  (i) *New-onset hypertension* defined as a sustained BP ≥140/90 mmHg in a previously normotensive woman (a prior definition included an elevation in systolic BP ≥30 or diastolic BP ≥15 mmHg over first trimester BP, but these criteria have now been dropped).
  (ii) *New-onset significant proteinuria* defined as >300 mg/24 hours or ≥1+ on a clean-catch urine in the absence of urinary tract infection.

(iii) *New-onset non-dependent oedema* (i.e. swelling of face and hands), which is not required for the diagnosis.
NOTE: a definitive diagnosis of preeclampsia should only be made after 20 weeks' gestation. Evidence of gestational proteinuric hypertension prior to 20 weeks should raise the possibility of an underlying molar pregnancy, drug withdrawal, or (rarely) chromosomal abnormality in the fetus.
- *Classification:* (*opposite*). Preeclampsia is classified as 'mild' or 'severe.' There is no category of 'moderate' preeclampsia.
- *Aetiology:* the cause of preeclampsia is not known. Theories include an abnormal maternal immunological response to the fetal allograft, an underlying genetic abnormality, an imbalance in the prostanoid cascade, and the presence of circulating toxins and/or endogenous vasoconstrictors. What is known is that the blueprint for the development of preeclampsia is laid down early in pregnancy. The primary event is likely to be a failure of the second wave of trophoblast invasion from 8–18 weeks that is responsible for destruction of the muscularis layer of the spiral arterioles in the myometrium adjacent to the developing placenta. As pregnancy progresses and the metabolic demand of the fetoplacental unit increases, the spiral arterioles are therefore unable to accommodate the necessary increase in blood flow. This then leads to the development of 'placental dysfunction' that manifests clinically as preeclampsia. Although attractive, this hypothesis remains to be validated. Whatever the placental abnormality, the end result is widespread vasospasm and endothelial injury.
- *Complications:* (*opposite*). Eclampsia—defined as one or more generalized convulsions or coma in the setting of preeclampsia and in the absence of other neurological conditions—was thought to be the end stage of preeclampsia, hence the nomenclature. It is now clear, however, that seizures are but one clinical manifestation of 'severe' preeclampsia. 50% of eclampsia occurs preterm. Of those at term, 75% occur either intrapartum or within 48 hours of delivery.
- *Management.* Delivery is the only effective treatment for preeclampsia, and is recommended:
  (i) in women with 'mild' preeclampsia once a favourable gestational age has been reached (>35–36 weeks);
  (ii) in all women with 'severe' preeclampsia regardless of gestational age (with the exception of 'severe' preeclampsia due to proteinuria alone or IUGR remote from term with good fetal testing). There has also been a recent trend towards expectant management of 'severe' preeclampsia by BP criteria alone <32 weeks' gestation.
- There is no proven benefit to routine delivery by caesarean. However, the probability of vaginal delivery in a patient with preeclampsia remote from term with an unfavourable cervix is only 15–20%.
- BP control is important to prevent cerebrovascular accident (usually associated with BP ≥170/120), but does not affect the natural course of preeclampsia.
- Intravenous magnesium sulfate should be given intrapartum and for at least 24 hours postpartum to prevent eclampsia.
- *Prevention.* Despite promising early studies, low-dose aspirin (acetylsalicylic acid (ASA)) and/or supplemental calcium does not prevent preeclampsia in either high- or low-risk women.
- *Prognosis.* Preeclampsia and its complications always resolve following delivery (with the exception of cerebrovascular accident). Diuresis (>4 L/day) is the most accurate clinical indicator of resolution. Fetal prognosis is dependent largely on gestational age at delivery and problems related to prematurity.

42 Diabetes mellitus in pregnancy

MATERNAL COMPLICATIONS OF PREGESTATIONAL DIABETES

- preeclampsia (12%)
- chronic hypertension (10%)
- diabetic ketoacidosis (8%)
- polyhydramnios (18%)
- preterm labour (8%)
- caesarean delivery (20–60%)

- other obstetric emergencies (hypoglycaemia, coma)
- genetic transmission (infants of mothers with type I diabetes have a 4–5% risk of acquiring diabetes; infants of mothers with type II diabetes have a 25–50% risk of diabetes)

FETAL COMPLICATIONS OF PREGESTATIONAL DIABETES

Complications

- Congenital abnormalities
- Spontaneous abortion (↑ 2–3 x)
- Diabetic ketoacidosis (50–90% fetal mortality)
- Intrauterine growth restriction
- Late intrauterine fetal demise
- Fetal macrosomia (with or without birth injury)
- Delayed organ maturation
  - respiratory distress syndrome (RDS)
  - neonatal hypoglycaemia
  - neonatal hypocalcaemia
  - neonatal hypomagnesaemia
  - polycythaemia/hyperviscosity
  - neonatal hyperbilirubinaemia (40%)

- incidence of major anomalies is 5–10% (↑ 2–3 x) compared with controls
- accounts for 50% of all perinatal deaths
- incidence is related to HbA1c (if <8.5%, 3% anomalies; if ≥8.5%, 22% anomalies)

HbA1c (%)

13	330
12	300
11	270
10	240
9	210
8	180
7	150
6	120
5	90
4	60

Average blood glucose (mg/dL)

Congenital anomalies in infants of diabetic mothers

Cardiac
- atrial septal defect
- ventricular septal defect
- coarctation of aorta
- transposition of great vessels

Other
- single umbilical artery

Gastrointestinal
- anorectal atresia
- duodenal atresia
- tracheo-oesophageal fistula

Skeletal and central nervous system
- anencephaly
- caudal regression syndrome (very rare, but highly specific for diabetes mellitus)
- microcephaly
- neural tube defect

Renal
- hydronephrosis
- renal agenesis
- ureteral duplication
- polycystic kidneys

RECOMMENDATIONS FOR ANTEPARTUM MANAGEMENT OF PREGESTATIONAL DIABETES

Strict glucose control using:
- diabetic diet (36 kcal/kg or 15 kcal/lb of ideal body weight + 100 kcal per trimester given as 40–50% carbohydrate, 20% protein, 30–40% fat to avoid protein catabolism)
- insulin (use humulin. Insulin therapy should be individualized, but a common regimen is 0.7–1.0 units/kg/day given 2/3 in AM (60% NPH, 4% regular) and 1/3 in PM (50% NPH, 50% regular))
- goal: fasting blood glucose <95 mg/dL; 1 h postprandial blood glucose <140 mg/dL
- home monitoring of blood sugar 4 x per day

Ophthalmological examination every trimester
Detailed sonographic fetal structural survey at 18–22 weeks' gestation (including fetal echocardiogram)
Consider checking thyroid functions (6% have co-existing thyroid disease), baseline preeclampsia blood tests, 24-hour urinary protein and creatinine clearance
HbA1c (opposite)
Fetal testing (NST, ultrasound for growth) after 32 weeks given risk of intrauterine growth restriction and fetal demise

Extent and duration of action of various types of insulin

Neutral protamine hagadom (NPH) insulin — Regular insulin — Protamine zinc insulin (PZI)

Semilente insulin — Lente insulin — Ultralente insulin

Gestational diabetes

Physiology
Pregnancy is a 'diabetogenic state' with increased insulin resistance and reduced peripheral uptake of glucose (due to placental hormones with anti-insulin activity). In this way, the fetus has a continuous supply of glucose.

Incidence
3–5% of pregnancies.

Maternal complications
- Gestational diabetes poses little risk to the mother. Such women are not at risk of diabetic ketoacidosis (DKA), which is a disease resulting from an absolute deficiency of insulin.
- Care should be taken to avoid iatrogenic hypoglycaemia due to excessive insulin administration.
- Gestational diabetes is a good screening test for insulin resistance; 50% will develop gestational diabetes in a subsequent pregnancy, and 40–60% will develop diabetes later in life.

Fetal complications

Fetuses of women with gestational diabetes are exposed to high concentrations of glucose and, as a result, grow large. Fetal macrosomia (Chapter 48) is associated with an increased risk of caesarean delivery and birth injury (Chapter 59).

Screening

• *Glucose load test* (GLT) is used to screen for gestational diabetes. In the UK, screening is recommended only for high-risk women at approximately 28 weeks, gestation. Risk factors include women with a family history of diabetes, sustained glycosuria, obesity, or a history of gestational diabetes, fetus macrosomia, or unexplained fetal demise. US practice favours screening all pregnant women at 24–28 weeks, and high-risk women at 16–20 weeks and again at 24–28 weeks, if necessary.

• GLT is a non-fasting test, but women should not eat after their 50 g glucose load until a venous blood sample is drawn 1 hour later. A positive test should be followed by a *glucose tolerance test* (GTT). A GLT cut-off of ≥7.8 mmol/L (≥140 mg/dL) will detect 80% of women with gestational diabetes with a false-positive rate of 14–18%; a cut-off of ≥7.2 mmol/L (≥130 mg/dL) will detect 90% with a false-positive rate of 20–25%.

• A definitive diagnosis of gestational diabetes requires a GTT; there is no GLT cut-off that is diagnostic. In the UK, a 2-hour 75-g GTT is used. Fasting glucose >5.5 mmol/L (>100 mg/dL) and 2 hours > 7.9 mmol/L (>140 mg/dL) will confirm the diagnosis. In the US, a GTT involves three days of carbohydrate loading followed by a 100 g glucose load administered after an overnight fast. Venous plasma glucose is measured fasting and at 1, 2, and 3 hours. Gestational diabetes requires two or more abnormal values, defined by the NDDG as ≥105 [≥5.8], ≥190 [≥10.5], ≥165 [≥9.1], and ≥145 mg/dL [≥8.0 mmol/L], respectively.

Antepartum management

• The primary aim is to prevent fetal macrosomia and its complications by maintaining blood glucose at desirable levels (defined as fasting, <95 mg/dL (<5.2 mmol/L); 1 hour postprandial, <140 mg/dL (<7.8 mmol/L); 2 hours postprandial, <120 mg/dL [<6.6 mmol/L]).

• A diabetic diet is recommended for all such women.

• Insulin may be required. If fasting glucose levels are >95 mg/dL (>5.2 mmol/L), insulin therapy can be initiated right away because 'you cannot diet more than fasting'. The use of oral hypoglycemic agents for the treatment of gestational diabetes in pregnancy is controversial.

Intrapartum management

• Caesarean delivery may be appropriate if the estimated fetal weight is excessive because of the risk of birth injury (Chapter 48).

• Since the primary source of anti-insulin hormones is the placenta, no further management is required in the immediate postpartum period.

• All women with gestational diabetes should have a standard (non-pregnant) 75 g GTT 6–8 weeks postpartum, because such women are at increased risk of developing diabetes in later life.

Pregestational diabetes
Pathophysiology

Results from either an absolute deficiency of insulin (type I, insulin-dependent diabetes mellitus (IDDM)) or increased peripheral resistance to insulin (type II, non-insulin-dependent diabetes mellitus (NIDDM)).

Incidence

Less than 1% of women of childbearing age.

Classification

• The age of onset and duration of diabetes (White classification) does not correlate with pregnancy outcome.

• Poor prognostic features include DKA, poor compliance, hypertension, pyelonephritis, and vasculopathy.

Complications

In contrast with gestational diabetes, pregestational diabetes is associated with significant maternal and perinatal mortality and morbidity (*opposite*).

Antepartum management (*opposite*)

• Diabetic women should ideally be seen prior to conception. Pregnancy complications such as fetal congenital anomalies and spontaneous abortion correlate directly with the degree of diabetic control at conception.

• Intense antepartum management can reduce perinatal mortality from 20% to 3–5%.

• Approximately 5% of maternal haemoglobin is glycosylated (bound to glucose), known as haemoglobin A1 (HbA1). HbA1c refers to the 80–85% of HbA1 that is irreversibly glycosylated. Since red blood cells have a life span of 120 days, HbA1c measurements reflect the degree of glycaemic control over the prior 3 months. HbA1c measurements should be checked prior to conception, at first prenatal visit, and every 4–6 weeks throughout pregnancy.

Intrapartum and postpartum management

• If metabolic control is good, spontaneous labour at term can be awaited. Because of the risk of unexplained fetal demise, women with pregestational diabetes should be delivered by 39–40 weeks.

• If the estimated fetal weight is excessive (likely ≥4500 g), elective caesarean may be appropriate to avoid birth injury.

• Women may not eat during labour. As such, intravenous glucose should be administered (5% dextrose at 75–100 mL/h) and blood glucose levels checked every 1–2 hours. Regular insulin should be given by subcutaneous injection or intravenous infusion to maintain blood glucose levels at 100–120 mg/dL (5.5–6.6 mmol/L).

• During the first 48 hours postpartum, women may have a 'honeymoon period' during which their insulin requirement is decreased. Blood glucose levels of 150–200 mg/dL (8.2–11.0 mmol/L) can be tolerated during this period. Once a woman is able to eat, she can be placed back on her regular insulin regimen.

MANAGEMENT OF SPECIFIC CARDIAC LESIONS IN PREGNANCY

Septal defects
- if lesions are small, patients are usually asymptomatic and require no specific treatment.
- large ventricular septal defects (VSD) are associated with aortic insufficiency, congestive cardiac failure, arrhythmias, pulmonary hypertension.
- air filters on all IV lines to prevent paradoxical air embolism

Right-to-left shunts
- due to pulmonary hypertension with shunting of blood away from lungs
- in pregnancy, decreased systemic vascular resistance worsens shunt with increased hypoxia
- management: avoid hypotension, maintain preload, oxygen, air filters on IV lines

Mitral/aortic valve stenosis
- such lesions are particularly dangerous in pregnancy because of the fixed cardiac output and left atrial dilatation (which can result in arrhythmias and/or thrombus formation)
- management: maintain preload, avoid tachycardia. Consider β-blockers for persistent heart rate ≥90–100 bpm. Adequate pain relief in labour to minimize tachycardia
- autotransfusion immediately postpartum can precipitate pulmonary oedema

Mitral valve prolapse
- patients are generally asymptomatic
- treat symptomatic prolapse with β-blocker
- bacterial endocarditis prophylaxis (check echo)

Prophylaxis against bacterial endocarditis
- vaginal delivery is associated with 2–3% risk of bacteraemia. Antibiotic use is controversial. Should be given at caesarean delivery in patients at risk

RA, LA, RV, LV

Prosthetic valves
- risks include embolization, valvular dysfunction, and infection (bacterial endocarditis)
- management: therapeutic anticoagulation for any mechanical valve, antibiotic prophylaxis against endocarditis

Cardiomyopathy
- presents with left ventricular dysfunction and global dilatation
- increased cardiac output in pregnancy may lead to decompensation
- management: avoid hypotension, careful volume replacement, inotropic support to maximize cardiac output if needed

Regimens for endocarditis prophylaxis during labour and delivery

Low risk regimen	Amoxicillin, 3 g p.o. 1 h before procedure or at onset of labour Repeat 1.5 g p.o q.6 h until after delivery
Standard regime	Ampicillin, 2 g i.v. plus gentamicin, 1.5 mg/kg i.v. (do not exceed 80 mg) 30 min before procedure or at onset of labour. Repeat above q.8 h until after delivery
Penicillin-allergic standard regimen	Substitute vancomycin, 1 g i.v. over 1 h q.12 h for ampicillin

DIAGNOSIS OF DEEP VEIN THROMBOSIS

Pregnancy predisposes to thromboembolism

Virchow's triad describes the underlying principles of clot formation

Venous stasis — Vessel wall damage — Hypercoagulable state

CLINICAL FEATURES OF DEEP VEIN THROMBOSIS

History: unilateral swelling and/or pain in the calf or thigh

Examination: may confirm unilateral swelling with or without calf tenderness or a tender 'cord' of thrombus. Homan's sign (ipsilateral calf pain on passive dorsiflexion of the foot) is only 30–40% predictive of DVT

Diagnosis must be confirmed by one or more imaging studies

RADIOLOGICAL STUDIES TO CONFIRM DEEP VEIN THROMBOSIS

Study	Accuracy	Comment
Doppler ultrasound*		Non-invasive, cheap, but poor for the detection of distal thrombosis
Proximal veins	85–95%	
Calf veins	≤50%	
Impedance plethysmography		Non-invasive, cheap, but poor for the detection of distal thrombosis
Proximal veins	90–95%	
Calf veins	<30%	
Venography		Accurate, but invasive with a risk of haemorrhage
Proximal veins	95–99%	
^{125}I fibrinogen		Accurate, contraindicated in pregnancy
Distal to mid-thigh	80–90%	

*also known as lower extremity non-invasive (LENI) test

DIAGNOSIS OF PULMONARY EMBOLISM

Clinical features

History: tachycardia, shortness of breath, tachypnoea, pleuritic chest pain, cough, and/or haemoptysis

Examination: may show cyanosis, pulmonary rales, and/or a friction rub. The most sensitive sign of PE is unexplained tachycardia

Labs: EKG may show right-heart strain (S_1, Q_3, T_3 with right axis deviation). Although useful to evaluate response to treatment, arterial blood gas (ABG) is not useful in the diagnosis of PE. 70% of women with PE will have evidence of DVT on LENI.

Ventilation-perfusion (V/Q) scan
- V/Q scans are interpreted as normal, intermediate, or abnormal with a low, moderate or high probability of PE
- if the perfusion scan is normal, PE can be reliably excluded
- data from the 'prospective investigation of pulmonary embolism diagnosis' (PIOPED) study show that overall abnormal studies are sensitive (96%), but not specific (10%)
- a high-probability scan (one showing mismatched perfusion defects) is highly specific (97%)

Pulmonary angiography
- the most accurate test for PE, but is invasive with a number of potentially serious side-effects (haemorrhage, acute renal failure, pneumothorax)

Assessing need for pulmonary angiography

V/Q scan category	Clinical suspicion		
	High	Intermediate	Low
High	96%	88%	56% *
Intermediate	66% *	28% *	16%
Low	40% *	16%	4%

* pulmonary angiography indicated

Maternal heart disease in pregnancy

Incidence: 1% of pregnancies.

Aetiology
• Congenital lesions account for >50% of heart disease in pregnancy.
• Other common causes include coronary artery disease, hypertension and thyroid dysfunction. Rare causes include myocarditis, cor pulmonale, cardiomyopathy, constrictive pericarditis, and cardiac dysrhymias. Historically, rheumatic fever accounted for 90% of heart disease in pregnancy, but is now rarely seen in industrialized countries.

Prognosis depends on four factors.
(i)   *Cardiac function.* A clinical classification was developed by the New York Heart Association (NYHA) in 1928 (*below*):
(ii) *Clinical conditions* that may further increase cardiac output (multiple gestation, anaemia, thyroid disease).
(iii) *Medications.*
(iv) The specific nature of the *cardiac lesion* (*opposite*).

Management (*opposite*)
• Allow spontaneous labour at term. Scheduled induction is indicated for women requiring invasive cardiac monitoring. • Adequate pain relief (regional analgesia is preferred). • Left lateral positioning with supplemental oxygen. • Maternal pulse oximetry and ECG monitoring. • Fluid intake and output monitoring. • Consider invasive haemodynamic monitoring for women with NYHA class III and IV disease. • Consider elective shortening of the second stage of labour.

Maternal mortality associated with specific heart lesions

Group 1 (mortality <1%)		Atrial septal defect
		Ventricular septal defect
		Patent ductus arteriosus
		Tetralogy of Fallot (surgically corrected)
		Bioprosthetic valve
		Pulmonary/tricuspid valve disease
		Mitral stenosis (NYHA class I and II)
Group 2 (mortality 5–10%)	2A	Aortic stenosis
		Mitral stenosis (NYHA class III & IV)
		Coarctation of aorta (no valvular involvement)
		Tetralogy of Fallot (uncorrected)
		Previous myocardial infarction
	2B	Marfan syndrome with normal aorta
		Mitral stenosis with atrial fibrillation
		Artificial valve
Group 3 (mortality 25–50%)		Pulmonary hypertension
		Coarctation of aorta (with valvular involvement)
		Marfan syndrome with aortic involvement

NYHA clinical classification of maternal heart disease

Class I	Uncompromised	No limitation of normal physical activity
Class II	Slightly compromised	Slight limitation of normal physical activity
Class III	Markedly compromised	Symptoms with normal activity
Class IV	Severely compromised	Symptoms at rest

Thromboembolic disease in pregnancy

Incidence
• The leading obstetric cause of maternal mortality.
• Deep vein thrombosis (DVT) complicates 0.05–0.3% of all pregnancies. It is 3- to 5-fold more common in the puerperium, and 3- to 16-fold more common after caesarean delivery. If untreated, 15–25% of patients with DVT will have a pulmonary embolus (PE) as compared with 4–5% of treated patients.

Aetiology
• Pregnancy is a thrombogenic state. Thromboembolic events are 5-fold more common in pregnancy than in non-pregnant women. Other predisposing factors include trauma (surgery), infection, obesity, and underlying thrombophilia (*below*).

Treatment
• *Unfractionated heparin* is the treatment of choice for acute thromboembolism. It must be given intravenously or subcutaneously to keep the PTT (partial thromboplastin time) at 1.5–2.0 × normal. Heparin does not cross the placenta and, as such, is not teratogenic. Adverse effects include haemorrhage (5–10%), thrombocytopaenia (2%), and osteoporosis (dose-related). In the setting of acute haemorrhage, protamine sulfate can be given to reverse heparin action.
• *Low molecular weight heparin* (LMWH) is replacing unfractionated heparin in non-pregnant women. Although safe, its efficacy in pregnancy is not well validated. Because of its long half-life and resistance to reversal by protamine sulfate, most authorities recommend converting LMWH to unfractionated heparin at 35–36 weeks.
• Treatment should be continued for the duration of pregnancy and for 6–12 weeks postpartum. After delivery, anticoagulation with oral warfarin (which is teratogenic and should therefore be avoided in pregnancy) can be used. Women on warfarin can breast-feed.
• Alternative therapies (fibrinolytic agents, surgical intervention) are best avoided.

Prophylaxis
• Women with prior unexplained DVT have a 5–12% incidence of recurrence in a subsequent pregnancy. In women with a documented thrombophilic disorder (below), antepartum *prophylactic* heparin is indicated (5000–10000 units SQ b.i.d.). PTT will not increase. Anti-factor Xa activity should be 0.1–0.3 U/mL. The management of women with a prior DVT but no thrombophilic disorder is controversial. In the UK, such women are generally given prophylactic anticoagulation in the postpartum period only for at least 6 weeks. US practice favours *prophylactic* anticoagulation throughout pregnancy and postpartum.
• In women with a prior PE, *therapeutic* anticoagulation is indicated throughout pregnancy. Maintain PTT at 60–80 s (2.0–2.5 × control) or anti-factor Xa activity at 0.6–1.0 U/mL. Postpartum anticoagulation is indicated for at least 6 weeks.

Thrombophilic disorders predisposing to thromboembolism in pregnancy

Condition	Is test reliable in pregnancy?
Factor V Leiden deficiency	Yes (genetic test)
Prothrombin gene defect	Yes (genetic test)
Protein C deficiency	No (levels may increase in pregnancy)
Protein S deficiency	No (levels decrease in pregnancy)
Antithrombin III deficiency	No (levels may increase in pregnancy)
Lupus anticoagulant	Yes (test for circulating antibodies)
Anticardiolipin antibodies	Yes (test for circulating antibodies)

44 Thyroid disease in pregnancy

THYROID PHYSIOLOGY

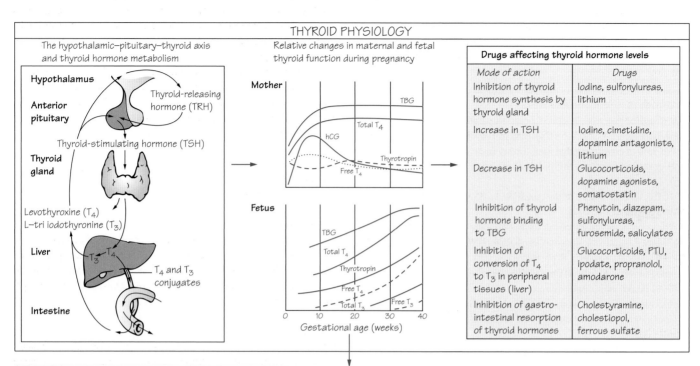

The hypothalamic–pituitary–thyroid axis and thyroid hormone metabolism

Relative changes in maternal and fetal thyroid function during pregnancy

Mother — TBG, Total T$_4$, hCG, Thyrotropin, Free T$_4$

Fetus — TBG, Total T$_4$, Thyrotropin, Free T$_4$, Total T$_3$, Free T$_3$

Gestational age (weeks) 0 10 20 30 40

Drugs affecting thyroid hormone levels	
Mode of action	Drugs
Inhibition of thyroid hormone synthesis by thyroid gland	Iodine, sulfonylureas, lithium
Increase in TSH	Iodine, cimetidine, dopamine antagonists, lithium
Decrease in TSH	Glucocorticoids, dopamine agonists, somatostatin
Inhibition of thyroid hormone binding to TBG	Phenytoin, diazepam, sulfonylureas, furosemide, salicylates
Inhibition of conversion of T$_4$ to T$_3$ in peripheral tissues (liver)	Glucocorticoids, PTU, ipodate, propranolol, amodarone
Inhibition of gastro-intestinal resorption of thyroid hormones	Cholestyramine, cholestiopol, ferrous sulfate

DIAGNOSIS OF MATERNAL THYROID DYSFUNCTION IN PREGNANCY

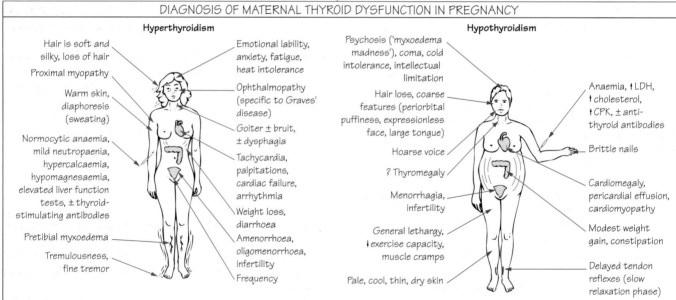

Hyperthyroidism

- Hair is soft and silky, loss of hair
- Proximal myopathy
- Warm skin, diaphoresis (sweating)
- Normocytic anaemia, mild neutropaenia, hypercalcaemia, hypomagnesaemia, elevated liver function tests, ± thyroid-stimulating antibodies
- Pretibial myxoedema
- Tremulousness, fine tremor
- Emotional lability, anxiety, fatigue, heat intolerance
- Ophthalmopathy (specific to Graves' disease)
- Goiter ± bruit, ± dysphagia
- Tachycardia, palpitations, cardiac failure, arrhythmia
- Weight loss, diarrhoea
- Amenorrhoea, oligomenorrhoea, infertility
- Frequency

Hypothyroidism

- Psychosis ('myxoedema madness'), coma, cold intolerance, intellectual limitation
- Hair loss, coarse features (periorbital puffiness, expressionless face, large tongue)
- Hoarse voice
- ? Thyromegaly
- Menorrhagia, infertility
- General lethargy, ↓exercise capacity, muscle cramps
- Pale, cool, thin, dry skin
- Anaemia, ↑LDH, ↑cholesterol, ↑CPK, ± anti-thyroid antibodies
- Brittle nails
- Cardiomegaly, pericardial effusion, cardiomyopathy
- Modest weight gain, constipation
- Delayed tendon reflexes (slow relaxation phase)

SYMPTOMS/SIGNS MAY SUGGEST THYROID DYSFUNCTION, BUT DEFINITIVE DIAGNOSIS REQUIRES THYROID FUNCTION TESTING

Thyroid function test	Units	Normal non-pregnant values (range)	Normal pregnant values (range)		Hyperthyroidism (range)	Hypothyroidism
Thyroid-stimulating hormone (TSH)	mU/L	0.2–4.0	0.8–1.3	No change	Markedly decreased	Markedly decreased
Thyroid-binding globulin (TBG)	mg/L	11–21	23–25	Increased	No change	No change
Total levothyroxine (T$_4$)	μg/dL	3.9–11.6	10.7–11.5	Increased	Increased	Decreased
Free levothyroxine (T$_4$)	ng/dL	0.8–2.0	1.0–1.4	No change	Increased	Decreased
Total L-triiodothyronine (T$_3$)	ng/dL	91–208	205–233	Increased	Markedly increased	Normal to decreased
Free L-triiodothyronine (T$_3$)	pg/dL	190–710	250–330	No change	Increased	Decreased

Thyroid physiology (opposite)

- Circulating levothyroxine (T_4) and L-triiodothyronine (T_3) are bound primarily to thyroxine-binding globulin (TBG) with <1% circulating as free (biologically active) hormone.
- Iodine is required for thyroid hormone production and fetal thyroid function is dependent on iodine from the mother.
- Non-thyroid medical illnesses and select drugs can affect thyroid function.

Thyroid function during pregnancy

- Oestrogen has two effects on thyroid function in pregnancy:
  (i)   it increases circulating TBG concentrations resulting in elevated levels of total T_4 and T_3;
  (ii)   it increases TBG sialylation which reduces hepatic clearance of T_4 and T_3.
  Despite these changes, levels of free T_4 and T_3 remain essentially unchanged.
- <0.1% of thyroid hormone crosses the placenta. As such, tests of fetal thyroid function (although rarely, if ever, indicated) are reliable and independent of maternal thyroid status.
- Thyroid hormone can be measured in fetal blood as early as 12 weeks gestation.

Maternal hyperthyroidism (thyrotoxicosis)
Incidence
0.05–0.2% of pregnancies.

Diagnosis
A definitive diagnosis requires thyroid function testing (opposite).

Aetiology
- *Graves' disease* is the most common cause of maternal hyperthyroidism in pregnancy (95%). It results from the presence of circulating thyroid-stimulating antibodies. Eye signs (ophthalmopathy) are specific to Graves' disease. Since IgG antibodies cross the placenta, the fetus is at risk of thyroid dysfunction.
- *Toxic multinodular goiter* is characterized by hyperthyroidism and the presence of a large, palpable thyroid gland.
- *Hyperemesis gravidarum* is often associated with elevated hCG levels. 50–70% of women will have biochemical studies suggestive of hyperthyroidism, but no symptoms or signs.
- Hyperthyroidism in the setting of *gestational trophoblastic neoplasia* is probably secondary to elevated levels of hCG.
- Metastatic *follicular cell carcinoma* of the thyroid (rare).
- *Exogenous* T_3 or T_3.
- *De Quervain's thyroiditis* (rare) is acute and painful.

Complications
- *Maternal complications*: infertility, recurrent pregnancy loss, cardiac failure (10–20%), thyroid storm (<0.1%).
- *Fetal complications*: preterm delivery, intrauterine growth restriction (IUGR), increased perinatal mortality.

Management
- The goal during pregnancy is to control thyrotoxicosis while avoiding fetal and/or transient neonatal hypothyroidism.
- *Antithyroid drugs* are the treatment of choice during pregnancy. Propylthiouracil (PTU) is preferred because it blocks the release of hormone from the thyroid gland and – unlike carbimazole – blocks peripheral conversion of T_4 to T_3. Carbimazole has also been associated with a rare congenital abnormality (aplasia cutis congenita). PTU treatment is initiated at 100–150 mg t.i.d., but it takes 3–4 weeks before a clinical response is seen. Thyroid-stimulating hormone (TSH) levels should be checked every 4–6 weeks and treatment adjusted accordingly.
- Radioactive iodine to ablate the thyroid gland is absolutely contraindicated in pregnancy.
- Surgery is best avoided during pregnancy but, if indicated for failed medical therapy, is best performed in the second trimester.
- Regular fetal testing is recommended after 32 weeks to look for evidence of fetal thyroid dysfunction. Fetal tachycardia (>160 bpm) is a sensitive index of fetal hyperthyroidism.

Maternal hypothyroidism
Incidence
0.6% of all pregnancies.

Diagnosis (opposite)
- Thyroid function testing is required for a definitive diagnosis.
- Subclinical maternal hypothyroidism during pregnancy may be associated with long-term cognitive deficits in the offspring. However, routine TSH screening of all pregnant women is not as yet recommended.

Aetiology
- *Hashimoto's thyroiditis* (chronic lymphocytic thyroiditis) is characterized by hypothyroidism, a firm goitre, and the presence of circulating antithyroglobulin or antimicrosomal antibodies. In women with existing Hashimoto's disease, pregnancy may result in a transient improvement of symptoms.
- Women *previously treated* for hyperthyroidism may manifest with hypothyroidism and require thyroid hormone replacement.
- *Infectious (suppurative) thyroiditis* is characterized by fever and a painful, swollen thyroid gland.
- *Subacute thyroiditis* is similar to suppurative thyroiditis with a painful, swollen thyroid with or without fever. It is usually the result of a viral infection, and is self-limiting.
- *Iodine deficiency* (rare).

Management
- Early diagnosis is essential to avoid antepartum complications (placental abruption, IUGR, stillbirth) and impaired neonatal and childhood development (cretinism).
- Levothyroxine (thyroxine) treatment should be initiated at 100–150 µg daily. TSH levels should be measured every 4–6 weeks, and the dose adjusted accordingly.
- Women on thyroxine prior to conception should have their TSH levels monitored every 4–6 weeks. Most women will need to increase their dose by 30–50% during pregnancy.

Postpartum thyroiditis
- *Incidence:* 4–10% of all postpartum women.
- *Aetiology:* unknown, but may be an autoimmune phenomenon.
- *Clinical features:* characterized by a transient hyperthyroid state occurring 2–3 months postpartum (with dizziness, fatigue, weight loss, palpitations) or a transient hypothyroid state 4–8 months postpartum (with fatigue, weight gain, and depression).
- *Treatment:* therapy may be indicated to control symptoms, and can usually be tapered within 1 year.

Other medical and surgical conditions in pregnancy

Neurological diseases in pregnancy
Headache
• A common complaint during pregnancy.
• *Causes:* migraine, tension headache, depression. Less common causes include sinusitis, pseudotumour cerebri, cerebrovascular disease, cerebral tumours, temporal arteritis, infection (meningitis, encephalitis), preeclampsia, and 'spinal' headache (seen in up to 30% of women within the first week after spinal analgesia, usually mild and self-limiting).
• The majority of headaches represent benign conditions. Headaches that disturb sleep, are exertional in nature, or are associated with focal neurological findings are suggestive of an underlying structural lesion.

Seizure disorders
• *Incidence:* 0.3–0.6% of pregnancies. The most frequently encountered major neurological condition in pregnancy.
• *Classification:* primary (idiopathic, epilepsy) or secondary (to trauma, infection, tumours, cerebrovascular disease, drug withdrawal, or metabolic disorders). Seizures in pregnancy should be regarded as preeclampsia until proven otherwise.
• *Effect of seizure disorder on pregnancy.* Obstetric complications include an increased risk of hyperemesis gravidarum, preterm delivery, preeclampsia, caesarean delivery, placental abruption, and perinatal mortality. However, the majority of women with seizure disorders will have an uneventful pregnancy.
• *Effect of pregnancy on seizure disorder* is variable. Oestrogen lowers the seizure threshold, while progesterone raises it. Seizure frequency is increased in 45% of pregnant women, reduced in 5%, and unchanged in 50%. If seizures are well controlled prior to pregnancy, there is little risk of deterioration. However, if poorly controlled, an increase in seizure frequency can be expected. Due to a number of factors (delayed gastric emptying, increase in plasma volume, altered protein binding, accelerated hepatic metabolism), the pharmacokinetics of anticonvulsant drugs change during pregnancy.
• *Effects on fetus and neonates.* Women with epilepsy have a 2- to 3-fold increased incidence of fetal anomalies even off treatment. Moreover, anticonvulsant drugs are teratogenic (Chapter 46). The incidence of fetal anomalies increases with the number of anticonvulsant drugs: 3–4% with one, 5–6% with two, 10% with three, and 25% with four. Monotherapy is thus recommended. *Valproic acid* is associated with neural tube defect (NTD) in 1% of cases. Risk is greatest from days 17–30 postconception (days 31–44 from LMP). Folic acid (4 mg daily) may decrease the incidence of NTD. 10–30% of women on *phenytoin* will have infants with one or more of the following features: craniofacial abnormalities (cleft lip, epicanthic folds, hypertelorism), cardiac anomalies, limb defects (hypoplasia of distal phalanges, nail hypoplasia), or IUGR. 'Fetal hydantoin syndrome' is characterized by all of the above features, and is rare. Exposure to other antiepileptic drugs (trimethadione, phenobarbitol, carbamazepine) can produce similar anomalies.
• *Management of seizure disorder during pregnancy.* Discontinuation of medication prior to conception should be considered in women who have been seizure-free for ≤2 years, although 25–40% will have recurrence of their seizures in pregnancy.
• Seizures may cause maternal hypoxemia with resultant fetal injury.

The aim of therapy is to control convulsions with a single agent using the lowest possible dose.
• Labour and delivery is usually uneventful. Benzodiazepines should be used with caution in labour, because they may cause maternal and neonatal depression.
• All anticonvulsant medications cross into breast milk to some degree. The amount of transmission varies with the drug (2% for valproic acid; 30–45% for phenytoin, phenobarbital, and carbamazepine; 90% for ethosuximide). However, the use of such medications is not a contraindication to breast-feeding.

Neurological emergencies in pregnancy
Status epilepticus
• *Definition:* repeated convulsions with no intervals of consciousness.
• A medical emergency for both mother and fetus.
• *Management:* as for non-pregnant women. Maintain maternal vital functions, control convulsions, prevent subsequent seizures. Transient fetal bradycardia is common. Resuscitate the fetus *in utero* before making a decision about delivery. Prolonged seizure activity may be associated with placental abruption.

Disorders of consciousness
• Disorders of *content* (confusion) and *level* of consciousness (coma).
• *Differential diagnosis:* similar to that in non-pregnant women, but also includes eclampsia.
• *Management:* treat underlying aetiology. Supportive care.

Psychiatric disorders in pregnancy
• Psychiatric medications should be continued in pregnancy. In general, the risk of a clinical relapse poses a greater threat to pregnancy than continued medication.
• Guidelines for drug treatment:
  (i) use the lowest effective dose;
  (ii) consider delaying treatment until after the first trimester to minimize the risk of teratogenicity (Chapter 46);
  (iii) avoid sedating agents immediately prior to delivery to minimize neonatal sedation;
  (iv) electroconvulsant therapy (ECT) is generally avoided in pregnancy, but is considered safe for the fetus.

Postpartum depression
• *Incidence:* 8–15% of all postpartum women.
• *Risk factors:* prior depression (30% risk), prior postpartum depression (70–85%).
• Peak onset of symptoms is 2–3 months postpartum, and usually resolves spontaneously within 6–12 months.
• Supportive care and monthly follow-up is necessary.

Postpartum psychosis
• *Incidence:* 1–2 per 1000 live births.
• *Risk factors:* primiparity, personal or family history of mental illness, prior postpartum psychosis (25–30% risk).

- Peak onset of symptoms is 10–14 days postpartum.
- Hospitalization, pharmacological therapy, ECT as needed.

Pulmonary disease in pregnancy
Asthma
- *Incidence:* 1–4% of all pregnancies.
- Pregnancy has a variable effect on asthma (25% improve, 25% worsen, 50% are unchanged). In general, women with mild, well-controlled asthma tolerate pregnancy well. Women with severe asthma are at risk of symptomatic deterioration.
- *Management:* as for non-pregnant women. Hospitalization, steroids, and/or intubation may be required.
- *Complications:* IUGR, stillbirth, maternal death.

Amniotic fluid embolism
- An obstetric emergency with 80–90% maternal mortality.
- *Risk factors:* multiparity, prolonged labour, fetal demise, 'excessive' oxytocin augmentation, placental abruption, caesarean delivery.
- Characterized by acute onset of dyspnoea, hypotension, and hypoxaemia. Therapy is primarily supportive.

Pulmonary oedema
- Classified as cardiogenic or non-cardiogenic.
- *Risk factors:* fluid overload, infection, preeclampsia, tocolytic therapy.
- *Management:* as for non-pregnant women. LMNOP: *l*asix (diuresis), *m*orphine, Na^{2+} and water restriction, *o*xygen, and *p*osition upright. Consider antibiotics.and ionotropic support, if indicated.

Renal disease in pregnancy
Asymptomatic bacteriuria
- *Incidence:* 4–7% of all pregnancies, which is similar to that in non-pregnant women.
- In pregnancy, asymptomatic bacteriuria is more likely to progress to pyelonephritis (20–30%).
- *Escherichia coli* is the most common causative organism.

Chronic renal failure
- *Complications:* infertility (usually due to chronic anovulation), spontaneous abortion, preeclampsia, IUGR, fetal death, and preterm birth.
- Pregnancy outcome is dependent on baseline renal function (below) and presence and severity of hypertension. The degree of proteinuria does not correlate with pregnancy outcome.
- In women with end-stage renal disease, renal transplantation offers the best chance of a successful pregnancy (especially if renal function is stable for 1–2 years and there is no hypertension). Triple-agent immunosuppression (cyclosporin, azathioprine, prednisone) should be continued in pregnancy.

Autoimmune diseases in pregnancy
Systemic lupus erythematosus
- Systemic lupus erythematosus (SLE) does not generally worsen in pregnancy. Pregnancy outcome is related primarily to the severity of underlying renal disease.
- *Complications:* preeclampsia, IUGR, preterm birth.

Immune (idiopathic) thrombocytopaenic purpura
- Immune thrombocytopaenic purpura (ITP) is a maternal disease characterized by the presence of circulating antiplatelet antibodies. It should be distinguished from **alloimmune thrombocytopaenia (ATP)** in which maternal platelet counts are normal, but antiplatelet antibodies (usually anti-PLA1/2) cross the placenta to cause fetal thrombocytopaenia and possibly intraventricular haemorrhage. ATP is analogous to Rh disease of platelets.
- *Differential diagnosis:* pre-eclampsia, coagulopathy, drugs, gestational thrombocytopaenia.
- *Complications:* IgG can cross the placenta and cause fetal thrombocytopaenia. However, the correlation between maternal and fetal platelet counts is poor. Fetal intraventricular haemorrhage in the setting of ITP is rare.
- *Management:* corticosteroids may be necessary if maternal thrombocytopaenia is severe. IVIg, plasmapharesis, and splenectomy are rarely necessary in pregnancy. Caesarean delivery has not been shown to improve perinatal outcome.

Rheumatoid arthritis
- Improves in 75% of pregnancies, but >90% of women will relapse within 6 months of delivery.
- Corticosteroids are safe in pregnancy. Gold salts, cytotoxic agents, penicillamine and antimalarials may have adverse fetal effects, but may be used if indicated.

Maternal anti-Ro and anti-La antibodies
- Associated with complete fetal heart block in 5–10% of cases.

Surgical conditions in pregnancy
- *Incidence:* 2–3 per 1000 pregnancies.
- *Indications:* appendicitis, biliary disease, ovarian disease.
- *Complications:* haemorrhage, anaesthetic complications, infection, preterm delivery. Complications can be minimized if surgery is performed in the second trimester.
- *Technical considerations:*
  (i)   left lateral tilt if ≥20 weeks to improve venous return;
  (ii) continuous fetal monitoring ≥24 weeks' gestation;
  (iii) avoidance of teratogenic agents (Chapter 46);
  (iv) specific anaesthetic considerations (Chapter 60).

Appendicitis
- *Incidence.* The incidence of appendicitis is not increased (1 in 1500 pregnancies), but an infected appendix is more likely to rupture in pregnancy.
- *Diagnosis.* Symptoms and signs are similar to that in non-pregnant women, except that the appendix moves up in pregnancy.
- *Management.* Surgical removal through a right paramedian incision is generally recommended (which can be extended if the appendix cannot be located or if caesarean delivery is indicated).

Pregnancy outcome in women with chronic renal disease			
	Category of chronic renal disease		
	Mild	Moderate	Severe
Serum creatinine (μmol/L)	120–150	150–250	>250
(mg/dL)	<1.4	1.4–2.5	>2.5
Complications	20%	40%	85%
Viable delivery	95%	90%	50%
Long-term sequelae	<5%	25%	55%

UNITED STATES FOOD AND DRUG ADMINISTRATION (FDA) RISK CATEGORIES FOR DRUGS IN PREGNANCY

Category	Definition	Examples
A	Controlled studies in women fail to demonstrate a risk to the fetus and the possibility of fetal harm appears remote	Vitamin C, folate, L-thyroxine
B	Either animal studies have not demonstrated a fetal risk but there are no controlled studies in pregnant women, or animal studies have shown an adverse effect that was not confirmed in controlled studies in women	Hydrochlorothiazide, α-methyldopa, ampicillin
C	Either studies in animals have revealed adverse effects on the fetus and there are no controlled studies in women, or there are no controlled studies in animals or women. Only use if potential benefit justifies risk to fetus	Theophylline, nifedipine, digoxin, β-blockers, verapamil, zidovudine (AZT), acyclovir
D	Positive evidence of human fetal risk, but the benefits from use in pregnant women may be acceptable despite the risk	Cytoxan, spironolactone, ACE inhibitors, methotrexate, phenytoin
X	Positive evidence of animal or human fetal abnormalities, or the risk of the use of the drug in pregnant women clearly outweighs any possible benefit. Contraindicated in women who are or may become pregnant	Aminopterin, isotretinoin (vitamin A), radioisotopes, oral contraceptives

DRUGS NOT CONSIDERED TERATOGENS

- acetaminophen
- acyclovir
- antiemetics (e.g. phenothiazines)
- antihistamines (e.g. doxylamine)
- aspirin
- caffeine
- hairspray
- marijuana
- metronidazole
- minor tranquilizers (e.g. fluoxetine)
- occupational chemical agents
- oral contraceptives
- pesticides
- trimethoprim/sulfamethoxazole
- vaginal spermicides
- zidovudine (AZT)

DRUGS WITH PROVEN BENEFIT IN PREGNANCY

- folic acid (folate)—4 mg/day (10 × RDA) begun 4 weeks prior to conception will reduce the incidence of neural tube defects by 70–80%
- zidovudine (AZT)—decreases vertical transmission of HIV from 25% to 8%
- acyclovir—200 mg p.o. t.i.d. after 36 weeks' gestation to women with frequent recurrent genital herpes infection or first episode primary herpes infection in pregnancy will reduce the need for caesarean delivery for active herpes in labour
- iron supplementation—prevents anaemia
- anaesthetic agents—pain relief in labour

DRUGS WITH PROVEN TERATOGENIC EFFECTS IN HUMANS

Androgens	Virilization of female, advanced genital development in males	Effects are dose dependent. Given before 9 weeks, labio-scrotal fusion can occur. Cliteromegaly can occur any time
Angiotensin-converting enzyme (ACE) inhibitors	Fetal renal tubular dysgenesis, oligohydramnios, neonatal renal failure, lack of cranial ossification, IUGR	Incidence of fetal morbidity ~ 30%, especially with second and third trimester exposure
Anticholinergic drugs	Neonatal meconium ileus	–
Antithyroid drugs	Fetal and neonatal goitre, hypothyroidism	Propylthiouracil (PTU) is preferred over methimazole because of the association with aplasia cutis
Coumarin derivatives (e.g. warfarin)	Warfarin embryopathy (nasal hypoplasia, stippled bone epiphysis, shortened phalanges, optic atrophy, mental retardation, microcephaly), IUGR, developmental delay	15–25% of fetuses exposed to warfarin prior to 9 weeks will have some anomalies, although the embryopathy syndrome only occurs in 5–8% of cases. Later exposure is associated with optic atrophy, developmental delay, placental abruption, fetal haemorrhage
Carbamazepine (tegretol)	Neural tube defects (NTD), microcephaly, IUGR, fetal hydantoin-like syndrome	0.5% risk of NTD
Cyclophosphamide	CNS malformations	–
Folic acid antagonists (aminopterin, methotrexate)	CNS and limb malformations	All cytotoxic drugs are potentially teratogenic. Associated with increased rate of abortion. Of fetuses who survive after first trimester exposure, ~ 30% will have some anomaly
Diethylstilbestrol (DES)	Clear-cell adenocarcinoma of vagina or cervix, abnormalities of cervix and uterus, possibly infertility in males	Vaginal adenosis is seen in 50% of women whose mothers took DES before 9 weeks' gestation. Risk for vaginal adenocarcinoma is low
Lithium	Congenital heart disease (?Ebstein anomaly)	Risk of cardiac anomaly is low. Exposure in last month of gestation may be toxic to thyroid, kidneys, CNS
Phenytoin	IUGR, mental retardation, microcephaly, dysmorphic craniofacial features, cardiac defects, nail and distal phalangeal hypoplasia	The full fetal hydantoin syndrome is seen in <10% of fetuses exposed in the first trimester, but ~ 30% of fetuses will have some manifestations. The effect may depend on whether the fetus inherits a mutant gene for epoxide hydrolase, an enzyme necessary to decrease the teratogenic metabolite phenytoin epoxide
Streptomycin and kanamycin	Hearing loss, eighth-nerve damage	No ototoxicity reported with gentamicin or vancomycin
Tetracycline	Hypoplasia of tooth enamel, permanent yellow-brown discoloration of deciduous teeth, ? weakening of long bones	Effects are limited to exposure in second or third trimester
Thalidomide	Bilateral limb deficiencies, microtia/anotia, cardiac and gastrointestinal anomalies	~ 20% of fetuses have anomalies if exposed between 35 and 50 days of gestation
Trimethadione and paramethadione	Cleft palate, cardiac defects, IUGR, mental retardation, microcephaly, facial dysmorphism	~ 60–80% risk of anomaly or abortion with first trimester exposure
Valproic acid	Minor facial defects, NTD	~ 1% risk of NTD, especially open spina bifida
Vitamin A and its derivatives (e.g. isotretinoin and retinoids)	Increased spontaneous abortion, microtia, CNS defects, mental retardation, craniofacial dysmorphism, cardiac defects, cleft lip and palate, thymic agenesis	Isotretinoin is not stored, but anomalies can occur long after the drug is discontinued. Teratogenic dose >8000 μg/day (RDA = 800 μg/day). The risk of topical retin A is not known

Drugs in pregnancy

Incidence
- 20–25% of women report using medications on a regular basis throughout pregnancy.
- Major congenital anomalies occur in 3–4% of live births and 70% of such anomalies have no known cause. It is estimated that 2–3% are due to medications and 1% to environmental toxins.

Drug trials in pregnancy
- Drug trials are difficult to carry out in pregnancy because of concern over the fetus. As such, many drugs have not been validated for use or safety in human pregnancy.
- Recommendations often rely on data from animal models. The occurrence of thalidomide-associated embryopathy has led to the belief that human teratogenicity cannot be predicted by animal studies. However, every drug that has since been found to be teratogenic in humans has caused similar effects in animals.

Pharmacokinetics during pregnancy
- Pharmacokinetics is the study of how a drug moves through the body.
- Drug *absorption* is altered in pregnancy. Gastric emptying and gastric acid secretion is reduced. Intestinal motility is decreased. Pulmonary tidal volume is increased which may affect the absorption of inhaled drugs.
- The volume of *distribution* changes in pregnancy. Plasma volume rises by 40%, total body water increases 7–8 L, and body fat increases 20–40%. Despite these changes (which would be expected to decrease drug levels), albumin concentrations decline and free fatty acid and lipoprotein values rise. As a result, protein binding of many drugs is lower in pregnancy leading to an increase in circulating free (biologically active) drug levels.
- *Metabolism* and *elimination* are also altered in pregnancy. High steroid hormone levels affect hepatic metabolism and prolong the half-life of some drugs. Glomerular filtration rate rises 50–60% thereby increasing the renal clearance of other drugs.

Teratogenicity
- Teratogenicity is the study of abnormal fetal development, and refers to both structural and functional abnormalities.
- With the exception of large molecules (such as heparin), all drugs given to the mother cross the placenta to some degree.
- The effect of a given drug on a fetus depends on dose, time and duration of exposure, and as yet poorly defined genetic and environmental factors which interact to determine the susceptibility of any individual fetus for structural injury. A fetus is at highest risk for injury during embryogenesis (days 17–54 postconception).
- Paternal exposure has never been shown to be teratogenic.

Risk categories for drugs in pregnancy *(opposite)*
The Food and Drug Administration (FDA) in the USA has defined five risk categories for drug use in pregnancy (A, B, C, D, X). Individual agents are assigned to a risk category according to their risk/benefit ratio (*opposite*). For example, although oral contraceptives are not teratogenic, they are classified as category X because there is no benefit to being on the pill once you are pregnant.

Principles of drug use in pregnancy
- Only use medications if absolutely indicated.
- If possible, avoid initiating therapy during the first trimester.
- Select a safe medication (preferably an older drug with a proven track record in pregnancy).
- Use the lowest effective dose.
- Single agent therapy is preferable.
- Discourage the use of over-the-counter drugs.

Illicit and social drug use

Cocaine
- Cocaine is associated with intrauterine fetal growth restriction (IUGR), cerebral infarction, and placental abruption. Reported congenital anomalies (limb reduction defects, porencephalic cysts, microcephaly, bowel atresias, necrotizing enterocolitis, and long-term behavioural effects) may be secondary to cocaine-induced vasospasm.
- Maternal complications include uterine rupture, hypertension, seizures, and death.

Alcohol
- Fetal alcohol syndrome is characterized by facial abnormalities (midfacial hypoplasia), central nervous system dysfunction (microcephaly, mental retardation), and growth restriction. Renal and cardiac defects may also occur.
- The risk of anomalies is related to the extent of alcohol use: 10% with rare use, 15% with moderate use, and 30–40% with heavy use (>6 drinks per day). There is no absolute safe level of alcohol use in pregnancy.

Marijuana
- No known teratogenic effect.
- Weak association with preterm delivery and IUGR.

Cigarette smoke (nicotine and thiocyanate)
- 20–30% of women continue to smoke during pregnancy.
- Adverse effects include decreased fertility as well as increased spontaneous abortion, preterm birth, perinatal mortality, and low-birth-weight infants (200 g decrease in birth weight for every 10 cigarettes smoked per day).
- Neonatal exposure is associated with sudden infant death syndrome, asthma, respiratory infections, and attention deficit disorder.

Caffeine
- No known teratogenic effect.
- Weak association with spontaneous abortion.

Environmental toxins

Radiation
- Associated with spontaneous abortion, mental retardation, microcephaly, and (possibly) malignancy in later life.
- Fetal exposure of >5–10 Rad is required for any adverse effect (estimated fetal exposure from common radiological procedures is ≤1 mRad).

Heat
- Weak association with spontaneous abortion and neural tube defects.

Electromagnetic field
- No known teratogenic effect.

47 Disorders of amniotic fluid volume

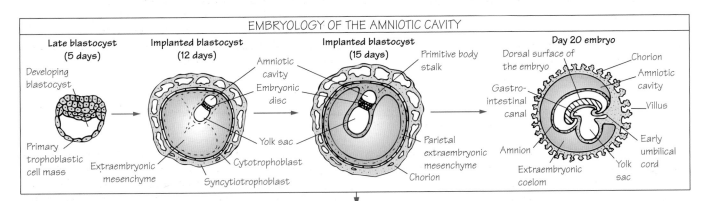

EMBRYOLOGY OF THE AMNIOTIC CAVITY

Late blastocyst (5 days)
- Developing blastocyst
- Primary trophoblastic cell mass

Implanted blastocyst (12 days)
- Amniotic cavity
- Embryonic disc
- Yolk sac
- Cytotrophoblast
- Syncytiotrophoblast
- Extraembryonic mesenchyme

Implanted blastocyst (15 days)
- Primitive body stalk
- Parietal extraembryonic mesenchyme
- Chorion

Day 20 embryo
- Dorsal surface of the embryo
- Gastro-intestinal canal
- Amnion
- Extraembryonic coelom
- Chorion
- Amniotic cavity
- Villus
- Early umbilical cord
- Yolk sac

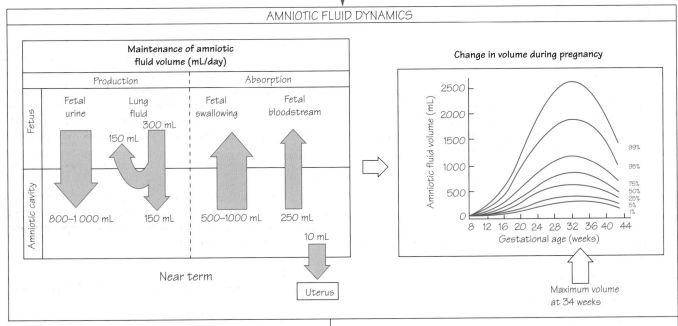

AMNIOTIC FLUID DYNAMICS

Maintenance of amniotic fluid volume (mL/day)

Near term

	Production		Absorption	
Fetus	Fetal urine	Lung fluid 300 mL	Fetal swallowing	Fetal bloodstream
Amniotic cavity	800–1 000 mL	150 mL / 150 mL	500–1000 mL	250 mL

10 mL → Uterus

Change in volume during pregnancy

(graph: Amniotic fluid volume (mL) vs Gestational age (weeks), 8–44 weeks; percentile curves 99%, 95%, 75%, 50%, 25%, 5%, 1%)

Maximum volume at 34 weeks

CAUSES OF OLIGOHYDRAMNIOS (LOW FLUID)

Increased absorption or loss of fluid

1 Premature rupture of membranes (PROM) accounts for 50% of cases of oligohydramnios. Perinatal outcome is dependent upon gestational age at which rupture occurs and severity of oligohydramnios

Decreased production of amniotic fluid

2 Congenital renal anomalies (renal agenesis, renal dysplasia) and exposure to ACE inhibitors will diminish fetal renal output. Bladder outlet or urethral obstruction will similarly decrease urine output

3 Uteroplacental insufficiency (caused by placental abruption, preeclampsia, postmaturity syndrome) will decrease renal perfusion and thus fetal urine output

4 Other causes include congenital infection, fetal cardiac defects, neural tube defects, twin–twin transfusion syndrome, non-steroidal anti-inflammatory drugs

CAUSES OF POLYHYDRAMNIOS (EXCESS FLUID)

1 Idiopathic (no known causes) accounts for 50–60% of cases

2 Maternal causes include isoimmunization (leading to immune hydrops fetalis) and diabetes mellitus (volume of amniotic fluid is dependent on degree of glycaemic control)

3 Fetal causes (10–15%) include non-immune hydrops fetalis (due, for example, to cardiac defect), multifetal gestation (with or without twin–twin transfusion), structural anomalies (gastrointestinal tract obstruction, cystic adenomatoid lung deformity), fetal diabetes insipidis, and defects of fetal swallowing (achalasia, oesophageal obstruction, trache-oesophageal fistula, or central nervous system abnormalities)

4 Placental causes (rare) including placental chorioangioma

Embryology of the amniotic cavity (opposite)

The *amnion* is a thin fetal membrane that begins to form on the 8th post-conceptional day as a small sac covering the dorsal surface of the embryonic disc. The amnion gradually encircles the growing embryo. *Amniotic fluid* fills the amniotic cavity.

Amniotic fluid dynamics (opposite)

Maintenance of amniotic fluid volume is a dynamic process that reflects a balance between fluid production and absorption.

Fluid production

• Prior to 8 weeks, amniotic fluid is produced by passage of fluid across the amnion and fetal skin (transudation).
• At 8 weeks, the fetus begins to urinate into the amniotic cavity. Fetal urine quickly becomes the primary source of amniotic fluid production. Near term, 800–1000 mL of fetal urine is produced each day.
• The fetal lungs produce some fluid (300 mL per day at term), but much of it is swallowed before entering the amniotic space.

Fluid absorption

• Prior to 8 weeks' gestation, transudative amniotic fluid is passively reabsorbed.
• At 8 weeks' gestation, the fetus begins to *swallow*. Fetal swallowing quickly becomes the primary source of amniotic fluid absorption. Near term, 500–1000 mL of fluid are absorbed each day by fetal swallowing.
• A lesser amount of amniotic fluid is absorbed through the fetal membranes and enters the fetal bloodstream. Near term, 250 mL of amniotic fluid is absorbed by this route every day.
• Small quantities of amniotic fluid cross the amnion and enter the maternal bloodstream (10 mL per day near term).

Changes in volume during pregnancy (opposite)

Amniotic fluid volume is maximal at 34 weeks (750–800 mL) and decreases thereafter to 600 mL at 40 weeks. The amount of fluid continues to decrease beyond 40 weeks.

The role of amniotic fluid

Amniotic fluid has a number of critical functions:
(i)   cushioning the fetus from external trauma;
(ii) protecting the umbilical cord from compression;
(iii) allowing unrestricted fetal movement, thereby promoting the development of the fetal musculoskeletal system;
(iv) contributing to fetal pulmonary development;
(v)   lubricating the fetal skin;
(vi) preventing maternal chorioamnionitis and fetal infection through its bacteriostatic properties;
(vii) assisting in fetal temperature control.

Measurement of amniotic fluid volume

Ultrasonography is a more accurate method of estimating amniotic fluid than measurement of fundal height. Several techniques are described:
(i)   subjective assessment of amniotic fluid volume;
(ii) measurement of the single deepest pocket (free of umbilical cord);
(iii) amniotic fluid index (AFI) is a semiquantitative method for estimating amniotic fluid volume which minimizes inter- and intra-observer error. AFI refers to the sum of the maximum vertical pocket of amniotic fluid (in cm) in each of the four quadrants of the uterus. Normal AFI beyond 20 weeks' gestation ranges from 5 to 20 cm.

Clinical importance of amniotic fluid volume

• Amniotic fluid volume is a marker of *fetal well-being*.
• Normal amniotic fluid volume suggests that uteroplacental perfusion is adequate. Abnormal amount of amniotic fluid volume is associated with an unfavourable perinatal outcome.

Oligohydramnios

• *Definition:* an abnormally small amount of amniotic fluid around the fetus.
• *Incidence:* 5–8% of all pregnancies.
• *Diagnosis.* Oligohydramnios should be suspected if the fundal height is significantly less than expected for gestational age. It is defined sonographically as a total amniotic fluid volume <300 mL, the absence of a single 2 cm vertical pocket, or an AFI <5 cm at term or <5th percentile for gestational age.
• *Causes:* (opposite).
• *Management.* Antepartum treatment options are limited, unless a structural defect (such as posterior urethral valve in a male infant) is amenable to *in utero* surgical repair. The timing of delivery depends on gestational age, aetiology, and fetal well-being. During labour, infusion of crystalloid solution into the amniotic cavity (*amnioinfusion*) may improve abnormal fetal heart rate patterns, decrease caesarean delivery rate, and (possibly) minimize the risk of neonatal meconium aspiration syndrome.
• *Outcome.* Oligohydramnios is associated with increased perinatal morbidity and mortality at any gestational age.
• *Complications.* Amniotic band syndrome (adhesions between the amnion and fetus causing serious deformities, including limb amputation) or musculoskeletal deformities due to uterine compression (such as clubfoot) may develop in some cases.

Polyhydramnios

• *Definition:* an abnormally large amount of amniotic fluid surrounding the fetus.
• *Incidence:* 0.5–1.5% of all pregnancies.
• *Diagnosis.* Polyhydramnios should be suspected if the fundal height is significantly more than expected for gestational age. It is defined sonographically as a total amniotic fluid volume >2 L, a single vertical pocket ≥10 cm, or an AFI >20 cm at term or >95th percentile for gestational age.
• *Causes:* (opposite).
• *Management.* Antepartum treatment options are limited. Non-steroidal anti-inflammatory drugs (indomethacin) can decrease fetal urine production, but may cause premature closure of the fetal ductus arteriosus. Removal of fluid by amniocentesis is only transiently effective. During labour, controlled amniotomy may reduce the incidence of complications resulting from rapid decompression (placental abruption, cord prolapse).
• *Outcome.* Polyhydramnios has been associated with increased maternal morbidity as well as perinatal morbidity and mortality.
• *Complications.* Uterine overdistension may result in maternal dyspnea or refractory oedema of the lower extremities and vulva. During labour, polyhydramnios can result in fetal malpresentation, dysfunctional labour, and/or postpartum haemorrhage.

Disorders of fetal growth

CAUSES OF INTRAUTERINE GROWTH RESTRICTION (IUGR)

Fetal causes
Genetic factors (5–15%)
- fetal chromosomal anomalies (2–5%) including trisomies (18 >13 >21) and sex chromosome abnormalities. Most chromosomally abnormal IUGR fetuses have associated structural abnormalities, but 2% do not.
- single gene defects (3–10%) such as phenylketonuria, dwarfism
- confined placental mosaicism (rare)

Fetal structural anomalies (1–2%)
- cardiovascular anomalies
- bilateral renal agenesis

Multiple pregnancy (2–3%)
- risk of IUGR increases with fetal number
- worse in poly/oligo sequence (twin–twin transfusion syndrome)

Uteroplacental causes
Uteroplacental insufficiency (25–30%)
- chronic hypertension, preeclampsia
- antiphospholipid antibody syndrome (25% of chromosomally and structurally normal IUGR fetuses have LAC or ACA positive mothers)
- unexplained chronic proteinuria (23% risk of IUGR)
- chronic placental abruption

Velamentous insertion of umbilical cord

Maternal causes
Drug and/or toxin exposure
- illicit drugs (cocaine)
- heavy cigarette smoking (effect is most pronounced in older mothers)

Malnutrition (especially gestational malnutrition superimposed on poor prepregnancy nutritional status)

Maternal medical conditions
- poorly controlled hyperthyroidism
- haemoglobinopathies
- chronic pulmonary disease
- cyanotic heart disease
- anaemia

Infections (5–10%)
- malaria (the **single greatest cause** of IUGR worldwide)
- rubella
- cytomegalovirus
- ? varicella

RISK FACTORS FOR IUGR
- hypertension (both chronic and pregnancy-induced hypertension)
- multifetal pregnancies
- prior IUGR infant
- poor maternal weight gain
- severe maternal anaemia
- antiphospholipid antibody syndrome
- diabetes with vascular disease
- maternal drug/cigarette abuse
- discrepancy between fundal height measurement and gestational age >3–4 cm

Note: maternal risk factors identify only 50% of cases of IUGR

DIAGNOSIS OF IUGR
- suspect the diagnosis in patients at high risk
- clinical examination will fail to identify >50% of IUGR fetuses
- confirm the diagnosis by ultrasound:
  (i) estimated fetal weight <3rd percentile (2 standard deviations from the mean) for gestational age
  OR
  (ii) estimated fetal weight <10th percentile for gestational age with evidence of fetal compromise (oligohydramnios, abnormal umbilical artery Doppler blood flow)
- serial ultrasound examinations are more useful than a single scan to confirm the diagnosis of IUGR, to follow fetal growth, and to detect oligohydramnios or umbilical Doppler abnormalities

MANAGEMENT OF IUGR
1. Attempt to determine aetiology (ultrasound for fetal anomalies, check karyotype, exclude infectious aetiology)
2. Regular (usually twice weekly) fetal testing
3. Consider delivery once a favourable gestational age is reached (>34 weeks), once fetal lung maturity is documented, or for worsening fetal testing (deterioration in biophysical profile, the development of reversed end-diastolic flow on umbilical Doppler velocimetry)
4. 50–80% of IUGR fetuses will develop fetal distress in labour requiring caesarean delivery
5. Send placenta/fetal membranes to pathology after delivery to look for evidence of vasculopathy

PATHOPHYSIOLOGY OF UTEROPLACENTAL IUGR

Compromise in uteroplacental blood flow
↓
Decreased nutrients (glucose, oxygen, amino acids, ? growth factors) to fetus
↓
Fetal growth begins to diminish in a fixed sequence (subcutaneous tissue → axial skeleton → vital organs such as brain, heart, liver, kidney)
↓
Nutrient, oxygen and energy demands of the growing fetoplacental unit begin to exceed supply leading to hypoxia, acidosis, and death

Changes in antepartum fetal testing reflect the pathophysiological changes (in sequence):
1. Umbilical systolic/diastolic ratio increases as placental vascular resistance increases
2. Fetal growth on ultrasound slows or stops
3. Oligohydramnios develops due to diminished perfusion of fetal kidneys
4. Loss of fetal heart rate variability + decelerations
5. Fetus dies

Definitions
- *Low birth weight* (LBW) refers to infants with an absolute birth weight <2500 g regardless of gestational age.
- *Small-for-gestational-age* (SGA) fetuses are <10th percentile for gestational age. Fetuses >90th percentile are termed *large for gestational age* (LGA). Fetuses between the 10th and 90th percentile are referred to as *appropriate for gestational age* (AGA). Correct assignment of fetal weight category is dependent on accurate dating of the pregnancy since birth weight is a function of both gestational age and rate of fetal growth.

Intrauterine growth restriction
(opposite)
- *Definition*. Intrauterine growth restriction (IUGR) refers to any fetus that fails to reach its full growth potential.
- *Incidence:* 4–8% of fetuses are diagnosed with IUGR.
- *Classification*. IUGR can be classified as *symmetric* (in which the fetus is proportionally small suggesting long-term compromise) or *asymmetric* (in which the fetal head is proportionally larger than the body suggesting short-term compromise with 'sparing' of the brain). This distinction, however, is of little clinical value.
- *Causes*. IUGR represents the clinical end-point of many different fetal, uteroplacental and maternal conditions. An attempt should be made to determine the cause prior to delivery in order to provide counselling, perform ultrasonographic evaluation for fetal growth and delineation of anatomy, and to obtain neonatal consultation. Frequently, the cause is readily apparent.
- *Risk factors*. Numerous preexisting and acquired conditions predispose the fetus to IUGR.
- *Diagnosis*. The clinical diagnosis of IUGR is unreliable, but a fundal height measurement significantly less than expected (3–4 cm) for gestational age may suggest the diagnosis. IUGR is confirmed by sonographic measurements.
- *Pathophysiology*. IUGR most commonly results from compromise of uteroplacental blood flow.
- *Prevention*. Bed rest and low-dose aspirin have been used in an attempt to prevent IUGR in women at high risk with variable results.
- *Management*. Principles of management include:
  (i)   the identification of women at high risk for IUGR;
  (ii) early antepartum diagnosis;
  (iii) determination of aetiology;
  (iv) regular (usually weekly) fetal testing with CTG (NST) (Chapter 49);
  (v) appropriate timing of delivery.
- *Complications*. IUGR infants have higher rates of perinatal morbidity and mortality at any given gestational age, but have a better prognosis than infants with the same birth weight delivered at earlier gestational ages. Unfortunately, neonatal morbidity (meconium aspiration syndrome, hypoglycaemia, polycythaemia, pulmonary haemorrhage) will be present in 50% of IUGR neonates. Long-term studies show a 38-fold increase in the incidence of cerebral dysfunction (ranging from minor learning disabilities to cerebral palsy) in term IUGR infants and more if the infant was born preterm.

Fetal macrosomia
- *Definition*. Fetal macrosomia is defined as an estimated weight (not birth weight) of ≥4500 g.
- *Incidence*. In developing countries, 5% of infants weigh >4000 g at delivery and 0.5% weigh >4500 g.
- *Risk factors*. Although a number of factors have been associated with macrosomia, most women with risk factors have normal weight babies.
  (i)   *Maternal diabetes* (35–40% of all macrosomic infants) is the most common risk factor.
  (ii) *Post-term pregnancy* (10–20%) is another common risk factor. Of all infants born at or beyond 42 weeks, 2.5% weigh >4500 g.
  (iii) *Maternal obesity* (10–20%), defined as a pre-pregnancy weight >90 kg, predisposes to fetal macrosomia. Moreover, clinical and ultrasound estimates of fetal weight in obese women are more difficult.
  (iv) *Other risk factors* include multiparity, a prior macrosomic infant, a male infant, increased maternal height, advanced maternal age, and Beckwith–Wiederman syndrome (pancreatic islet cell hyperplasia).
- *Diagnosis*. Clinical estimates of fetal weight based on Leopold's manouevres or fundal height measurements are often unreliable. Ultrasound is generally used to estimate fetal weight (Chapter 38). However, currently available ultrasonographic techniques are accurate only to within 15–20% of actual fetal weight.
- *Prevention*. Meticulous control of maternal diabetes throughout pregnancy reduces the incidence of fetal macrosomia.
- *Management*.
  (i)   *Antepartum:* women at high risk for having a macrosomic infant or who have a known LGA fetus should be followed with serial ultrasound examinations at 3–4 weeks to chart fetal growth.
  (ii) *Induction of labour*. Because of the association between macrosomia and both birth trauma and caesarean delivery, early induction of labour is often recommended with a view to maximizing the probability of a vaginal delivery. However, induction of labour for 'impending macrosomia' does not decrease the caesarean rate. As such, this approach should not be encouraged.
  (iii) To prevent birth trauma, *elective (prophylactic) caesarean delivery* should be offered to diabetic women with an estimated fetal weight >4500 g and non-diabetic women with estimated fetal weight >5000 g.
  (iv) *Vaginal delivery* of a macrosomic infant should take place in a controlled fashion, with immediate access to anaesthesia staff and a neonatal resuscitation team. It is prudent to avoid assisted vaginal delivery in this setting.
- *Fetal morbidity and mortality*. Macrosomic fetuses have an increased risk of intrauterine and neonatal death (Chapter 51) and birth trauma, especially shoulder dystocia and brachial plexus palsy (Chapter 59). Other neonatal complications include hypoglycaemia, polycythaemia, hypocalcaemia, and jaundice.
- *Maternal morbidity*. The increased maternal morbidity associated with the birth of a macrosomic infant is due primarily to a higher incidence of caesarean delivery. Other maternal complications include postpartum haemorrhage, perineal trauma, and puerperal infection.

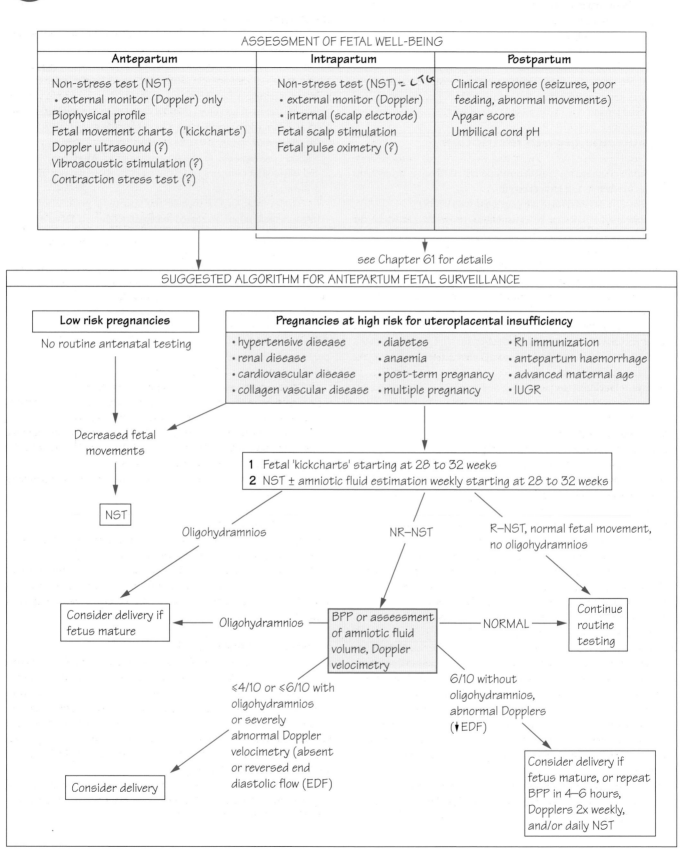

ASSESSMENT OF FETAL WELL-BEING

Antepartum	Intrapartum	Postpartum
Non-stress test (NST) • external monitor (Doppler) only Biophysical profile Fetal movement charts ('kickcharts') Doppler ultrasound (?) Vibroacoustic stimulation (?) Contraction stress test (?)	Non-stress test (NST) = CTG • external monitor (Doppler) • internal (scalp electrode) Fetal scalp stimulation Fetal pulse oximetry (?)	Clinical response (seizures, poor feeding, abnormal movements) Apgar score Umbilical cord pH

see Chapter 61 for details

SUGGESTED ALGORITHM FOR ANTEPARTUM FETAL SURVEILLANCE

Low risk pregnancies

No routine antenatal testing

Pregnancies at high risk for uteroplacental insufficiency

- hypertensive disease
- renal disease
- cardiovascular disease
- collagen vascular disease
- diabetes
- anaemia
- post-term pregnancy
- multiple pregnancy
- Rh immunization
- antepartum haemorrhage
- advanced maternal age
- IUGR

Decreased fetal movements

NST

1 Fetal 'kickcharts' starting at 28 to 32 weeks
2 NST ± amniotic fluid estimation weekly starting at 28 to 32 weeks

Oligohydramnios

NR–NST

R–NST, normal fetal movement, no oligohydramnios

Consider delivery if fetus mature ← Oligohydramnios — BPP or assessment of amniotic fluid volume, Doppler velocimetry — NORMAL → Continue routine testing

≤4/10 or ≤6/10 with oligohydramnios or severely abnormal Doppler velocimetry (absent or reversed end diastolic flow (EDF)

Consider delivery

6/10 without oligohydramnios, abnormal Dopplers (↓EDF)

Consider delivery if fetus mature, or repeat BPP in 4–6 hours, Dopplers 2x weekly, and/or daily NST

Introduction

- Obstetric care-providers have two patients: the mother and fetus. Assessment of maternal well-being is relatively easy, but fetal well-being is far more difficult to assess. Several tests have been developed to confirm fetal well-being prior to labour and delivery (*opposite*).

Goal

- There are many causes of irreversible neonatal cerebral injury, including congenital abnormalities, intracerebral haemorrhage, hypoxia, infection, drugs, trauma, hypotension, and metabolic derangements (hypoglycaemia, thyroid dysfunction).
- Antenatal fetal testing cannot predict or reliably detect all of these causes. The goal of antepartum fetal surveillance (*opposite*) is early identification of a fetus at risk for preventable morbidity or mortality due specifically to uteroplacental insufficiency.
- Antenatal fetal tests make the following assumptions:
  (i) that pregnancies may be complicated by progressive fetal asphyxia which can lead to fetal death or permanent handicap;
  (ii) that current antenatal tests can adequately discriminate between asphyxiated and non-asphyxiated fetuses;
  (iii) that detection of asphyxia at an early stage can lead to an intervention which is capable of reducing the likelihood of an adverse perinatal outcome.

It is not clear whether any of these assumptions are true. At most, 15% of cerebral palsy is due to birth asphyxia.

NOTE: all antepartum fetal tests should be interpreted in light of the gestational age, the presence or absence of congenital anomalies, and underlying clinical risk factors.

Antepartum fetal tests

Non-stress test (NST)

- Also known as cardiotocography (CTG).
- NST refers to changes in the fetal heart rate pattern with time (Chapter 61). It reflects maturity of the fetal autonomic nervous system. NST is non-invasive, simple to perform, readily available, and inexpensive. Interpretation is largely subjective.
- *Is a 'reactive' NST (R-NST) reassuring?* R-NST is defined as an NST with normal baseline heart rate (110–160 bpm), moderate variability, and at least two accelerations in 20 minutes each lasting ≥15 seconds and peaking at ≥15 bpm above baseline (≥10 bpm for ≥10 seconds if <32 weeks). Weekly R-NST after 32 weeks gestation has been shown to decrease perinatal mortality. R-NST is therefore reassuring.
- *Is a non-reactive NST (NR-NST) worrisome?* NR-NST should be interpreted in light of gestational age: 65% of fetuses will have R-NST by 28 weeks; 95% will have R-NST by 32 weeks. Once R-NST has been documented in a given pregnancy, it should remain so throughout delivery. NR-NST at term is associated with poor perinatal outcome in only 20% of cases. The significance of NR-NST depends on the clinical end-point. If the end-point is a 5-min Apgar score <7, NR-NST at term has a sensitivity of 57%, positive predictive value of 13%, negative predictive value of 98% (assuming a prevalence of 4%). If the end-point is permanent cerebral injury, then NR-NST at term has a 99.8% false-positive rate.
- *Is there a place for vibroacoustic stimulation?* Refers to the response of the fetal heart rate to a vibroacoustic stimulus. An acceleration on NST (≥15 bpm for ≥15 seconds) is a positive result. It is a useful adjunct to decrease the time to achieve R-NST and to decrease the proportion of NR-NST at term, thereby precluding the need for further testing.

Biophysical profile

- Biophysical profile (BPP) refers to a sonographic scoring system designed to assess fetal well-being.
- The five variables described in the original BPP were: NST, fetal movement, fetal tone, amniotic fluid volume, and fetal breathing. Two points are awarded if the variable is present or normal; 0 points if absent or abnormal. Amniotic fluid volume is the most important variable. More recently, BPP is interpreted without the NST.
- Recommended management based on the original BPP:

Score	Interpretation	Recommended management
8–10	Normal	No intervention.
6	Suspect asphyxia	Repeat in 4–6 hours. Consider delivery for oligohydramnios.
4	Suspect asphyxia	≥36 weeks or mature pulmonary indices, deliver. <36 weeks, repeat in 4–6 hours vs. delivery with mature pulmonary indices. If persistently ≤4, deliver.
0–2	High suspicion of asphyxia	Evaluate for immediate delivery.

Fetal movement charts ('kickcharts')

- Maternal appreciation of fetal movement is reliable.
- Fetal movement decreases with advancing gestational age, oligohydramnios, smoking, and antenatal corticosteroid therapy.
- 'Kickcharts' involve either counting all fetal movements in 1 hour or counting the time it takes the fetus to kick 10 times ('count-to-ten'). Measurements should be repeated at least twice daily.
- Use of 'kickcharts' in high-risk pregnancies can decrease perinatal mortality 4-fold.

Doppler velocimetry

- Umbilical artery Doppler velocimetry measurements reflect resistance to blood flow from the fetus to the placenta.
- Absent or reversed diastolic flow is associated with poor perinatal outcome in the setting of IUGR, and urgent delivery should be considered. It is unclear how to interpret these data in the setting of a normally grown fetus.

Contraction stress test (CST)

- CST refers to the response of the fetal heart rate to artificially induced uterine contractions. A minimum of three contractions in 10 minutes are required to interpret the test. A negative CST (no decelerations with contractions) is reassuring. A positive CST (severe variable or late decelerations with ≥50% of contractions) is associated with adverse perinatal outcome in 35–40% of cases. However, the false-positive rate exceeds 50%. An equivocal CST should be repeated in 24–72 hours. >80% of repeat tests will be negative.
- Because this test is time consuming, requires skilled nursing care, and may precipitate 'fetal distress' requiring emergent caesarean delivery, it is rarely used in clinical practice.

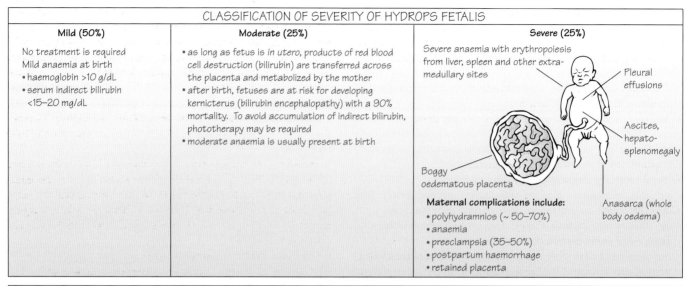

CLASSIFICATION OF SEVERITY OF HYDROPS FETALIS

Mild (50%)	Moderate (25%)	Severe (25%)
No treatment is required Mild anaemia at birth • haemoglobin >10 g/dL • serum indirect bilirubin <15–20 mg/dL	• as long as fetus is *in utero*, products of red blood cell destruction (bilirubin) are transferred across the placenta and metabolized by the mother • after birth, fetuses are at risk for developing kernicterus (bilirubin encephalopathy) with a 90% mortality. To avoid accumulation of indirect bilirubin, phototherapy may be required • moderate anaemia is usually present at birth	Severe anaemia with erythropoiesis from liver, spleen and other extra-medullary sites

Pleural effusions

Ascites, hepato-splenomegaly

Anasarca (whole body oedema)

Boggy oedematous placenta

Maternal complications include:
• polyhydramnios (~ 50–70%)
• anaemia
• preeclampsia (35–50%)
• postpartum haemorrhage
• retained placenta

EVALUATION AND MANAGEMENT OF Rh ISOIMMUNIZATION IN PREGNANCY

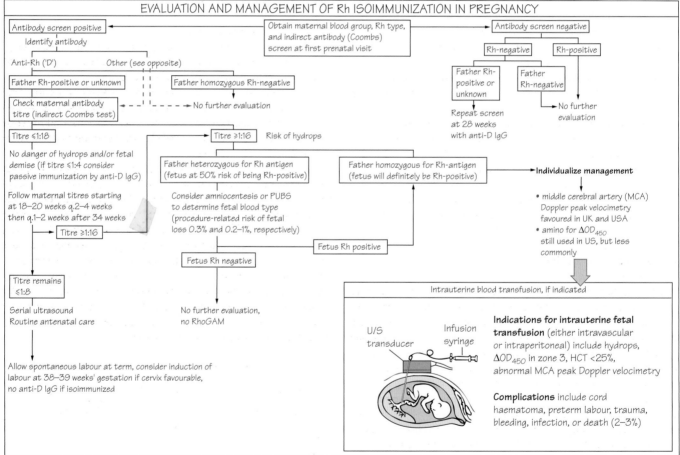

Obtain maternal blood group, Rh type, and indirect antibody (Coombs) screen at first prenatal visit

Antibody screen positive
Identify antibody

Anti-Rh ('D') | Other (see opposite)

Father Rh-positive or unknown | Father homozygous Rh-negative → No further evaluation

Check maternal antibody titre (indirect Coombs test)

Titre ≤1:18
No danger of hydrops and/or fetal demise (if titre ≤1:4 consider passive immunization by anti-D IgG)

Follow maternal titres starting at 18–20 weeks q.2–4 weeks then q.1–2 weeks after 34 weeks

Titre ≥1:16

Titre remains ≤1:8

Serial ultrasound
Routine antenatal care

Allow spontaneous labour at term, consider induction of labour at 38–39 weeks' gestation if cervix favourable, no anti-D IgG if isoimmunized

Titre ≥1:16 Risk of hydrops

Father heterozygous for Rh antigen (fetus at 50% risk of being Rh-positive)

Consider amniocentesis or PUBS to determine fetal blood type (procedure-related risk of fetal loss 0.3% and 0.2–1%, respectively)

Fetus Rh negative

No further evaluation, no RhoGAM

Father homozygous for Rh-antigen (fetus will definitely be Rh-positive)

Fetus Rh positive

Antibody screen negative

Rh-negative | Rh-positive

Father Rh-positive or unknown | Father Rh-negative

Repeat screen at 28 weeks with anti-D IgG

No further evaluation

Individualize management
• middle cerebral artery (MCA) Doppler peak velocimetry favoured in UK and USA
• amino for ΔOD_{450} still used in US, but less commonly

Intrauterine blood transfusion, if indicated

U/S transducer | Infusion syringe

Indications for intrauterine fetal transfusion (either intravascular or intraperitoneal) include hydrops, ΔOD_{450} in zone 3, HCT <25%, abnormal MCA peak Doppler velocimetry

Complications include cord haematoma, preterm labour, trauma, bleeding, infection, or death (2–3%)

Definition
• Latin for 'oedema of the fetus'.
• Refers to an abnormal accumulation of fluid in more than one fetal extravascular compartment.

Incidence
<1% of pregnancies.

Diagnosis
• Hydrops fetalis is a sonographic diagnosis requiring the presence of

an abnormal accumulation of fluid in more than one fetal extravascular compartment, including ascites, pericardial effusion, pleural effusion, subcutaneous oedema, or placental oedema. Polyhydramnios is seen in 50–75% of cases.

- A search for the underlying cause should include:
  (i) a detailed history (for example, of recent maternal infection);
  (ii) serological screening (blood type and antibody screen, antibody screen for toxoplasmosis, rubella, cytomegalovirus, herpes ('TORCH titers'));
  (iii) Kleihauer–Betke test (an acid elution test to estimate the total volume of fetal–maternal haemorrhage);
  (iv) ultrasound survey with or without fetal karyotype.

Prognosis
- Depends on gestational age, severity, and aetiology.
- Overall perinatal mortality rate exceeds 50%.

Classification
Non-immune fetal hydrops (90%)
- *Definition:* hydrops fetalis without an immune aetiology.
- *Incidence:* 1 in 2000 live births. Since the introduction of anti-D immunoglobin G (IgG), non-immune hydrops is the most common cause of hydrops fetalis.
- *Aetiology.* The major causes of non-immune hydrops include:
  (i) idiopathic (no known cause) (50–60%);
  (ii) cardiac abnormalities (20–35%) including congenital dysrhythmias and structural anomalies;
  (iii) chromosomal anomalies (15%) such as Turner syndrome;
  (iv) haematological aberrations (10%) such as α-thalassemia, fetal anaemia;
  (v) other causes (fetal structural anomalies, infection, twin–twin transfusion, vascular malformations, placental anomalies, congenital metabolic disorders).
- *Management:* depends on gestational age, severity, and aetiology. Pregnancy termination is an option prior to fetal viability. Ultrasound may be useful to confirm diagnosis, determine severity (*opposite*), and monitor progression. Moderate or severe hydrops may be an indication for immediate delivery regardless of gestational age.

Immune fetal hydrops (10%)
- Also known as erythroblastosis fetalis or haemolytic disease.
- *Aetiology.* Immune hydrops occurs when fetal erythrocytes express a protein(s) which is not present on maternal erythrocytes. The maternal immune system can become sensitized and produce antibodies against these 'foreign' proteins. IgG antibodies can cross the placenta and destroy fetal erythrocytes, leading to fetal anaemia and high-output cardiac failure. Immune fetal hydrops is associated usually with a fetal haematocrit <15% (normal, 50%). The most antigenic protein on the surface of erythrocytes is D, also known as rhesus (Rh) factor. Other antigens which can cause severe immune hydrops include Kell ('Kell kills'), E, c, and Duffy ('Duffy dies'). Antigens causing less severe hydrops include ABO, e, C, Fy^a, Ce, k, and s. Lewis^{a,b} incompatibility can cause mild anaemia but not hydrops because they are primarily IgM (immunoglobin M) antibodies ('Lewis lives'). 60% of immune hydrops is currently due to ABO incompatibility.

- *Screening.* Blood type and antibody screening is recommended for all women at their first prenatal visit.
- *Rh isoimmunization* (*opposite*). D (Rh) antigen is expressed only on primate erythrocytes. It is evident by 38 days of intrauterine life. Mutation in the D gene on chromosome 1 results in lack of expression of D antigen on circulating erythrocytes. Such individuals are regarded as Rh-negative. This mutation arose first in the Basque region of Spain, and the difference in prevalence of Rh-negative individuals between the races may reflect the amount of Spanish blood in their ancestry (Caucasians, 15%; African-Americans, 8%; African, 4%; Native American, 1%; Asian, ≪1%).
- If the fetus of an Rh-negative woman is itself Rh-negative, Rh sensitization will not occur. However, 60% of Rh-negative women will have an Rh-positive fetus.
- Exposure of Rh-negative women to as little as 0.25 mL of Rh-positive blood may induce an antibody response (*below*). Since the initial immune response is IgM (which does not cross the placenta), the index pregnancy is rarely affected. However, immunization in subsequent pregnancies will trigger an IgG response which will cross the placenta and cause haemolysis.
- *Risk factors* for Rh sensitization include:
  (i) mismatched blood transfusion (95% sensitization rate);
  (ii) ectopic pregnancy (<1%);
  (iii) abortion (3–6%);
  (iv) amniocentesis (1–3%);
  (v) pregnancy (16–18% sensitization rate following normal pregnancy without anti-D IgG, 1.3% with anti-D IgG at delivery, 0.13% with anti-D IgG at delivery and at 28 weeks).
- *Prevention.* Passive immunization with anti-D IgG can destroy fetal erythrocytes before they evoke a maternal immune response. Anti-D IgG should be given within 72 hours of potential exposure. 300 µg (US) or 500 IU (UK) given intramuscularly will cover up to 30 mL fetal whole blood or 15 mL fetal red cells.
- *Management.* Immune-mediated fetal haemolysis results in release of bile pigment into amniotic fluid that can be measured as the change in optical density at wavelength 450 nm (ΔOD_{450}). Traditionally, the degree of haemolysis was measured by serial amniocentesis. Amniotic fluid ΔOD_{450} measurements were plotted against gestational age in an attempt to predict fetal outcome. If the ΔOD_{450} rose into the upper 80% of zone 2 or into zone 3 of the Liley curve, prompt intervention was indicated. More recently, measurements of peak velocity in the middle cerebral artery of the fetus using non-invasive Doppler ultrasound has been shown to accurately identify fetuses with severe anaemia requiring intervention. Depending on gestational age, this may include immediate delivery or fetal blood transfusion.

Transfusion volume	Incidence at delivery	Risk of isoimmunization*
Unmeasurable	50%	Minimal
<0.1 mL	45–50%	3%
>5 mL	1%	20–40%
>30 mL	0.25%	60–80%

* Without anti-D IgG

51 Intrauterine fetal demise

COMPLICATIONS OF INTRAUTERINE FETAL DEMISE

Consumptive coagulopathy

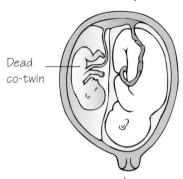

Dead fetus

↓

Transplacental leakage of thromboplastin and thromboplastin-like material into the maternal circulation

↓

Consumption of coagulation factors including factors V, VIII, prothrombin, and platelets

↓

Clinical manifestations of disseminated intravascular coagulopathy (DIC)

Multicystic encephalomalacia

Dead co-twin

↓

Embolization of thromboplastic material from the dead fetus via placental vascular communications to the surviving fetus with or without dramatic haemodynamic changes (hypotension) at the time of fetal demise

↓

Infarction and cellular injury in the brain (known as multicystic encephalomalacia, diagnosis confirmed by echoencephalography), bowel, kidney, lung

IDENTIFICATION OF THE CAUSE OF INTRAUTERINE FETAL DEMISE

Tests which should be sent to help determine the aetiology of the fetal death

Maternal conditions
- random glucose
- maternal complete blood count
- urine toxicology
- thyroid function testing
- Rh antibody status

Placenta/fetal membrane complications
- pathological examination of the placenta, fetal membranes, umbilical cord
- histological examination

Infections
- VDRL or RPR
- CMV titers
- bacterial/viral cultures
- histological examination of placenta/fetal membranes

Antiphospholipid antibody syndrome
- lupus anticoagulant
- anticardiolipin antibody ('positive' high titres IgG)
- other antiphopholipid antibodies (anti-La, anti-Rho, anti-phosphatidylcholine, anti-phosphatidylethanolamine, anti-phosphatidylserine)

Fetal-maternal haemorrhage
- Kleihauer–Betke test (the only test which must be sent immediately after delivery as fetal cells will rapidly disappear from the maternal circulation)

Chromosomal anomalies
- fetal karyotype
- fetal autopsy (including X-rays)

Definition

Intrauterine fetal demise (IUFD) (stillbirth) refers to fetal demise prior to delivery.

Incidence

In developing countries, the stillbirth rate has decreased from 15–16 per 1000 total births in the 1960s to 7–8 per 1000 births in the 1990s.

Risk factors

Include extremes of maternal age, multifetal pregnancy, post-term pregnancy, male fetus, and fetal macrosomia (defined as estimated fetal weight ≥4500 g).

Diagnosis

• *Symptoms.* If fetal demise occurs early in pregnancy, there may be no symptoms aside from cessation of the usual symptoms of pregnancy (nausea, frequency, breast tenderness). Later in pregnancy, fetal demise should be suspected if there is a prolonged period without fetal movement.

• *Signs.* The inability to identify fetal heart tones at a prenatal visit beyond 12 weeks' gestation and/or the absence of uterine growth may suggest the diagnosis.

• *Laboratory tests.* Declining levels of human chorionic gonadotropin (hCG) may aid in the diagnosis early in pregnancy.

• *Radiological studies.* Historically, abdominal X-ray was used to confirm IUFD. The three X-ray findings suggestive of fetal death include overlapping of the fetal skull bones (Spalding sign), an exaggerated curvature of the fetal spine, and gas within the fetus. However, X-rays are no longer used. Ultrasound is now the gold standard to confirm IUFD by documenting the absence of fetal cardiac activity beyond 6 weeks' gestation. Other sonographic findings include scalp oedema and fetal maceration.

Singleton IUFD
Natural history

Latency (the period from fetal demise to delivery) varies depending on the underlying cause and gestational age. The earlier the gestational age, the longer is the latency period. Overall, >90% of women will go into spontaneous labour within 2 weeks of fetal death.

Complications (*opposite*)

About 20–25% of women who retain a dead fetus for longer than 3 weeks will develop *disseminated intravascular coagulopathy* (DIC) due to excessive consumption of clotting factors.

Management

• Every effort should be made to avoid caesarean delivery. As such, expectant management is often recommended. However, many women find the prospect of carrying a dead fetus distressing and want the pregnancy terminated as soon as possible.

• Early pregnancies can be terminated surgically by dilatation and evacuation. After 20 weeks, the safest method of pregnancy termination is induction of labour. Cervical ripening may be necessary.

• Parents should be allowed to grieve for their lost child. Individualization of patient care is important, but parents should be encouraged to hold their child, give him/her a name, and should be involved in the decision regarding disposal of remains.

• Identification of a cause for the fetal demise (*opposite*) may help in the grieving process and in future counselling. An autopsy is the single most useful step in identifying the cause of fetal death.

Aetiology

• 50% of fetal deaths are *idiopathic* (have no known cause).

• *Maternal medical conditions* (hypertension, preeclampsia, diabetes mellitus) are associated with an increased incidence of fetal death. Early detection and appropriate management will reduce the risk of IUFD.

• *Placental complications* (placenta previa, abruption) may cause fetal death. Cord accident is impossible to predict, but is most commonly seen in monochorionic/monoamniotic twin pregnancies prior to 32 weeks' gestation.

• Fetal karyotyping should be considered in all cases of fetal death to identify *chromosomal abnormalities*, particularly in cases with documented fetal structural abnormalities. The success of cytogenetic analysis decreases as latency increases. On occasion, amniocentesis is performed to salvage viable amniocytes for cytogenetic analysis.

• *Fetal–maternal haemorrhage* (transplacental passage of red blood cells from fetus to mother) can cause fetal death. It occurs in all pregnancies, but is usually minimal (<0.1 mL). In rare instances, fetal–maternal haemorrhage may be massive. The Kleihauer–Betke (acid elution) test allows an estimate of the volume of fetal blood in the maternal circulation.

• *Antiphospholipid antibody syndrome.* The diagnosis requires the correct clinical setting (≥3 first trimester or ≥1 second trimester unexplained pregnancy losses, unexplained venous thromboembolic event, and/or autoimmune thrombocytopenia) and one or more confirmatory laboratory tests (*opposite*).

• *Intra-amniotic infection* resulting in fetal death is usually evident on clinical examination. Placental culture and histological examination of the fetus, placenta/fetal membranes, and umbilical cord may be useful.

IUFD of one twin
Prognosis

• The prognosis for the surviving twin following demise of its co-twin is dependent on the cause of death, gestational age, degree of shared fetal circulation (chorionicity), and time interval between death of the first twin and delivery of the second.

• Dizygous twin pregnancies do not share circulation (Chapter 52). As such, death of one twin has little impact on the surviving twin. The dead twin may be resorbed completely or become compressed and incorporated into the membranes (*fetus papyraceus*). DIC in the mother is exceptionally rare.

• Some degree of shared circulation can be demonstrated in 99% of monozygous twin pregnancies. In this setting, death of one fetus often results in immediate death of the other. If, by chance, the second fetus survives, it is at high risk of developing *multicystic encephalomalacia*.

Management

• Management of a surviving co-twin depends on chorionicity and gestational age.

• Fetal well-being (kickcharts, non-stress testing, biophysical profile) should be assessed on a regular basis. In the setting of 'fetal distress'/non-reassuring fetal testing, immediate delivery is indicated.

• Delivery should be considered once pulmonary maturity is documented or a favourable gestational age is reached.

52 Multiple pregnancy

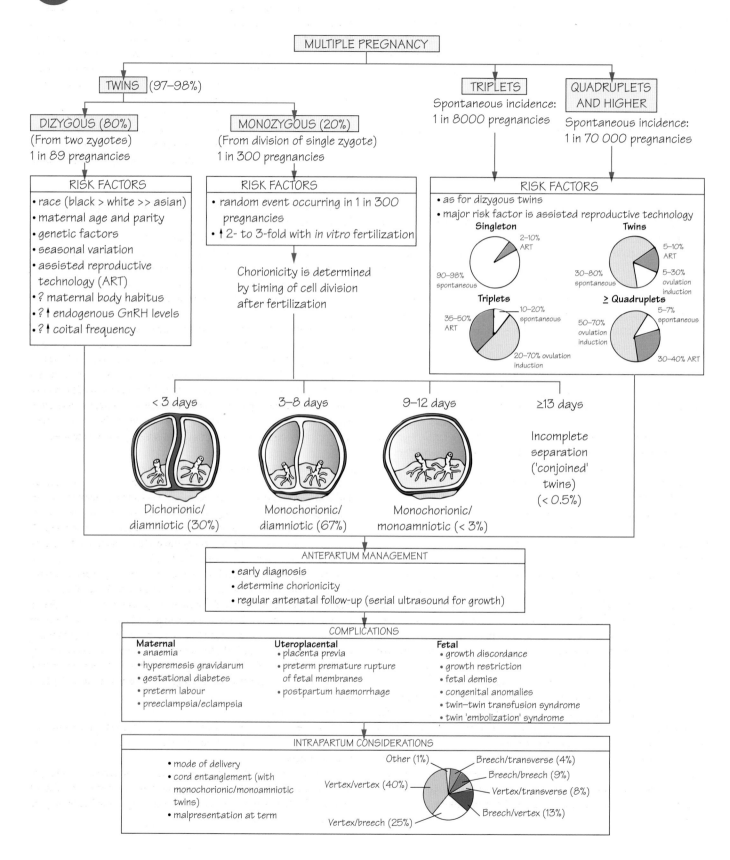

MULTIPLE PREGNANCY

TWINS (97–98%)

TRIPLETS
Spontaneous incidence:
1 in 8000 pregnancies

QUADRUPLETS
AND HIGHER
Spontaneous incidence:
1 in 70 000 pregnancies

DIZYGOUS (80%)
(From two zygotes)
1 in 89 pregnancies

MONOZYGOUS (20%)
(From division of single zygote)
1 in 300 pregnancies

RISK FACTORS
- race (black > white >> asian)
- maternal age and parity
- genetic factors
- seasonal variation
- assisted reproductive technology (ART)
- ? maternal body habitus
- ? ↑ endogenous GnRH levels
- ? ↑ coital frequency

RISK FACTORS
- random event occurring in 1 in 300 pregnancies
- ↑ 2- to 3-fold with *in vitro* fertilization

Chorionicity is determined by timing of cell division after fertilization

RISK FACTORS
- as for dizygous twins
- major risk factor is assisted reproductive technology

Singleton
2–10% ART
90–98% spontaneous

Twins
5–10% ART
5–30% ovulation induction
30–80% spontaneous

Triplets
10–20% spontaneous
35–50% ART
20–70% ovulation induction

≥ Quadruplets
5–7% spontaneous
50–70% ovulation induction
30–40% ART

< 3 days
Dichorionic/ diamniotic (30%)

3–8 days
Monochorionic/ diamniotic (67%)

9–12 days
Monochorionic/ monoamniotic (< 3%)

≥13 days
Incomplete separation ('conjoined' twins) (< 0.5%)

ANTEPARTUM MANAGEMENT
- early diagnosis
- determine chorionicity
- regular antenatal follow-up (serial ultrasound for growth)

COMPLICATIONS

Maternal
- anaemia
- hyperemesis gravidarum
- gestational diabetes
- preterm labour
- preeclampsia/eclampsia

Uteroplacental
- placenta previa
- preterm premature rupture of fetal membranes
- postpartum haemorrhage

Fetal
- growth discordance
- growth restriction
- fetal demise
- congenital anomalies
- twin–twin transfusion syndrome
- twin 'embolization' syndrome

INTRAPARTUM CONSIDERATIONS
- mode of delivery
- cord entanglement (with monochorionic/monoamniotic twins)
- malpresentation at term

Other (1%)
Vertex/vertex (40%)
Vertex/breech (25%)
Breech/transverse (4%)
Breech/breech (9%)
Vertex/transverse (8%)
Breech/vertex (13%)

Incidence

- 1–2% of all deliveries.
- The majority (97–98%) are twins pregnancies. 80% of twin pregnancies are dizygous (derived from two separate embryos).
- Multiple pregnancies are becoming increasingly common, primarily as a result of assisted reproductive technology (ART). This is especially true of higher-order multiple pregnancies (triplets and up) which now constitute 0.1–0.3% of all births.

Diagnosis

- Multiple pregnancy should be suspected in women with risk factors (*opposite*), excessive symptoms of pregnancy, or uterine size greater than expected.
- Ultrasound will confirm the diagnosis.

Chorionicity *(opposite)*

- Chorionicity refers to the arrangement of membranes in multiple pregnancies. It has important prognostic implications.
- Perinatal mortality is higher with monozygous (30–50%) than with dizygous twins (10–20%), and is especially high with monochorionic/monoamniotic twins (65–70%).
- Chorionicity is determined most accurately by examination of the membranes after delivery. Antenatal diagnosis is more difficult. Identification of separate sex fetuses or two separate placentae confirms dichorionic/diamniotic placentation.

Complications

Antepartum complications develop in 80% of multiple pregnancies as compared with 30% of singleton pregnancies.

1 Multiple pregnancies account for 10% of all *perinatal deaths.*

2 *Preterm delivery* increases as fetal number increases: the average length of gestation is 40 weeks in singletons, 37 weeks in twins, 33 weeks in triplets, and 29 weeks in quadruplets.

3 *Preterm premature rupture of membranes* occurs in 10–20% of multiple pregnancies (Chapter 56).

4 *Fetal growth discordance* (defined as a ≥25% difference in estimated fetal weight between fetuses) occurs in 5–15% of twins and 30% of triplets. Perinatal mortality is increased 6-fold.

5 *Intrauterine demise* of one twin (Chapter 51).

6 *Twin polyhydramnios/oligohydramnios sequence* results from an imbalance in blood flow from the 'donor' twin to the 'recipient.' Both twins are at risk for adverse events. Twin–twin transfusion is a subset of polyhydramnios/oligohydramnios sequence seen in 15% of monochorionic pregnancies, and is due to vascular communications between the fetal circulations. Following delivery, a difference in birth weight of ≥20% or a difference in hematocrit of ≥5 g/dL confirms the diagnosis. Prognosis depends on gestational age, severity, and underlying aetiology. Overall perinatal mortality is 40–80%. Treatment options include expectant management, serial amniocentesis, indomethacin (to decrease fetal urine output), laser obliteration of the placental vascular communications, or selective fetal reduction.

7 *'Stuck-twin' syndrome* is an ultrasound diagnosis with severe oligohydramnios of the affected fetus which appears 'vacuum-packed' in its membranes. In 40% of cases, this represents severe polyhydramnios/oligohydramnios sequence. Perinatal mortality is very high.

8 *Twin reversed arterial perfusion (TRAP) sequence* is a rare complication of monozygotic twinning (1 in 35,000 deliveries) in which vascular communications within the umbilical cord or placenta cause blood to flow from one twin retrograde up the umbilical arteries to its co-twin before returning to the placenta. As a result, the co-twin (known as the 'acardiac' twin) develops multiple congenital anomalies, including absent head and trunk regions, absent cardiac structures, and reduction anomalies in other organ systems. Prognosis for the normal twin may be improved if the acardiac twin is removed.

9 *Cord entanglement* is rare (1 in 25,000 births), but may occur in up to 70% of monochorionic/monoamniotic pregnancies and account for >50% of perinatal mortality in this subgroup. As such, delivery is usually by caesarean. The risk of death due to cord entanglement appears to decrease after 32 weeks.

Management issues specific to multiple pregnancy

Selective fetal reduction

- 10–15% of higher-order multiple pregnancies will reduce spontaneously during the first trimester. For those that do not reduce, selective fetal reduction to twins at 13–15 weeks has been recommended.
- The procedure-related loss rate prior to 20 weeks is 15% (range, 5–35%), which is comparable to the background risk for higher-order multiple pregnancies.
- The benefits of selective reduction include increased gestational length, increased birth weight, and reduced prematurity and perinatal mortality. For quadruplet pregnancies and upward, the benefits of selective reduction clearly outweigh the risks. In the absence of fetal anomaly, no clear benefit has been demonstrated for reduction of twins to a singleton. Whether triplet pregnancies benefit from selective reduction to twins, however, remains controversial. Overall, reduction of triplets to twins seems to result in a more satisfactory pregnancy outcome.

Screening for congenital anomalies

- Second trimester maternal serum analyte screening for aneuploidy and/or MS-AFP alone for open neural tube defect is available for twins (not triplets) as it is for singletons at 15–20 weeks' gestation. *First trimester aneuploidy screening* (nuchal translucency + serum PAPP-A and free β-hCG) is rapidly becoming the preferred aneuploidy screening test for multiple pregnancies (Chapter 37).
- In dizygous twin pregnancies, the risk of *aneuploidy* (genetic abnormality) is independent for each fetus. As such, the chance that one or both fetuses has a karyotypic abnormality is greater than for a singleton. US practice favours offering amniocentesis when the probability of aneuploidy is equal to or greater than the procedure-related pregnancy loss rate (quoted as 1 in 270). In singleton pregnancies, this balance is reached at a maternal age at delivery of 35 years. In twin pregnancies, this balance is reached at a maternal age at delivery of around 32 years.

Route of delivery

- Recommended route of delivery of twins depends on presentation (*opposite*), gestational age (or estimated fetal weight), and maternal and fetal well-being.
- Caesarean delivery has traditionally been recommended for multiple pregnancies in which the presenting fetus is not vertex and for all higher-order multiple pregnancies, although vaginal delivery may be appropriate in selected patients.

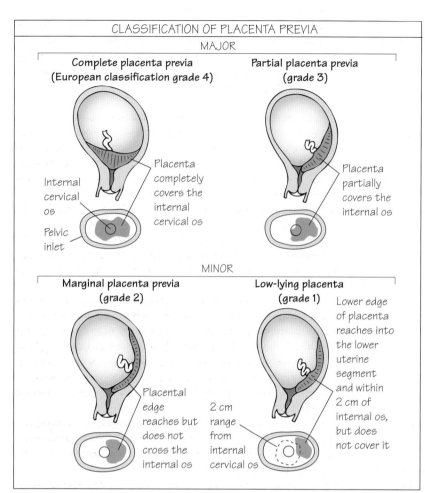

CLASSIFICATION OF PLACENTA PREVIA

MAJOR

Complete placenta previa (European classification grade 4)

Internal cervical os

Pelvic inlet

Placenta completely covers the internal cervical os

Partial placenta previa (grade 3)

Placenta partially covers the internal os

MINOR

Marginal placenta previa (grade 2)

Placental edge reaches but does not cross the internal os

Low-lying placenta (grade 1)

2 cm range from internal cervical os

Lower edge of placenta reaches into the lower uterine segment and within 2 cm of internal os, but does not cover it

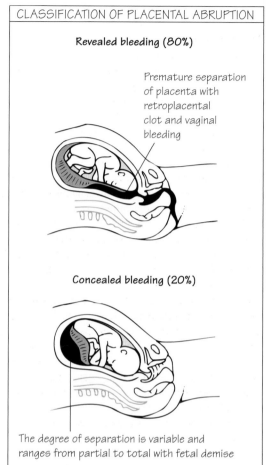

CLASSIFICATION OF PLACENTAL ABRUPTION

Revealed bleeding (80%)

Premature separation of placenta with retroplacental clot and vaginal bleeding

Concealed bleeding (20%)

The degree of separation is variable and ranges from partial to total with fetal demise

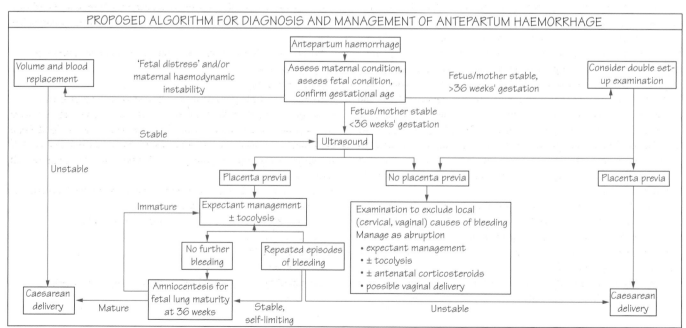

PROPOSED ALGORITHM FOR DIAGNOSIS AND MANAGEMENT OF ANTEPARTUM HAEMORRHAGE

Antepartum haemorrhage

Assess maternal condition, assess fetal condition, confirm gestational age

'Fetal distress' and/or maternal haemodynamic instability

Volume and blood replacement

Fetus/mother stable, >36 weeks' gestation

Consider double set-up examination

Fetus/mother stable <36 weeks' gestation

Stable

Unstable

Ultrasound

Placenta previa

No placenta previa

Placenta previa

Immature

Expectant management ± tocolysis

Examination to exclude local (cervical, vaginal) causes of bleeding
Manage as abruption
• expectant management
• ± tocolysis
• ± antenatal corticosteroids
• possible vaginal delivery

No further bleeding

Repeated episodes of bleeding

Caesarean delivery

Mature

Amniocentesis for fetal lung maturity at 36 weeks

Stable, self-limiting

Unstable

Caesarean delivery

Definition

Vaginal bleeding after 24 weeks' gestation and before labour.

Incidence

4–5% of all pregnancies.

Differential diagnosis

Placenta previa (20%)

• *Definition.* Implantation of the placenta over the cervical os in advance of the fetal presenting part.

• *Incidence:* 1 in 200 pregnancies.

• *Risk factors:* multiparity, advanced maternal age, prior placenta previa, prior caesarean delivery, smoking.

• *Classification* (*opposite*).

• *Diagnosis.* Characterized clinically by painless, bright-red vaginal bleeding. Bleeding is of maternal origin. Fetal malpresentation is common because the placenta prevents engagement of the presenting part. May be an incidental finding on ultrasound.

NOTE: when a woman presents with antepartum haemorrhage, pelvic examination should be avoided until placenta previa is excluded.

• *Ultrasound.* Ultrasound is accurate at diagnosing placenta previa. Only 5% of placenta previa identified by ultrasound in the second trimester persist to term.

• *Antepartum management.* The goal is to maximize fetal maturation while minimizing risk to mother and fetus. 'Fetal distress' and excessive maternal haemorrhage are contraindications to expectant management, and may necessitate immediate caesarean irrespective of gestational age. However, most episodes of bleeding are not life-threatening. With careful monitoring, delivery can be safely delayed in most cases. Outpatient management may be an option for women with a single small bleed if they can comply with restrictions on activity and maintain proximity to a hospital. Placenta previa may resolve with time, thereby permitting vaginal delivery.

• *Intrapartum management.* Elective caesarean delivery is recommended at 36–38 weeks' gestation. Vaginal delivery is rarely appropriate, but may be indicated in the setting of intrauterine fetal demise, fetal malformation(s) incompatible with life, advanced labour with engagement of the fetal head and minimal vaginal bleeding, or an indicated delivery with a previable fetus. A *double set-up examination* in labour may be appropriate when ultrasound cannot exclude placenta previa and the patient is strongly motivated for vaginal delivery. This procedure is performed in the operating room with surgical anaesthesia and two surgical teams. One team is scrubbed and ready for immediate caesarean in the event of haemorrhage or 'fetal distress'. The other team then performs a gentle bimanual examination initially of the vaginal fornices and then the cervical os. If a previa is present, immediate caesarean is indicated. If no placenta is palpated, amniotomy can be performed and labour induced.

• *Maternal complications.* Placenta accreta (abnormal attachment of placental villi to the uterine wall) is rare (1 in 7000 pregnancies), but complicates 5% of pregnancies with placenta previa, 10–25% with placenta previa and one prior caesarean, and >50% with placenta previa and two or more prior caesareans.

• *Neonatal complications:* preterm birth, malpresentation. Placenta previa is not associated with IUGR.

Placental abruption (30%)

• *Definition:* premature separation of the placenta from the uterine sidewall.

• *Incidence:* 1 in 120 pregnancies.

• *Risk factors:* hypertension, prior placental abruption, trauma, smoking, cocaine, uterine anomaly or fibroids, multiparity, advanced maternal age, preterm premature rupture of the membranes, bleeding diathesis, and rapid decompression of an overdistended uterus (multiple pregnancy, polyhydramnios).

• *Classification* (*opposite*).

• *Diagnosis:* presents clinically with vaginal bleeding (80%), uterine contractions (35%), and abdominal tenderness (70%) with or without 'fetal distress' (50%). Uterine tenderness suggests extravasation of blood into the myometrium (Couvelaire uterus). The amount of vaginal bleeding may not be a reliable indicator of the severity of the haemorrhage since bleeding may be concealed. Serial measurements of fundal height and abdominal girth are useful to monitor large retroplacental blood collections.

• *Ultrasound.* A retroplacental collection of ≥300 mL is necessary for sonographic visualization. Only 2% of abruptions can be visualized on ultrasound. Port-wine discoloration of the amniotic fluid is highly suggestive of abruption.

• *Antepartum management.* Hospitalization is indicated to evaluate maternal and fetal condition. Mode and timing of delivery depends on the condition and gestational age of the fetus, condition of the mother and state of the cervix. In the setting of haemodynamic instability, invasive monitoring and immediate caesarean may be necessary. If the abruption is mild and pregnancy is remote from term, expectant management may be appropriate. Placental abruption is a relative contraindication to tocolysis.

• *Maternal complications.* Maternal mortality (due to haemorrhage, cardiac failure, or renal failure) ranges from 0.5 to 5%. Aggressive volume and blood replacement should be initiated. Clinically significant coagulopathy occurs in 10% of cases.

• *Fetal complications.* Fetal demise occurs in 10–35% of cases due to fetal hypoxia, exsanguination, or complications of prematurity. Abruption is also associated with an increased rate of congenital anomalies and IUGR.

• *Recurrence:* 10% after one abruption, 25% after two abruptions.

Vasa previa (rare)

• *Definition:* bleeding from the umbilical vessels (fetal blood).

• *Diagnosis.* Apt test (haemoglobin alkaline elution test) involves the addition of 2–3 drops of an alkaline solution to 1 mL of blood. Fetal erythrocytes are resistant to rupture, and the mixture will remain red. If the blood is maternal, erythrocytes will rupture and the mixture will turn brown.

• *Complications:* bleeding is fetal in origin. As such, fetal mortality is >75% due primarily to fetal exsanguination.

• *Treatment:* emergency caesarean if the fetus is viable.

Other causes (50%)

• Early labour.

• Lesions of the lower genital tract (cervical polyps, erosion).

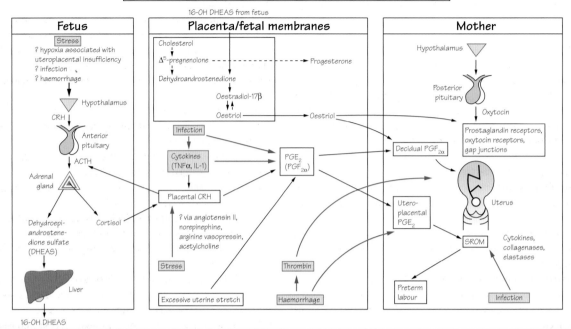

PATHOPHYSIOLOGY OF PRETERM LABOUR

PHARMACOLOGICAL MANAGEMENT OF PRETERM LABOUR

Tocolytic agent	Route of administration (dosage)	Efficacy[†]	Major maternal side-effects	Major fetal side-effects
Calcium channel blockers • nifedipine	Oral (20–30 mg q.4–8 h)	Effective	Hypotension, reflex tachycardia, headache, nausea, flushing, potentiates the cardiac depressive effect of magnesium sulfate, hepatotoxicity	-
β-Adrenergic agonists • terbutaline sulfate	i.v. (2 µg/min infusion, max 80 µg/min) SC (0.25 mg q.20 min) Oral maintenance (2.5–5 mg q.4–6 h) i.v. pump (0.02 mL/h)	Effective Effective Not effective Not effective	Jitteriness, anxiety, restlessness, rash, nausea, vomiting, rash, cardiac dysrythmias, chest pain, myocardial ischemia, palpitations, hypotension, tachycardia, pulmonary oedema, paralytic ileus, hypokalaemia, hyperglycaemia, acidosis	Fetal tachycardia, hypotension, ileus, hyper-insulinaemia, hypoglycaemia, hyperbilirubinaemia, hypocalcaemia, ? hydrops fetalis
• ritodrine hydrochloride	i.v. (50 mg/min infusion, max 350 µg/min i.m. (5–10 mg q.2–4 h) Oral maintenance (10–20 mg q.3–4 h)	Effective Effective Not effective		
Oxytocin antagonists • atosiban	i.v. (1 µM/min infusion, max 32 µM/min)	Effective	Nausea, headache, chest pain, arthralgia	?
Prostaglandin inhibitors • indomethacin	Oral (25–50 mg q.4–6 h) Rectal (100 mg q.12 h)	Effective Effective	Gastrointestinal effects (nausea, heartburn), headache, rash, interstitial nephritis, increased bleeding time	Transient oliguria, oligohydramnios, premature closure of the neonatal ductus arteriosus and persistent pulmonary hypertension, ? necrotizing enterocolitis, intraventricular haemorrhage
Magnesium sulfate	i.v. (4–6 g bolus, 2–3 g/h infusion) Oral maintenance (100–120 mg q.4 h)	Effective Not effective	Nausea, vomiting, ileus, headache, weakness, hypotension, pulmonary oedema, cardio-respiratory arrest, ? hypocalcaemia	Decreased fetal heart rate variability, neonatal drowsiness, hypotonia, ? ileus, ? congenital ricketic syndrome (with treatment >3 weeks)
Othersl • nitroglycerine	TD (10–50 mg q. day) i.v. (100 µg bolus, then 1–10 µg/kg/min)	Unproven Unproven	Hypotension, headache	Fetal tachycardia

† Efficacy is defined as proven benefit in delaying delivery by 24–48 hours as compared with placebo or standard control
i.m., intramuscular; i.v.; intravenous; SC, subcutaneous; TD, transdermal

Definition

Premature (preterm) labour refers to the onset of labour prior to 37 weeks' gestation.

Incidence

• 7–10% of all deliveries
• Accounts for 85% of all perinatal morbidity and mortality.

Pathophysiology

Preterm labour represents either a breakdown in the mechanisms responsible for maintaining uterine quiescence throughout pregnancy or a short-circuiting or overwhelming of the normal parturition cascade which triggers labour prematurely. Four discrete pathways are described, including stress, infection, stretch, and haemorrhage (*opposite*).

Aetiology

• Preterm labour represents a syndrome rather than a diagnosis since the aetiologies are varied.

• Of all preterm births, 20% are iatrogenic (performed for maternal or fetal indications), 30% are associated with infection, 20–25% are associated with preterm premature rupture of membranes (PPROM), and 20–25% result from spontaneous (idiopathic) preterm labour.

Prediction of preterm birth

• *Risk factors* for preterm birth have been identified (below). However, reliance on risk factors alone will fail to identify over 50% of pregnancies that deliver preterm.

• Although an increase in uterine activity is a prerequisite for preterm labour, *home uterine monitoring* has not been shown to decrease the incidence of preterm birth.

• Serial *cervical evaluation* is reassuring if the examination remains normal. However, an abnormal finding (dilatation or effacement) is associated with preterm delivery in only 4% of low-risk and 20% of high-risk women.

• There is a strong inverse correlation between sonographic *cervical length* and preterm delivery, but whether this can be prevented is not clear.

• *Vaginal infections* (bacterial vaginosis, *N. gonorrhoeae*, *C. trachomatis*, *T. vaginalis*) have been associated with preterm birth. However, routine screening and treatment of high-risk asymptomatic women does not appear to decrease this risk.

• *Intra-amniotic infection* is responsible for 30% of preterm labour. A positive amniotic fluid culture is necessary for a definitive diagnosis, but biomarkers of infection (high interleukin-6, low glucose, increase C-reactive protein, and high white cell count in amniotic fluid) may suggest the diagnosis.

• A number of *biochemical markers* have been associated with preterm delivery, but only cervicovaginal fetal fibronectin (fFN) has been established as a screening tool. The value of fFN lies in its negative predictive value: 99% of women with a negative fFN at 22–34 weeks will still be pregnant in 7 days. However, only 25% of women with a positive fFN will deliver prior to 35 weeks.

• A number of *endocrine assays* are also being developed to predict preterm labour. Elevated maternal salivary oestriol (≥2.1 ng/mL) is predictive of preterm delivery in high-risk populations. Other endocrine assays (relaxin, corticotropin-releasing hormone) are being developed.

Management

• A firm *diagnosis* of preterm labour is necessary before treatment is considered. Diagnosis requires the presence of both uterine contractions and cervical change (or an initial cervical examination ≥2 cm and/or ≥80% effacement in a nulliparous patient).

• A *cause* for preterm labour should always be sought.

• *Absolute contraindications* to tocolytic agents (drugs which inhibit uterine contractions) include intrauterine infection, 'fetal distress', vaginal bleeding, and intrauterine fetal demise. PPROM is a relative contraindication.

• Bed rest and hydration are commonly recommended, but without proven efficacy.

• Short-term *pharmacological therapy* (*opposite*) remains the cornerstone of management. However, there is no reliable data to suggest that any tocolytic agent is able to delay delivery for longer than 48 hours. No single agent has a clear therapeutic advantage. As such, the side-effect profile of each of the drugs will often determine which to use in a given clinical setting.

  (i) Calcium channel blockers (such as nifedipine) are effective, have few side-effects, and are rapidly becoming the first-line tocolytic agent of choice.

  (ii) β-Adrenergic agonists are also commonly used, but have a higher incidence of maternal adverse effects.

  (iii) Atosiban (oxytocin receptor antagonist) and nitroglycerine are used in some institutions in the UK.

  (iv) Magnesium sulfate (which acts as a physiological calcium antagonist and a general inhibitor of neurotransmission) has a wide margin of safety and is still commonly used as a first-line tocolytic agent in the US.

  (v) Indomethacin (a non-steroidal, anti-inflammatory drug) is an effective tocolytic agent, but is associated with a number of serious neonatal complications. As such, it is rarely used.

• Maintenance tocolysis beyond 48 hours has not consistently been shown to delay delivery and is associated with significant adverse effects. It is therefore not generally recommended. However, recent meta-analyses suggest that maintenance tocolysis with nifedipine may be beneficial.

• The concurrent use of two or more tocolytic agents has not been shown to be more effective than a single agent alone, and the additive risk of side-effects generally precludes this course of management.

• Recent data suggests that progesterone supplementation (not treatment) from 16–24 weeks through 34–36 weeks may prevent preterm delivery in some women at high-risk by virtue of a prior unexplained preterm birth. This approach is experimental. Studies are underway to better define which women will benefit, which formulation and dose to use, and when to start.

Risk factors	Relative risk
Intra-amniotic infection	50
Multiple gestation	40
Placental abruption	35
Third-trimester vaginal bleeding	10
Second-trimester vaginal bleeding	2
Prior preterm delivery	2–5
Uterine anomalies	5–7
Diethylstilbestrol (DES) exposure	4
Urinary tract infection	2
Smoking (≥10 cigarettes per day)	2
Illicit drug use (especially cocaine)	2
Maternal age >30 years	2–3
African-American race	2
Low socioeconomic status	1.5–2

RISK FACTORS FOR CERVICAL INSUFFICIENCY

Congenital
- congenital cervical hypoplasia
- *in utero* DES exposure

Acquired
- trauma to cervix (conization, amputation, obstetric laceration)
- ? forced cervical dilatation (may occur during elective pregnancy termination)

INDICATIONS FOR CERVICAL CERCLAGE

- history suggestive of cervical insufficiency
- ? higher-order multiple gestations
- ?? cervical shortening on ultrasound (<20mm)

ABSOLUTE CONTRAINDICATIONS TO CERVICAL CERCLAGE

Maternal
- uterine contractions/labour
- life-threatening maternal condition precluding anaesthesia

Uteroplacental
- rupture of fetal membranes
- unexplained vaginal bleeding (abruption)
- intrauterine/vaginal infection

Fetal
- intrauterine fetal demise
- major fetal anomaly not compatible with life
- gestational age ≥28 weeks

Elective (prophylactic) cerclage
- usually performed at 13–16 weeks
- complications rare
- efficacy relatively well established (estimated 25 cerclages needed to salvage one pregnancy)

— OR —

Expectant management
Serial clinical examinations and/or transvaginal ultrasound of the cervix every 1–2 weeks

Emergent (therapeutic) cerclage
i.e. after dilatation/effacement of the cervix
- usually performed at 18–23 weeks
- complications more common
- efficacy unproven

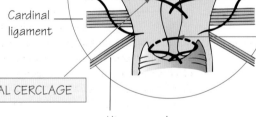
Internal os

Uterine artery

Cardinal ligament

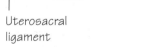

TRANSVAGINAL CERCLAGE

TRANSABDOMINAL CERCLAGE
- no proven benefit over transvaginal cerclage
- requires laparotomy and delivery by caesarean
- indicated only if transvaginal cerclage technically impossible or previously unsuccessful

Uterosacral ligament

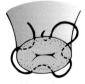
McDonald
- purse-string suture
- no dissection
- at level of external os

Shirodkar
- single suture
- dissection needed
- closer to internal os

Cervical insufficiency (also known as cervical incompetence)

Definition

Refers to an inability to support a pregnancy to term due to a functional defect of the cervix.

Incidence

- 0.05–1% of all pregnancies.

Clinical features

- Cervical insufficiency is characterized by acute, painless dilatation of the cervix usually in the mid-trimester culminating in prolapse and/or preterm premature rupture of the membranes (PPROM) with resultant preterm and often previable delivery.
- Symptoms may include watery vaginal discharge, pelvic pressure, vaginal bleeding, and/or PPROM in the mid-trimester, but most women are asymptomatic.

Diagnosis

- Cervical insufficiency is a clinical diagnosis. It should be suspected when an advanced cervical examination is noted at 16–24 weeks' gestation on pelvic (or sonographic) examination in the absence of uterine contractions. If uterine contractions are present, the diagnosis is more likely to be preterm labour.
- Several tests have been described in an attempt to confirm the diagnosis in non-pregnant women, but are of little clinical value.

Aetiology

- Cervical insufficiency is likely to be the clinical end-point of many pathological processes. In most cases, the precise aetiology is unknown.

Future pregnancies

- The probability of cervical insufficiency recurring in a subsequent pregnancy is 15–30%.
- The chance of carrying a pregnancy to term with a history of two consecutive mid-trimester pregnancy losses is 60–70%.

Cervical cerclage

Indications

- *Elective (prophylactic)* cerclage should be distinguished from emergent (therapeutic) cerclage *(opposite)*.
- A prior history of cervical insufficiency is the only clear indication for prophylactic cerclage.
- Prophylactic cerclage in women with a history of *in utero* diethylstilbestrol (DES) exposure or multiple pregnancy (in the absence of prior pregnancy loss) is controversial.

Contraindications

- *Absolute contraindications* are listed opposite.
- *Relative contraindications* include:
  (i) fetal membranes prolapsing through the cervical os (because of the high incidence of PPROM);
  (ii) elevated marks of inflammation in amniotic fluid (failure rate ≥90%);
  (iii) placenta previa;
  (iv) intrauterine fetal growth restriction;
  (v) ≥24 weeks' gestation (the limit of fetal viability).

Complications

- Complications increase with increasing gestational age and increasing cervical dilatation.
- *Short-term (<48 hours) complications*: excessive blood loss, PPROM, spontaneous pregnancy loss (3–20%).
- *Long-term complications*: cervical lacerations (3–4%), chorioamnionitis (4%), cervical stenosis (1%), other (placental abruption, migration of the suture, bladder discomfort).
- *Puerperal infection* occurs in 6% of patients with cerclage, twice as common as in women with no cerclage.

Types of cerclage

Transvaginal cervical cerclage *(opposite)*

Transvaginal cerclage remains the mainstay for the management of cervical insufficiency. Shirodkar and McDonald cerclage are probably equally efficacious.

1 Shirodkar cerclage is a single suture placed around the cervix at the level of the internal os after surgically reflecting the bladder anteriorly and the rectum posteriorly. The suture is secured either anteriorly or posteriorly, and the mucosal incisions are closed.

2 McDonald cerclage is one or more purse-string sutures placed around the cervix without dissection of the bladder or rectum.

Transabdominal cerclage *(opposite)*

Transabdominal cerclage has not been shown to be superior to transvaginal cerclage, and is a far more morbid procedure requiring a laparotomy and subsequent delivery by caesarean. It should therefore be reserved for women in whom a cerclage is indicated, but who have either failed previous transvaginal cerclages or in whom a transvaginal cerclage is technically impossible to place.

Technical considerations

- An ultrasound examination should be performed prior to cerclage placement to exclude gross structural anomalies (such as anencephaly) and/or fetal demise.
- Confirmation of fetal viability both immediately before and after the procedure (either by auscultation or by ultrasound).
- Regional anaesthesia is preferred.
- Prophylactic tocolysis may be used to inhibit transient uterine contractions associated with placement, but there is no objective evidence that this improves outcome.
- Prophylactic antibiotics are recommended in emergent cerclage because of the risk of chorioamnionitis. The routine use of antibiotics for elective cerclage, however, is controversial.
- If the fetal membranes are prolapsing through the external os, the risk of iatrogenic rupture of the membranes may be as high as 40–50%. Trendelenburg position, filling the bladder, and/or amnioreduction can be used to reduce the fetal membranes prior to cerclage placement.

Postoperative care

- Frequent (weekly or bi-weekly) visits for cervical checks.
- Bed rest and 'pelvic rest' (no coitus, tampons, or douching) until a favourable gestational age is reached.
- Remove cerclage electively at 37–38 weeks or with the onset of premature uterine contractions (to avoid cervical lacerations or uterine rupture).

56 Premature rupture of the membranes

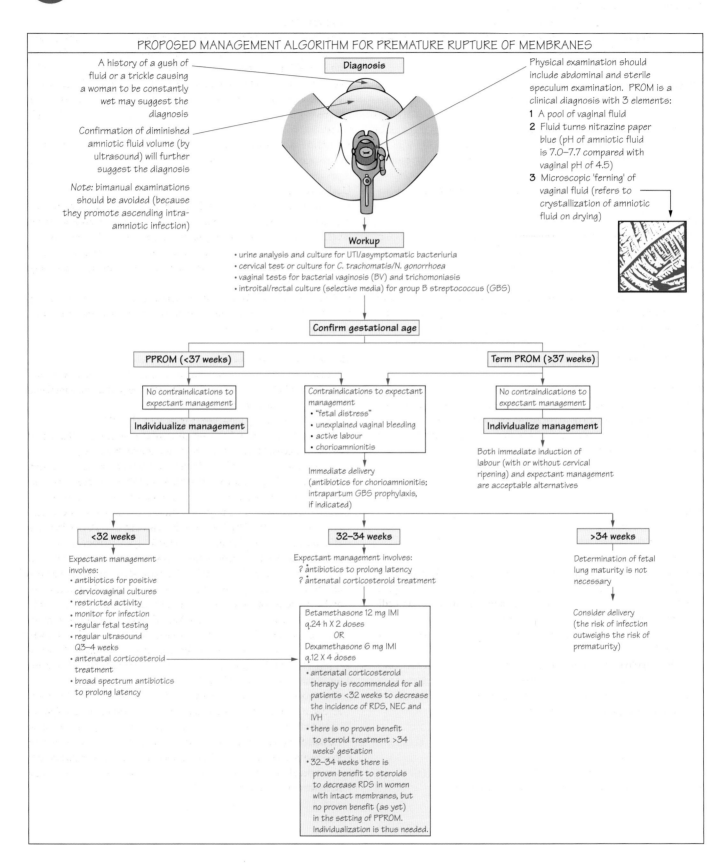

PROPOSED MANAGEMENT ALGORITHM FOR PREMATURE RUPTURE OF MEMBRANES

Diagnosis

A history of a gush of fluid or a trickle causing a woman to be constantly wet may suggest the diagnosis

Confirmation of diminished amniotic fluid volume (by ultrasound) will further suggest the diagnosis

Note: bimanual examinations should be avoided (because they promote ascending intra-amniotic infection)

Physical examination should include abdominal and sterile speculum examination. PROM is a clinical diagnosis with 3 elements:

1 A pool of vaginal fluid
2 Fluid turns nitrazine paper blue (pH of amniotic fluid is 7.0–7.7 compared with vaginal pH of 4.5)
3 Microscopic 'ferning' of vaginal fluid (refers to crystallization of amniotic fluid on drying)

Workup
• urine analysis and culture for UTI/asymptomatic bacteriuria
• cervical test or culture for *C. trachomatis*/*N. gonorrhoea*
• vaginal tests for bacterial vaginosis (BV) and trichomoniasis
• introital/rectal culture (selective media) for group B streptococcus (GBS)

Confirm gestational age

PPROM (<37 weeks)   **Term PROM (≥37 weeks)**

No contraindications to expectant management

Contraindications to expectant management
• "fetal distress"
• unexplained vaginal bleeding
• active labour
• chorioamnionitis

No contraindications to expectant management

Individualize management   **Individualize management**

Both immediate induction of labour (with or without cervical ripening) and expectant management are acceptable alternatives

Immediate delivery (antibiotics for chorioamnionitis; intrapartum GBS prophylaxis, if indicated)

<32 weeks   **32–34 weeks**   **>34 weeks**

Expectant management involves:
• antibiotics for positive cervicovaginal cultures
• restricted activity
• monitor for infection
• regular fetal testing
• regular ultrasound Q3–4 weeks
• antenatal corticosteroid treatment
• broad spectrum antibiotics to prolong latency

Expectant management involves:
? antibiotics to prolong latency
? antenatal corticosteroid treatment

Determination of fetal lung maturity is not necessary

Consider delivery (the risk of infection outweighs the risk of prematurity)

Betamethasone 12 mg IMI q.24 h X 2 doses
OR
Dexamethasone 6 mg IMI q.12 X 4 doses

• antenatal corticosteroid therapy is recommended for all patients <32 weeks to decrease the incidence of RDS, NEC and IVH
• there is no proven benefit to steroid treatment >34 weeks' gestation
• 32–34 weeks there is proven benefit to steroids to decrease RDS in women with intact membranes, but no proven benefit (as yet) in the setting of PPROM. Individualization is thus needed.

Definitions
• *Premature rupture of the membranes (PROM)* refers to rupture of the fetal membranes prior to the onset of labour.
• *Preterm PROM (PPROM)* refers to PROM <37 weeks.
• *Prolonged PROM* refers to PROM >24hours and is associated with an increased risk of intra-amniotic infection.

Diagnosis
• PROM is a clinical diagnosis (*opposite*).
• If equivocal, US practice favours an amnio/dye test ('tampon test') in which indigo carmine dye (not methylene blue because of an association with fetal methaemoglobinaemia) is instilled into the amniotic cavity and leakage into the vagina confirmed by staining of a tampon within 20–30 min.
• *Differential diagnosis*: leakage of urine, vaginal discharge.

Latency
• Latency refers to the interval between PROM and the onset of labour.
• 50% of women with PROM at term will go into labour within 12 hours, 70% within 24 hours, 85% within 48 hours, and 95% within 72 hours.
• Latency is influenced by gestational age (50% of women with PPROM will go into labour within 24–48 hours, and 70–90% within 7 days), severity of oligohydramnios (severe oligohydramnios is associated with shortened latency), and multiple pregnancy (twins have a shorter latency period than singletons).

Aetiology
• Near term, a focal weakness develops in the fetal membranes over the internal cervical os which predisposes to rupture at this site.
• Several pathological processes (including bleeding, infection) may predispose to PPROM.

Term premature rupture of the membranes
Incidence
8–10% of term pregnancies.

Management (*opposite*)
• In the absence of contraindications to expectant management (intra-amniotic infection, 'fetal distress'/non-reassuring fetal testing, vaginal bleeding, and active labour), both expectant management and immediate augmentation of labour are acceptable options.
• If the cervix is unfavourable, cervical ripening may be required (Chapter 57).
• Severe oligohydramnios may be associated with umbilical cord compression in labour leading to non-reassuring fetal testing and caesarean delivery. It is not clear whether intrapartum amnioinfusion can improve fetal testing and decrease the caesarean delivery rate.

Preterm premature rupture of the membranes
Incidence
• 2–4% of singleton and 7–10% of twin pregnancies.

• PPROM is associated with 30–40% of preterm births and 10% of all perinatal mortality.

Risk factors
• Risk factors include prior PPROM (recurrence risk, 20–30%), unexplained vaginal bleeding, placental abruption (seen in 15% of women with PPROM, but may be a result rather than a cause), cervical insufficiency, vaginal or intra-amniotic infection, amniocentesis, smoking, multiple pregnancy, polyhydramnios, chronic steroid treatment, connective tissue diseases, anaemia, low socioeconomic status, and single women.
• Factors not associated with PPROM include coitus, cervical examinations, maternal exercise, and parity.

Complications
• *Neonatal complications* are related primarily to prematurity, including respiratory distress syndrome (RDS), intraventricular haemorrhage (IVH), sepsis, pulmonary hypoplasia (especially with PPROM <22 weeks), and skeletal deformities (related to severity and duration of PPROM). Overall, PPROM is associated with a 4-fold increase in perinatal mortality.
• *Maternal complications* include increased caesarean delivery (due to malpresentation, cord prolapse), intra-amniotic infection (15–30%), and postpartum endometritis.

Management (*opposite*)
• Management of PPROM should be individualized. The risk of prematurity should be weighed against the risk of expectant management, primarily intra-amniotic infection.
• Areas of controversy in the management of PPROM.
  (i) *Tocolysis*. PPROM is a relative contraindication to the use of tocolytic agents (drugs which inhibit uterine contractions).
  (ii) *Antibiotics*. Prophylactic broad-spectrum antibiotics have been shown to prolong latency in the setting of PPROM. There is currently no evidence to recommend one antibiotic regime over another.
  (iii) *Steroids*. Antepartum glucocorticoid administration decreases the incidence of RDS by 50%. Maximal benefit is achieved 48 hours after the initial dose. This effect lasts for 7 days, but it is unclear what happens thereafter. Glucocorticoids also decrease the incidence of necrotizing enterocolitis and IVH. Intramuscular dexamethasone can also be used, but not prednisone (as it does not cross the placenta) or oral dexamethasone (because it has been associated with a 10-fold increase in neonatal infection and IVH). Of note, multiple (3 or more) courses of steroids may be associated with intrauterine growth restriction, smaller head circumference, and (in animals) abnormal myelination of the optic nerves. As such, repeat courses of steroids are not routinely recommended.
  (iv) *Fetus surveillance*. Following PPROM, fetuses are at risk for ascending infection, cord accident, placental abruption, and (possibly) uteroplacental insufficiency. It is generally accepted that some form of fetal monitoring is necessary, but the type and frequency of monitoring is controversial. Options include non-stress testing and/or biophysical profile (Chapter 49), but none have been shown to be superior to fetal kickcharts.

PATIENT ASSESSMENT PRIOR TO INDUCTION OF LABOUR

Confirm indication for induction
Review for contraindications to labour and/or vaginal delivery
Confirm gestational age
Estimate fetal weight (clinically or by ultrasound)
Determine fetal presentation
Assess shape and adequacy of bony pelvis (clinical pelvimetry)
Assess cervical examination (Bishop score)
Assess need for documentation of fetal lung maturity
Review risk and benefits of induction of labour

CONTRAINDICATIONS FOR INDUCTION OF LABOUR

Absolute contraindications

Maternal contraindications
  Active genital herpes
  Serious chronic medical conditions
Fetal contraindications
  Malpresentation
  "Fetal distress" non-reassuring fetal testing
Uteroplacental contraindications
  Cord prolapse
  Placenta previa
  Vasa previa
  Prior 'classical' caesarean section

Relative contraindications

Maternal contraindications
  Cervical carcinoma
  Pelvic deformities
Fetal contraindications
  Extreme fetal macrosomia
Uteroplacental contraindications
  Low-lying placenta
  Unexplained vaginal bleeding
  Cord presentation
  Myomectomy involving the uterine cavity

INDICATIONS FOR INDUCTION OF LABOUR AT TERM

Absolute indications

Maternal indications
Preeclampsia/eclampsia
Maternal medical problems
• diabetes mellitus
• chronic renal disease
• chronic pulmonary disease

Fetal indications
Chorioamnionitis
Abnormal antepartum testing
Intrauterine growth restriction
Post-term pregnancy (>42 weeks)
Isoimmunization

Uteroplacental indications
Placental abruption

Relative indications

Maternal indications
Chronic hypertension
Pregnancy-induced hypertension
Gestational diabetes
Logistic factors
• risk of rapid labour
 • distance from the hospital
 • psychosocial indications
Fetal indications
Premature rupture of membranes
Fetal macrosomia
Fetal demise
Previous stillbirth
Fetus with a major congenital anomaly
Uteroplacental indications
Unexplained oligohydramnios

ASSESSMENT OF CERVICAL STATUS BY BISHOP SCORE

	Score			
	0	1	2	3
Dilation (cm)	0	1–2	3–4	≥5
Effacement (%)	0–30	40–50	60–70	≥80
Station	–3	–2	–1 or 0	≥1+
Consistency	Firm	Medium	Soft	–
Cervical position	Posterior	Mid-position	Anterior	–

bishop score >6

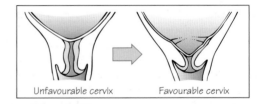

Unfavourable cervix → Favourable cervix

METHODS OF CERVICAL RIPENING AND INDUCTION OF LABOUR

Preinduction cervical ripening

Hormonal techniques
 Prostaglandins
 • PGE$_2$ (Dinoprostone)
 • PGE$_1$ (Misoprostol)
 Oxytocin
 Oestrogen
 RU486 (Mifepristone) (?) *progesterone ant.*
 Relaxin (?)
Amniotomy – *ARoM*
Membrane stripping
Mechanical dilators
 Hygroscopic dilators
 • laminaria (desiccated seaweed)
 • dilapan (polyacrilonitrile)
 • lamicel (magnesium sulphate in alcohol)
 Balloon catheter (alone, with traction, with infusion)

Initiation/augmentation of uterine contractility

Hormonal techniques
 Oxytocin
 Prostaglandins
 • PGE$_2$ (Dinoprostone)
 • PGE$_1$ (Misoprostol)
 • PGF$_{2\alpha}$ (Prostin) (?)
 RU486 (Mifepristone) (?)
Amniotomy

Induction of labour

Definition

• *Induction* refers to interventions designed to initiate labour prior to spontaneous onset with a view to achieving vaginal delivery.

• This should be distinguished from *augmentation* which refers to enhancement of uterine contractability in women in whom labour has already begun.

Patient assessment *(opposite)*

• The appropriate timing for induction is the point at which benefit to mother or fetus is greater if pregnancy is interrupted than if pregnancy is continued, and is gestational-age dependent.

• Indications and contraindications are detailed opposite.

Bishop score

• The success of induction depends in large part on the status of the cervix. In 1964, Bishop designed a cervical scoring system to prevent iatrogenic prematurity. This system has since been modified *(opposite)* and used to predict the success rate of induction. If the Bishop score is favourable (defined as ≥6), the likelihood of a successful induction and vaginal delivery is high. If unfavourable (<6), the probability of successful induction is reduced and pre-induction cervical 'ripening' (maturation) may be indicated.

• Cervical ripening describes a complex series of biochemical events that alter cervical collagen and ground substance composition resulting in a softer and more pliable cervix. A number of agents are available to facilitate this maturation *(opposite)*. Potential benefits include fewer failed inductions, shorter hospital stay, lower fetal and maternal morbidity, lower medical costs, and possibly lower caesarean delivery rates.

Methods *(opposite)*

The choice of induction regime should be individualized. A single technique is rarely effective on its own, and a combination of interventions may be required.

• *Prostaglandin E_2* (PGE$_2$) improves the rate of vaginal delivery, regardless of route of administration. Gastrointestinal side-effects are lower with vaginal administration. The rate of failed induction is only 1–6%. The most commonly used local PGE$_2$ preparation is dinoprostone gel (Prepidil®). PGE$_1$ analogues, such as misoprostol (Cytotec®), are cheaper, can be administered orally with few side-effects, and are as effective as PGE$_2$ for cervical ripening and labour induction. PGE$_2$ should be avoided in women with asthma, glaucoma, and severe renal, pulmonary, or hepatic disease. Prostaglandin induction of labour should be used cautiously in patients with a prior caesarean delivery, because of the fourfold increased risk of uterine rupture.

• *Oxytocin* infusion by any protocol (low-dose or high-dose, continuous or pulsatile) has been shown to be effective in pre-induction cervical ripening and labour induction. Continuous low-dose infusion is as effective as other protocols, while minimizing oxytocin requirements and adverse effects (especially maternal water intoxication due to an antidiuretic hormone-like effect). Advantages of oxytocin include cost and familiarity for the clinician. Fetal monitoring is required because of the risk of uterine tachysystole and 'fetal distress'.

• *Progesterone receptor antagonists* (RU 486 (Mifepristone®), ZK98299 (Onapristone®)) have been shown to promote cervical ripening and lower oxytocin requirements in labour.

• *Amniotomy* (artificial rupture of the membranes (AROM)) may be sufficient on its own to induce labour, but is more effective if used in combination with oxytocin. It shortens the interval from induction to delivery by 1–3 hours, but does not appear to lower the rate of caesarean delivery. Contraindications to amniotomy include HIV, active perineal herpes infection, and viral hepatitis.

• *Sweeping (stripping) of the membranes* refers to digital separation of the fetal membranes from the lower uterine segment prior to labour at term. It may accelerate the onset of labour by releasing endogenous prostaglandins. However, the majority of studies show no significant increase in the proportion of women going into labour within 7 days.

• *Mechanical dilators* have been shown to significantly shorten the induction to delivery interval as compared with no pre-induction ripening. Hygroscopic dilators rely on absorption of water to swell and forcibly dilate the cervix, and are as effective as PGE$_2$. A disadvantage of mechanical dilators is patient discomfort both at the time of insertion and with progressive cervical dilatation.

Augmentation of labour

Indications

Augmentation of uterine activity is indicated for failure to progress in labour in the presence of inadequate contractions and in the absence of absolute cephalopelvic disproportion (see Chapter 59).

Methods

Include amniotomy and/or oxytocin. It is still unclear whether such interventions improve obstetric outcome or merely produce the same outcome in a shorter period of time.

Active management of labour

• 'Active management' describes a protocol of clinical management based on the premise that enhancing uterine contractility in the first stage of labour will improve obstetric outcome. It applies only to nullipara in spontaneous labour with a cephalic presentation.

• Active management protocols rely on strict criteria for the diagnosis of labour, amniotomy within 1 hour of labour onset, and high-dose oxytocin if cervical dilatation is not maintained at ≥1.0 cm/hour. Other components include antenatal education, one-on-one nursing care, and close supervision by a senior obstetrician.

• The National Maternity Unit in Dublin, Ireland pioneered active management in 1968. Although the aim was to shorten the duration of nulliparous labour, it has attracted much attention for its apparent (but as yet unproven) ability to lower the caesarean delivery rate. Active management does decrease the duration of labour in nulliparas, but an improvement in obstetric outcome has yet to be conclusively demonstrated.

58 Normal labour and delivery

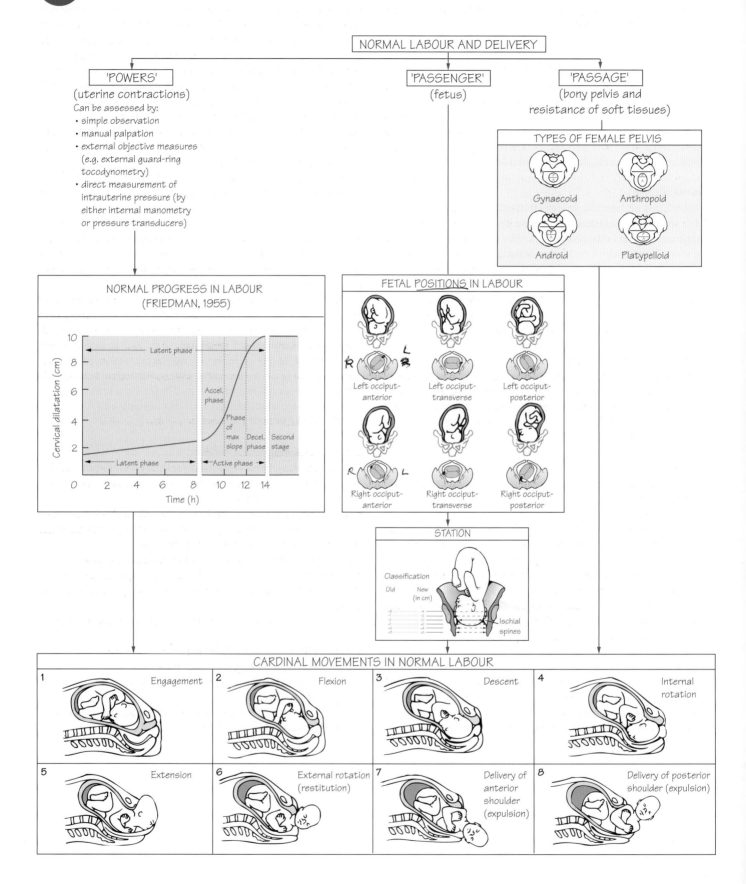

NORMAL LABOUR AND DELIVERY

'POWERS'
(uterine contractions)
Can be assessed by:
• simple observation
• manual palpation
• external objective measures
  (e.g. external guard-ring
  tocodynometry)
• direct measurement of
  intrauterine pressure (by
  either internal manometry
  or pressure transducers)

'PASSENGER'
(fetus)

'PASSAGE'
(bony pelvis and
resistance of soft tissues)

TYPES OF FEMALE PELVIS

Gynaecoid   Anthropoid

Android   Platypelloid

NORMAL PROGRESS IN LABOUR
(FRIEDMAN, 1955)

Latent phase

Cervical dilatation (cm)

Accel.
phase

Phase
of
max
slope   Decel.   Second
         phase   stage

Latent phase   Active phase

Time (h)

FETAL POSITIONS IN LABOUR

Left occiput-
anterior

Left occiput-
transverse

Left occiput-
posterior

Right occiput-
anterior

Right occiput-
transverse

Right occiput-
posterior

STATION

Classification

Old   New
       (in cm)

Ischial
spines

CARDINAL MOVEMENTS IN NORMAL LABOUR

1 Engagement
2 Flexion
3 Descent
4 Internal rotation
5 Extension
6 External rotation (restitution)
7 Delivery of anterior shoulder (expulsion)
8 Delivery of posterior shoulder (expulsion)

Definition

Labour is a clinical diagnosis with two elements: (i) uterine contractions increasing in frequency and intensity, and (ii) progressive effacement and dilatation of the cervix.

Stages of labour

For clinical purposes, labour is divided into three stages.

1 The *first stage* refers to cervical dilatation in preparation for passage of the fetus. It is further divided into phases according to the rate of cervical dilatation. The partogram (Friedman curve) is a graphical representation of the normal labour curve against which a patient's progress is plotted (*opposite*). Normal latent phase is <20 hours in nullipara and <14 hours in multipara. In the active phase, the cervix should dilate >1.2 cm/hour in nullipara (>1.5 cm/hour in multipara). A delay in cervical dilatation in the active phase of ≥2 hours over that expected suggests labour dystocia and requires further evaluation.

2 The *second stage* commences when the cervix achieves full dilatation (10 cm) and ends with delivery of the fetus. Prolonged second stage refers to >3 hours with or >2 hours without regional analgesia in a nullipara and >2 hours with or >1 hour without regional analgesia in a multipara.

3 The *third stage* refers to delivery of the placenta and fetal membranes and usually lasts ≤10 minutes. In the absence of excessive bleeding, up to 30 minutes may be allowed before intervention.

Mechanics of normal labour

The ability of the fetus to negotiate the pelvis is dependent on the interaction of three variables: powers, passenger, and passage. The 'powers' consist of the forces generated by the uterine musculature, the 'passenger' is the fetus, and the 'passage' consists of the bony pelvis and resistance provided by soft tissues.

Powers

• Several techniques are available to assess uterine activity (*opposite*). Uterine activity is characterized by frequency, amplitude, and duration of contractions.

• Despite technological advances, the definition of 'adequate' uterine activity remains unclear. Classically, 3–5 contractions in 10 minutes has been used to define adequate labour. This contraction pattern is seen in 95% of women in spontaneous labour at term. If an intrauterine pressure monitor is used, 150–200 Montevideo units (strength of contractions in mmHg multiplied by the frequency per 10 minutes) is deemed adequate. The ultimate barometer of uterine activity is the rate of cervical dilatation and descent of the presenting part.

Passenger

• Two main variables influence the course of labour: *attitude* (degree of flexion or extension of the head) and *fetal size*. When the fetal head is optimally flexed, the smallest possible diameter of the head (suboccipitobregmatic diameter, 9.5 cm) presents at the pelvic inlet.

• The lie, presentation, position and station of the fetus can be assessed on clinical examination. *Lie* refers to the long axis of the fetus relative to the long axis of the uterus, and can be longitudinal, transverse, or oblique. *Presentation* can be either cephalic or breech, referring to the pole of the fetus that overlies the pelvic inlet. *Position* refers to the relationship of a nominated site on the presenting part to a nominated location on the maternal pelvis, and can be assessed most accurately on bimanual examination. In a cephalic presentation, the nominated site is usually the occiput. In the breech, the nominated site is the sacrum. *Station* refers to the level of the presenting part relative to the maternal pelvis (specifically the ischial spines) as assessed on bimanual examination (*opposite*). The vertex is said to be *engaged* when the widest diameter has entered the pelvic inlet.

• *Fetal weight* can be estimated clinically or by ultrasound. When compared with absolute birth weight, both techniques have a 15–20% error.

Passage

• The bony pelvis is composed of the sacrum, ilium, ischium, and pubis. The shape of the pelvis can be classified into one or more of four broad categories: gynecoid, android, anthropoid, and platypelloid (*opposite*). The gynecoid pelvis is the classical female shape.

• Clinical pelvimetry can be used to estimate the shape and adequacy of the bony pelvis, but has not been shown to change clinical management.

• Pelvic soft tissues (cervix and pelvic floor musculature) can provide resistance in labour. In the second stage, the pelvic musculature may play an important role in facilitating rotation and descent of the head. Excessive resistance, however, may contribute to failure to progress in labour.

Cardinal movements in normal labour (*opposite*)

Clinical assistance at delivery

• As the fetal head crowns, the clinician's hand is used to control delivery thereby preventing precipitous expulsion (which has been associated with intracranial haemorrhage).

• Mouth and pharynx can be gently suctioned, although this manouevre has not been shown to change perinatal outcome. Vigorous suctioning can cause a vagal response and fetal bradycardia.

• If a nuchal cord is present, it should be reduced at this time.

• Following restitution of the fetal head, a hand is placed on each parietal eminence and the anterior shoulder delivered by gentle downward traction.

• The posterior shoulder and torso are then delivered by upward traction.

• The umbilical cord should be double clamped and cut.

• The infant should be supported at all times.

• The third stage of labour can be managed either passively or actively (Chapter 64).

• The placenta and fetal membranes should be examined, and the number of blood vessels in the umbilical cord recorded.

BREECH PRESENTATION

Definition: fetus presenting buttocks first (position of the breech is defined relative to the sacrum)

Diagnosis: by Leopold's manoeuvre, vaginal examination or ultrasound

Incidence: 3–4% at term

Risk factors:
- prematurity (28% breech at 28 weeks, 15% at 30 weeks)
- uterine anomaly
- polyhydramnios
- prior breech delivery
- multiple gestation
- placenta previa
- fetal anomalies (anencephaly, hydrocephalus)

Associated with:
- 2-fold ↑ risk of congenital abnormality
- ↑ risk of cord prolapse, preterm labour, birth trauma, maternal morbidity

Types of breech

Frank breech (70%)

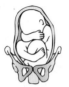

Complete breech (10%)

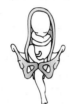

Footling or incomplete breech (20%)

External cephalic version (ECV)

- refers to attempted conversion of breech to vertex by manual manipulation through maternal abdomen
- performed after 36 weeks

Benefits: ↓ breech at term

Risks of ECV: "fetal distress", abruption, cord accident, rupture of fetal membranes, neurological injury

Contraindications to ECV may be absolute (uterine anomaly) or relative (prior caesarean, IUGR, twins, oligohydramnios, labour)

Predictors of success: Frank breech, normal amniotic fluid volume, operator experience, non-engaged breech, multiparous and thin mother, laterally located fetal spine

Techniques of ECV:
- >36 weeks, no labour, consent obtained, reactive NST anti-D IgG if needed
- under ultrasound guidance
- + epidural/β-mimetic tocolysis
- check NST after ECV

Success rate: 50–70%

Vaginal breech delivery

- preterm singleton breeches are best delivered by caesarean (because of risk of head entrapment)
- management of breech 2nd twin is addressed in Chapter 52
- term breech fetuses are most commonly delivered abdominally (because of the ↑ risk of head entrapment, cord prolapse, asphyxia, birth trauma with vaginal breech delivery)
- vaginal breech delivery may be a safe alternative to caesarean under the following conditions:
  - term frank breech
  - estimated fetal weight 2500–4000 g by ultrasound
  - no hyperextension of fetal head
  - capacity for emergent caesarean
  - experienced operator
  - adequate anaesthesia
  - adequate progress in labour
  - absence of "fetal distress"
  - preferably multiparous woman ('proven pelvis')

SHOULDER DYSTOCIA AND BRACHIAL PLEXUS INJURIES

Definition: impaction of the anterior shoulder of the fetus behind the pubic symphysis following delivery of the head

Risk factors:
- fetal macrosomia (EFW ≥4500g)
- history of prior shoulder dystocia
- diabetes mellitus
- midcavity operative vaginal delivery
- labour dystocia (2nd stage >60 min)
- post-term pregnancy
- obesity

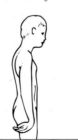

Brachial plexus

Ventral rami ('roots')
Trunk
Divisions
Lateral cord
Axillary artery
Axillary nerve

Posterior cord
Median cord
Pectoralis minor
Ulnar nerve
Median nerve
Radial nerve
Musculocutaneous nerve

C5
C6
C7
C8
T1

Klumpke's palsy (traction injury to C8/T1 only)

Erb's palsy
- traction injury to C5–C7 (± C8/T1)
- 2–5% cause permanent deformity

Management of shoulder dystocia

?? Prevention (difficult because it is almost impossible to predict)

↓

Identify problem immediately. Call for help. Note the time (you have ± 5 min to deliver the baby safely)

↓

Create space (empty bladder, consider generous episiotomy, remove the bottom of the bed)

↓

Perform McRoberts' manoeuvre ± suprapubic pressure

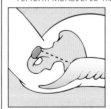
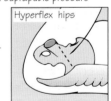

Hyperflex hips

If unsuccessful consider:
- suprapubic (not fundal) pressure
- Woods' Screw manoeuvre
- cut proctoepisiotomy
- deliver posterior arm
- ? break clavicle (pull outwards)
- ? Zavanelli manoeuvre (replace head, caesarean)
- ? symphysiotomy
- ? place patient in knee–chest position

Labour dystocia

- *Definition*: abnormal or inadequate progress in labour (Chapter 58).
- Also known as failure to progress, prolonged labour, failure of cervical dilatation, failure of descent of the fetal head.
- *Causes*: inadequate 'power' (uterine contractions), inadequate 'passage' (bony pelvis), or abnormalities of the 'passenger' (fetal macrosomia, hydrocephalus, malpresentation, extreme extension or asynclitism (lateral tilting) of the fetal head).
- *Cephalopelvic disproportion* (CPD) is classified as absolute (where the disparity between the size of the bony pelvis and the fetal head precludes vaginal delivery even under optimal conditions) or relative (where fetal malposition, asynclitism, or extension of the fetal head prevents delivery). Absolute CPD is an absolute contraindication to vaginal delivery.
- *Management*. Exclude absolute CPD. Confirm 'adequate' uterine activity (Chapter 58). If contractions are 'adequate', one of two events will occur: dilatation and effacement of the cervix with descent of the head, or worsening caput succedaneum (scalp oedema) and molding (overlapping of the skull bones). Proceed with timely caesarean delivery, if indicated.

Malpresentation
Breech *(opposite)*

Transverse (shoulder presentation) or oblique lie
- *Incidence:* 0.3% of term pregnancies.
- *Aetiology:* prematurity, placenta previa, grandmultiparity, multiple gestation, uterine anomalies (fibroids, bicornuate uterus).
- *Management*. Consider external cephalic version. Caesarean delivery if unsuccessful.

Other malpresentations
- Malpresentations can occur in a vertex fetus. Some can be delivered vaginally (such as occiput posterior, face with mentum (chin) anterior). In others (brow, face with mentum posterior), conversion to occiput anterior is necessary for vaginal delivery.
- *Compound presentation* (<0.1% of all deliveries) refers to the presence of a fetal extremity alongside the presenting part. It is associated with prematurity, polyhydramnios, and multiple gestations. Vaginal delivery can often be effected.
- *Funic presentation* refers to presentation of the umbilical cord below the head. It is rare. If identified in labour, caesarean delivery may be indicated because of the risk of cord prolapse.

Intrapartum complications
Cord prolapse
- An obstetric emergency characterized by prolapse of the umbilical cord into the vagina after rupture of the fetal membranes.
- *Incidence:* 0.4% of term cephalic pregnancies.
- *Risk factors:* malpresentation (breech, transverse lie), polyhydramnios, small fetus, prematurity.
- *Diagnosis:* palpation of a pulsatile cord on vaginal examination with or without fetal bradycardia.
- *Prevention*. Perform amniotomy only once the vertex is well applied to the cervix and always with fundal pressure.
- *Management*. Replace cord manually and expedite delivery immediately (usually by emergency caesarean).

Shoulder dystocia and brachial plexus injury *(opposite)*

- *Shoulder dystocia* is an obstetric emergency associated with neonatal birth trauma (neurological injury, fractures of the humerus, skull, clavicle) in up to 30% of cases. Immediate identification and prompt and appropriate intervention may prevent neonatal birth trauma in some cases. Shoulder dystocia complicates 0.2–2% of all vaginal deliveries. Although several risk factors are described, the majority of cases occur in women with no risk factors
- *Brachial plexus paralysis* is the second most common neurological birth injury (after facial nerve palsy) complicating 0.5–3 per 1000 deliveries. It results from 'excessive' lateral traction on the head and neck at delivery with resultant injury to the brachial plexus, usually to cervical nerve roots C5–C7 (Erb/Duchenne palsy). The lower brachial plexus (C8–T1) may also be involved. On examination, the arm hangs limply at the side of the body with the forearm extended and internally rotated, the classic 'waiter's tip' deformity (*opposite*). The function of the fingers is usually retained. Ninety-five per cent of brachial plexus injuries resolve completely within 2 years with the help of physical therapy. Elective caesarean delivery will prevent most (but not all) brachial plexus injuries. Given the difficulty in predicting shoulder dystocia, however, caesarean delivery cannot be recommended for all women with identifiable risk factors.

Other congenital neurological birth injuries
- *Facial nerve paralysis* results from pressure on the facial nerve as it exits the skull through the stylomastoid foramen. It is the most common neurological birth injury (0.1–8 per 1000 live births). It is more common after operative vaginal (forceps) delivery. Resolution is usually complete within a few days.
- *Injuries to the neck and spinal cord* may result from excessive traction at delivery with fracture or dislocation of the vertebrae. Such injuries may prove fatal. The true incidence of spinal injuries is not known.
- *Multicystic encephalomalacia* is a pathological condition specific to multiple pregnancy in which cerebral damage develops in the surviving fetus following intrauterine demise of its co-twin (Chapter 52). The mechanism of cerebral injury is not known. Unfortunately, immediate caesarean delivery does not appear to prevent neurological injury in the surviving twin.

Intracranial haemorrhage
- Bleeding into the fetal head can occur at several anatomic sites. Intraventricular haemorrhage (IVH), defined as bleeding into the germinal matrix within the ventricles, occurs most commonly.
- *Incidence:* 4–5% of term infants will have sonographic evidence of IVH unrelated to obstetric factors.
- *Risk factors:* prematurity, fetal bleeding diathesis, alloimmune thrombocytopenia. Birth trauma is an uncommon cause of intracranial haemorrhage.
- *Treatment:* primarily supportive. Surgery is rarely indicated.
- *Prognosis* depends on gestational age at delivery, the presence and extent of ventriculomegaly, and the extent and location of the haemorrhage (parenchymal and subdural haemorrhages have a poor prognosis in 90% of cases because the haemorrhage is often more excessive; IVH has a poor prognosis in 45% of cases; only grade 3 and 4 IVH are associated with long-term neurological sequelae).

60 Pain relief in labour

PAIN RELIEF IN LABOUR	
Techniques	Efficacy
Pharmacological techniques	
General endotracheal analgaesia	Very effective
Systemic analgaesia	
• opioid (narcotic) agonists (such as morphine, meperidine, fentanyl)	Effective
• partial opioid agonist/antagonists (such as nalbuphine, butorphanol)	Effective
• 'twilight sleep' (morphine plus scopolamine. historical interest only)	-
Regional analgaesia	
• pudendal block	Moderately effective
• epidural block	Very effective
• spinal block	Very effective
• caudal block (saddle block)	Very effective
Local analgaesia	
• field block (local infiltration)	Minimally effective
• paracervical block	Minimally effective
Inhalation analgaesia	
• ether (historical interest only)	-
• chloroform (historical interest only)	-
• nitrous oxide (alone, with air, with oxygen)	Moderately effective
Non-pharmacological techniques	
Acupuncture	Probably effective
Hypnosis	Probably ineffective
Aromatherapy	No data
Transcutaneous electrical nerve stimulation (TENS)	Probably ineffective
Psychoprophylaxis (pioneered by Lamaze in France)	Probably ineffective

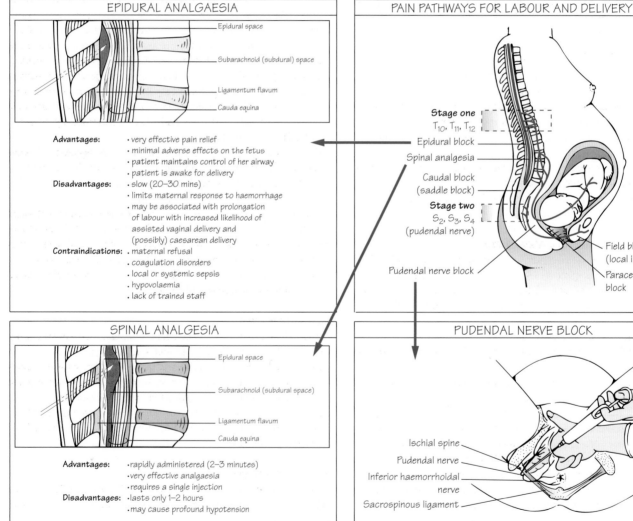

EPIDURAL ANALGAESIA

Epidural space
Subarachnoid (subdural) space
Ligamentum flavum
Cauda equina

Advantages:
• very effective pain relief
• minimal adverse effects on the fetus
• patient maintains control of her airway
• patient is awake for delivery

Disadvantages:
• slow (20–30 mins)
• limits maternal response to haemorrhage
• may be associated with prolongation of labour with increased likelihood of assisted vaginal delivery and (possibly) caesarean delivery

Contraindications:
. maternal refusal
. coagulation disorders
. local or systemic sepsis
. hypovolaemia
. lack of trained staff

PAIN PATHWAYS FOR LABOUR AND DELIVERY

Stage one
T_{10}, T_{11}, T_{12}
Epidural block
Spinal analgesia
Caudal block (saddle block)
Stage two
S_2, S_3, S_4 (pudendal nerve)
Pudendal nerve block
Field block (local infiltration)
Paracervical block

SPINAL ANALGESIA

Epidural space
Subarachnoid (subdural space)
Ligamentum flavum
Cauda equina

Advantages:
• rapidly administered (2–3 minutes)
• very effective analgaesia
• requires a single injection

Disadvantages:
• lasts only 1–2 hours
• may cause profound hypotension

PUDENDAL NERVE BLOCK

Ischial spine
Pudendal nerve
Inferior haemorrhoidal nerve
Sacrospinous ligament

- Pain during labour is generally severe, with only 2–4% of women reporting minimal pain in labour.
- Pain relief (analgesia; *opposite*) during normal labour is not mandatory. However, all women should be aware of the options available to them. There are no contraindications for pain relief in labour.
- Analgesia is strongly recommended for certain maternal conditions (select cardiac disorders, suspected difficult intubation) and in situations where intrapartum manipulation is likely (breech, multiple pregnancy).
- Adequate analgesia is mandatory for assisted vaginal delivery, perineal repair, manual removal of placenta, and caesarean delivery.

Pain pathways *(opposite)*
- During the *first stage* of labour, pain results from both cervical dilatation and uterine contractions (myometrial ischemia). Pain sensation travels from the uterus via visceral afferent (sympathetic) nerves that enter the spinal cord through the posterior segments of thoracic spinal nerves, T10–T12.
- Pain during the *second stage* of labour results primarily from distention of the pelvic floor, vagina, and perineum by the presenting part of the fetus and travels via sensory fibres of sacral nerves, S2–S4 (pudendal nerve). The sensation of uterine contractions also contributes, but is probably secondary.

Non-pharmacological techniques
- Acupuncture, hypnosis, and aromatherapy may have a place in clinical practice, but their efficacy is not yet proven.
- Transcutaneous electrical nerve stimulation (TENS) is thought to act by promoting endogenous enkephalin release within the spinal cord where it acts to inhibit the transmission of pain. Its efficacy is unproven.
- Warm baths, massage, relaxation, antenatal classes, breathing exercises, and the presence of a supportive 'doula' (midwife) have all been shown to decrease analgesic requirements in labour.

Pharmacological techniques
General endotracheal anaesthesia
- *Indications.* General anaesthesia should generally be avoided. It is best reserved for emergent caesarean or instrumental vaginal delivery (because of speed of administration) and for entrapment of the aftercoming head at vaginal breech delivery (because it relaxes the cervix).
- *Advantages:* rapidly administered, low incidence of hypotension, appropriate for women with hypovolemia and women at high-risk of haemorrhage.
- *Disadvantages.* Higher incidence of aspiration (because the patient is unable to protect her airway), neonatal depression, and postpartum haemorrhage (due to uterine relaxation).
- *Complications:* aspiration of gastric contents leading to pneumonia or pneumonitis (Mendelson syndrome), maternal hypoxic cerebral injury (due to failed intubation or obstructed endotracheal tube), injury to upper airway. Complications can be minimized by pre-operative starvation, intravenous fluid and antacid administration, cricoid pressure at intubation, and careful monitoring throughout the procedure.

Systemic analgesia
- *Opiate agonists* have good analgesic and sedative properties, but delay gastric emptying and can cause neonatal sedation and respiratory depression. A reversal agent (naloxone) should be available in the event of maternal or neonatal depression.
- *Partial opioid agonists/antagonists* have fewer side-effects, but are less effective analgesics.
- *Advantages:* readily available, easily administered, does not adversely affect the progress of labour.
- *Side-effects:* nausea and vomiting, respiratory depression, over-sedation, and decreased fetal heart rate variability.

Regional
- Regional blockade of the spinal sensory nerves can be achieved through a number of techniques.
  (i) *Epidural analgesia* (*opposite*) involves insertion of a cannula at L2/3 or L3/4. The cannula is left in place in the peridural fat which allows for administration of local analgesic agents by intermittent bolus injections or continuous infusion. Advantages and disadvantages are reviewed opposite. Epidural analgesia provides superior pain relief, but may prolong labour and limit a woman's ability to push. Moreover, epidural analgesia may be associated with an increased incidence of malpresentation (occiput posterior), instrumental vaginal delivery, severe perineal trauma, and (possibly) caesarean delivery. Complications include hypotension (which can usually be avoided by pre-loading with 500 mL crystalloid), accidental dural puncture (<1%), postdural puncture headache (5–25%), drug toxicity, direct neurological injury, and spinal haematoma (very rare). Maternal hypotension may be associated with fetal bradycardia which is usually short-lived and may be reversed by maternal ephedrine administration.
  (ii) *Spinal analgesia* (*opposite*) involves an injection of local anaesthetic into the subarachnoid space. It is usually reserved for caesarean, because its effect is limited to 1–2 hours.
  (iii) *Combined spinal–epidural analgesia.*
- *Pudendal nerve block* (*opposite*) is a regional block achieved through transvaginal infiltration of the pudendal nerves (S2–S4) bilaterally as they exit Alcock's canal and circumnavigate the ischial spines. It is most useful for outlet manipulations in the second stage of labour.
- *Caudal block* (saddle block) is a localized regional block of the cauda equina administered through the sacral hiatus.

Local analgesia
- *Field block* (infiltration of the nerve endings in the vulva) is used most often to repair perineal laceration or episiotomy.
- *Paracervical block* (bilateral infiltration of the sensory nerves leaving the uterus through the cardinal ligaments) is used most often to provide analgesia for the latter part of the first stage of labour.
- Local analgesic agents include bupivacaine, lidocaine, chloroprocaine. Prilocaine is generally avoided because of the risk of methaemoglobinaemia.

Inhalation analgesia
Inhalation analgesia, especially Entonox (50% oxygen/50% nitrous oxide), is widely used in Third World countries with good patient satisfaction.

ASSESSMENT OF FETAL WELL-BEING

Antepartum	Intrapartum	Postpartum
Non-stress test (NST) • external monitor (Doppler) only Biophysical profile Vibroacoustic stimulation Contraction stress test Fetal movement charts ('kickcharts') Doppler velocity (?)	Non-stress test (NST) • external monitor (Doppler) • internal (scalp electrode) Vibroacoustic stimulation Contraction stress test Fetal scalp sampling Biophysical profile (?) Fetal pulse oximetry (?)	Clinical response (seizures, poor feeding, abnormal movements) Apgar score Umbilical cord pH

see Chapter 49 for details

INTERPRETATION OF NON-STRESS TESTS

Accelerations

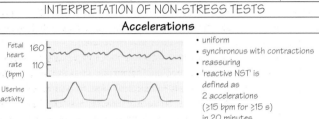

Fetal heart rate (bpm) 160 / 110

Uterine activity

- uniform
- synchronous with contractions
- reassuring
- 'reactive NST' is defined as 2 accelerations (≥15 bpm for ≥15 s) in 20 minutes

Decelerations

Early decelerations

Fetal heart rate (bpm) 160 / 110

Uterine activity

- uniform
- synchronous with contractions
- rarely falls below 110 bpm
- reflects head compression and is mediated through the parasympathetic nervous system (vagus nerve)
- not a sign of "fetal distress"

Variable decelerations

Fetal heart rate (bpm) 160 / 110

Uterine activity

- variable in appearance and timing
- may be associated with increased variability
- reflects umbilical cord compression
- may be a sign of "fetal distress"

Late decelerations

Fetal heart rate (bpm) 160 / 110

Uterine activity

- uniform
- starts after peak of contraction
- associated with decreased variability
- reflects a chemoreceptor response
- may indicate fetal hypoxaemia

Other fetal heart rate patterns

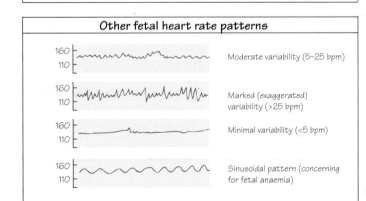

160 / 110 — Moderate variability (5–25 bpm)

160 / 110 — Marked (exaggerated) variability (>25 bpm)

160 / 110 — Minimal variability (<5 bpm)

160 / 110 — Sinusoidal pattern (concerning for fetal anaemia)

APGAR SCORING SYSTEM

	Score		
	0	1	2
Appearance	Blue, pale	Pink body, blue extremity	Pink all over
Heart rate (bpm)	Absent	<100	≥100
Grimace	No response	Some response	Cry, cough
Activity	Limp	Some flexion	Active motion
Respiratory effort	Absent	Slow	Strong cry

NORMAL FETAL ACID–BASE VALUES AT TERM

	pH	PO₂ (mmHg)	PCO₂ (mmHg)	Bicarbonate (mE/L)	O₂ saturation (%)
Umbilical vein	7.35 ± 0.05	29.2 ± 5.9	38.2 ± 5.6	20.4 ± 2.1	70
Umbilical artery	7.28 ± 0.05	18.0 ± 6.2	14.2 ± 8.4	22.3 ± 2.5	28
Fetal scalp blood					
• early first stage	7.33 ± 0.03	21.8 ± 2.6	44.0 ± 4.05	20.1 ± 1.2	
• late first stage	7.23 ± 0.02	21.3 ± 2.1	42.0 ± 5.1	19.1 ± 2.1	
• second stage	7.29 ± 0.04	16.5 ± 1.4	46.3 ± 4.2	17.0 ± 2.0	

DRUGS AFFECTING INTRAPARTUM FETAL HEART RATE TRACING

Effect on fetus	Drug
Fetal tachycardia	Adrenalin Atropine β-agonists (ritodrine, terbutaline)
Fetal bradycardia	Anti-thyroid agents (including propothiouracil) β-blockers (such as propranolol) Epidural anaesthesia (regardless of the agent used) Methergine (contraindicated prior to delivery) Oxytocin (if associated with excessive uterine activity)
Sinusoidal heart rate pattern	Narcotic analgesics (especially alphaprodine butorphamol, meperidine)
Diminished variability	Atropine Anticonvulsants (but not phenytoin) β-blockers Betamethasone Ethanol General anaesthesia Hypnotics (including diazepam) Insulin (if associated with hypoglycaemia) Magnesium sulfate Narcotic analgesics Promethazine (Phenergan)

Introduction

• Fetal morbidity and mortality can occur as a consequence of labour. A number of tests have been developed to assess fetus well-being (*opposite*).

• Attention has focused on *hypoxic ischaemic encephalopathy* (HIE) as a marker of birth asphyxia and a predictor of long-term outcome. HIE is a clinical condition that develops within the first hours or days of life. It is characterized by abnormalities of tone and feeding, alterations in consciousness, and convulsions. In order to attribute such a state to birth asphyxia, the following four criteria must all be fulfilled:

(i) profound metabolic or mixed acidaemia (pH < 7.00) on an umbilical cord arterial blood sample, if obtained;

(ii) Apgar score (*opposite*) of 0–3 for longer than 5 minutes;

(iii) neonatal neurological manifestations (seizures, coma);

(iv) multisystem organ dysfunction.

At most, only 15% of cerebral palsy and mental retardation can be attributed to HIE.

Intrapartum fetal monitoring

Non-stress test (NST) or fetal cardiotocography (CTG)

A fetal scalp electrode for the continuous monitoring of the fetal heart rate during labour was introduced by Hon and Lee in 1963. A year later, Doppler technology made external fetal heart analysis possible. Continuous intrapartum CTG is now recommended for all high-risk pregnancies and is commonly used in low-risk pregnancies too.

Characteristics of intrapartum fetal heart rate patterns

• *Baseline fetal heart rate* refers to the dominant reading taken over ≥10 minutes. Normal baseline fetal heart rate is 110–160 beats per minute (bpm). Bradycardia is a baseline rate <110 bpm. Tachycardia is a baseline rate >160 bpm.

• *Fetal heart rate variability* is classified as moderate (which refers to peak-to-trough excursions of 5–25 bpm around the baseline, and is a healthy sign), minimal (<5 bpm excursions, which is concerning for hypoxia and requires further evaluation), absent (0 bpm excursions, which is worrisome for hypoxia), or marked (>25 bpm excursions, which suggests hypoxia without acidosis).

• *Accelerations* are periodic, transient increases in fetal heart rate of ≥15 bpm for ≥15 seconds (or ≥10 bpm for ≥10 seconds for fetuses <32 weeks). Accelerations are often associated with fetal activity, and are a sign of a healthy fetus.

• *Decelerations* are periodic, transient decreases in fetal heart rate usually associated with uterine contractions. They can be further classified into early, variable, or late decelerations by their shape and timing in relation to contractions (*opposite*). Decelerations are regarded as 'repetitive' if they occur with more than 50% of contractions.

Interpretation of NST (*opposite*)

• Fetal heart rate patterns in labour are classified as:

(i) 'reactive' (defined as two or more accelerations in 20 minutes), which is considered reassuring;

(ii) suspicious or equivocal (indeterminate);

(iii) ominous or agonal (non-reassuring).

• Reassuring elements of the fetal heart rate include normal baseline, moderate variability and accelerations. Non-reassuring elements include bradycardia, tachycardia, minimal or absent variability, and/or repetitive severe variable or late decelerations.

• Non-reassuring patterns are seen in up to 60% of labours, suggesting that they are not specific to fetal hypoxia. Severely abnormal fetal heart rate patterns (specifically, repetitive severe variable or late decelerations), on the other hand, occur in only 0.3% of intrapartum fetal heart rate tracings.

• NST interpretation is largely subjective and should always take into account gestational age, the presence or absence of congenital anomalies, and underlying clinical risk factors. Fetuses who are premature or growth restricted are less likely to tolerate episodes of decreased placental perfusion and, as such, may be more prone to hypoxia and acidosis. Drugs can also affect heart rate and variability (*opposite*).

• Only two intrapartum fetal heart rate patterns have been associated with poor perinatal outcome, namely repetitive severe variable (defined as decreasing to <70 bpm and lasting for ≥60 seconds) and repetitive late decelerations.

• When compared with intermittent fetal heart rate auscultation, continuous fetal heart rate monitoring during labour is associated with a decrease in the incidence of seizures prior to 28 days of life, but no difference in other measures of short-term perinatal morbidity or mortality. Moreover, the increase in neonatal seizures does not translate into differences in long-term morbidity (cerebral palsy, mental retardation, or seizures after 28 days of life). However, continuous fetal heart rate monitoring is associated with a significant increase in obstetric intervention, including operative vaginal and caesarean delivery.

• Several unusual fetal heart rate patterns have been described:

(i) a *salutatory* pattern (in which there are large oscillations in baseline) is of unclear clinical significance. It may indicate intermittent cord occlusion;

(ii) a *lambda* pattern (an acceleration followed by a deceleration) is attributed to fetal movement. It is not felt to be of pathological significance;

(iii) a *sinusoidal* pattern (one with normal baseline, decreased variability, and a cyclic sinusoidal pattern with a frequency of 2–5 cycles per minute and amplitude of 5–15 bpm) is associated most strongly with fetal anaemia. It may also be seen in the setting of chorioamnionitis, impending fetal demise, and maternal drug administration (especially narcotic analgesics).

Fetal scalp sampling

• The pH of fetal capillary blood lies between that of fetal arterial and venous blood (*opposite*).

• Fetal scalp blood sampling was introduced by Saling in 1962. It is most useful in labour when alternative non-invasive tests are unable to confirm fetal well-being.

• Suggested management based on fetal scalp pH:

Scalp pH	Suggested management
>7.25	May manage expectantly, consider repeating in 1 hour if CTG still abnormal
7.20–7.25	Repeat at 30 minutes intervals
<7.20	Expedite delivery immediately

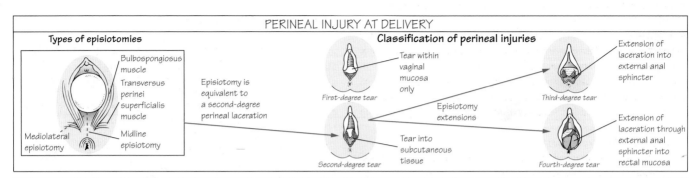

PERINEAL INJURY AT DELIVERY

Types of episiotomies

Bulbospongiosus muscle
Transversus perinei superficialis muscle
Mediolateral episiotomy
Midline episiotomy

Episiotomy is equivalent to a second-degree perineal laceration

Classification of perineal injuries

Tear within vaginal mucosa only
First-degree tear

Episiotomy extensions

Tear into subcutaneous tissue
Second-degree tear

Extension of laceration into external anal sphincter
Third-degree tear

Extension of laceration through external anal sphincter into rectal mucosa
Fourth-degree tear

OPERATIVE VAGINAL DELIVERY

INDICATIONS FOR OPERATIVE VAGINAL DELIVERY

Maternal indications
- maternal exhaustion
- inadequate maternal expulsive efforts (such as women with spinal cord injuries or neuromuscular diseases)
- need to avoid maternal expulsive efforts (such as women with certain cardiac or cerebrovascular diseases)

Fetal indications
- "fetal distress"/non-reassuring fetal testing

Other indications
- prolonged second stage of labour
  → nulliparous: 3 hours with regional analgesia or 2 hours without regional analgesia
  → parous: 2 hours with regional analgesia or 1 hour without regional analgesia

CRITERIA WHICH NEED TO BE FULFILLED PRIOR TO OPERATIVE VAGINAL DELIVERY

Maternal criteria
- adequate analgesia
- verbal and/or written consent
- lithotomy position
- bladder empty
- adequate clinical pelvimetry

Fetal criteria
- vertex presentation
- vertex engaged (i.e. biparietal diameter of the head has passed through the pelvic inlet)
- station (i.e. leading bony point of the head relative to the ischial spines) ≥ + 2/+ 5 cm
- position, attitude of fetal head as well as presence of caput or moulding is known

Uteroplacental criteria
- cervix fully dilated
- membranes ruptured
- no placenta previa

Other criteria
- an experienced operator
- capability to perform an emergency caesarean delivery if required

FORCEPS

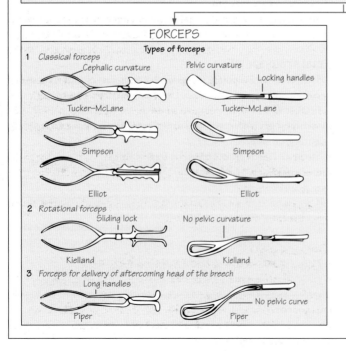

Types of forceps

1 *Classical forceps*
Cephalic curvature
Pelvic curvature
Locking handles
Tucker–McLane   Tucker–McLane
Simpson   Simpson
Elliot   Elliot

2 *Rotational forceps*
Sliding lock
No pelvic curvature
Kielland   Kielland

3 *Forceps for delivery of aftercoming head of the breech*
Long handles
No pelvic curve
Piper   Piper

VACUUM

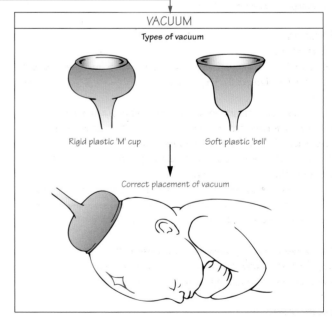

Types of vacuum

Rigid plastic 'M' cup   Soft plastic 'bell'

Correct placement of vacuum

Episiotomy

- *Definition:* a surgical incision made in the perineum to facilitate delivery.
- *Incidence.* It is still performed in >50% of vaginal deliveries, most often in nulliparous women.
- *Indications.* It may be performed in isolation or in preparation for operative vaginal delivery. It may also be used to facilitate delivery complicated by shoulder dystocia (Chapter 59).
- *Goal.* Episiotomy was introduced to reduce complications of pelvic floor trauma at delivery, including bleeding, infection, genital prolapse, and incontinence. However, there does not appear to be any benefit to the mother of elective episiotomy.
- *Types/extensions (opposite).*
  (i) *Midline episiotomy* refers to a vertical midline incision from the posterior forchette towards the rectum. It is effective in hastening delivery, but is associated with increased severe perineal trauma involving the external anal sphincter (3rd and 4th degree extensions). Used more commonly in USA.
  (ii) *Mediolateral episiotomy* is cut at 45° to the posterior forchette on one side. Such incisions appear to protect against severe perineal trauma, but have been associated with increased blood loss, wound infection, and worsened postpartum pain (none of which have been definitively demonstrated). Used more commonly in UK.
- *Episiotomy repair.* Primary approximation affords the best opportunity for functional repair, especially if there is rectal involvement. The external anal sphincter should be repaired by securing the cut ends using interrupted sutures.

Operative vaginal delivery

- Assisted vaginal delivery refers to any operative procedure designed to expedite vaginal delivery, and includes forceps delivery and vacuum extraction.
- There is no proven benefit of one instrument over another.
- The choice of which instrument to use is dependent largely on clinician preference and experience.

Forceps

Instruments

Since their introduction into obstetric practice by the Chamberlain family in the eighteenth century in Europe, the use of forceps has been controversial.

Forceps can be classified into three categories (*opposite*).
1 Classical forceps (such as Simpson forceps) which have a pelvic curvature, a cephalic curvature, and locking handles.
2 Rotational forceps (such as Kielland forceps) which lack a pelvic curvature and have sliding shanks.
3 Forceps designed to assist breech deliveries (such as Piper forceps) which lack a pelvic curve and have long handles on which to place the body of the breech while delivering the head.

Indications (*opposite*) and contraindications

Relative contraindications include prematurity, fetal macrosomia, and suspected fetal coagulation disorder.

Complications

- Increased maternal perineal injury, especially with rotational forceps delivery.

- Fetal complications include facial bruising and/or laceration. Facial nerve palsy, skull fractures, cervical spine injuries, and intracranial haemorrhage are rare.

Classification of forceps deliveries

Type of procedure	Criteria
Outlet forceps	Fetal head is at or on the perineum, scalp is visible at the introitus without separating the labia, sagittal suture is in the anteroposterior diameter or right or left occiput anterior or posterior position, rotation is ≤45
Low forceps	Leading point of the fetal skull is at ≥+2 cm but not on the pelvic floor, rotation may be: (a) ≤45° *or* (b) >45°
Mid-forceps	Station <+2 cm but head engaged
High forceps	(Not included in classification)

Vacuum

Instruments

- In 1954, Malmström developed the vacuum extractor ('ventouse') which now bears his name. The first (classical) Malmström vacuum extractor used a metal cup (the 'M' cup). Current instruments are plastic, polyethylene, or silicone.
- There are two general types (*opposite*): (i) a firm, mushroom-shaped cup similar to the 'M' cup (the rigid cup); (ii) a pliable, funnel-shaped cup (the soft cup).

Indications and contraindications

As for forceps delivery (*opposite*).

Technical considerations

- To promote flexion of the fetal head with traction, the suction cup is placed over the 'median flexing point' (symmetrically astride the sagittal suture with the posterior margin of the cup 1–3 cm anterior to the posterior fontanelle).
- Low suction (100 mmHg) is applied. After ensuring that no maternal soft tissue is trapped between the cup and fetal head, suction is increased to 500–600 mmHg and sustained downward traction applied along the pelvic curve in concert with uterine contractions. Suction is released between contractions.
- Ideally, episiotomy should be avoided as pressure of the perineum on the vacuum cup will help to keep it applied to the fetal head and assist in flexion and rotation.
- The procedure should be abandoned if the cup detaches three times or if no descent of the head is achieved.

Complications

- *Failed delivery* may be more common with the soft cup.
- *Fetal complications* include cephalohaematoma (bleeding into the scalp) and scalp lacerations ('cookie-cutter' injuries which result from the operator attempting to manually rotate the head with the vacuum). It remains unclear whether fetal intracerebral haemorrhage is increased with vacuum extraction.
- *Maternal* perineal injuries are not significantly increased.

63 Caesarean delivery

INDICATIONS FOR CAESAREAN DELIVERY		
	Absolute	**Relative**
Maternal	• failed induction of labour • failure to progress (labour dystocia) • cephalopelvic disproportion	• elective repeat caesarean • maternal disease (severe preeclampsia, cardiac disease, diabetes, cervical cancer)
Utero-placental	• previous uterine surgery (classical caesarean) • prior uterine rupture • outlet obstruction (fibroids) • placenta previa, large placental abruption	• prior uterine surgery (full-thickness myomectomy) • funic (cord) presentation in labour
Fetal	• "fetal distress"/non-reassuring fetal testing • cord prolapse • fetal malpresentation (transverse lie)	• fetal malpresentation (breech, brow, compound presentation) • macrosomia • fetal anomaly (hydrocephalus)

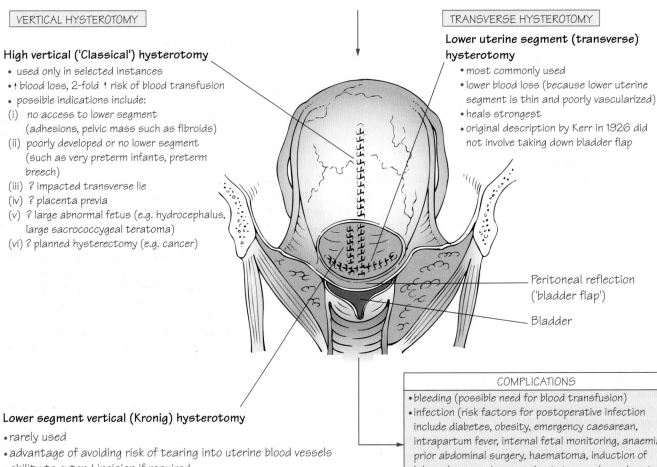

VERTICAL HYSTEROTOMY

TRANSVERSE HYSTEROTOMY

High vertical ('Classical') hysterotomy
- used only in selected instances
- ↑ blood loss, 2-fold ↑ risk of blood transfusion
- possible indications include:
  (i) no access to lower segment (adhesions, pelvic mass such as fibroids)
  (ii) poorly developed or no lower segment (such as very preterm infants, preterm breech)
  (iii) ? impacted transverse lie
  (iv) ? placenta previa
  (v) ? large abnormal fetus (e.g. hydrocephalus, large sacrococcygeal teratoma)
  (vi) ? planned hysterectomy (e.g. cancer)

Lower uterine segment (transverse) hysterotomy
- most commonly used
- lower blood loss (because lower uterine segment is thin and poorly vascularized)
- heals strongest
- original description by Kerr in 1926 did not involve taking down bladder flap

Peritoneal reflection ('bladder flap')

Bladder

Lower segment vertical (Kronig) hysterotomy
- rarely used
- advantage of avoiding risk of tearing into uterine blood vessels
- ability to extend incision if required
- by definition, incision should be confined to lower segment
- possible indications include:
  (i) multiple gestation
  (ii) malpresentation (especially transverse lie)
  (iii) delivery of very small premature infant
  (iv) planned/elective puerperal hysterectomy

COMPLICATIONS
• bleeding (possible need for blood transfusion) • infection (risk factors for postoperative infection include diabetes, obesity, emergency caesarean, intrapartum fever, internal fetal monitoring, anaemia, prior abdominal surgery, haematoma, induction of labour, lower socioeconomic status, prolonged rupture of fetal membranes) • injury to fetus • injury to adjacent organs (bowel, bladder, ureter, blood vessels) • possible need for further surgery (puerperal hysterectomy, bowel repair)

Definition

Delivery of a fetus via the abdominal route (laparotomy) requiring an incision into the uterus (hysterotomy).

Incidence

Caesarean delivery is the second most common surgical procedure (behind male circumcision) accounting for around 20–25% of all deliveries in the UK; 28% in the USA.

Indications (opposite)

• Most indications for caesarean are relative and rely on the judgement of the obstetric care provider.
• The most common indication for a primary (first) caesarean is failure to progress in labour. *labour dystocia*
• Absolute cephalopelvic disproportion (CPD) refers to the clinical setting in which the fetus is too large relative to the bony pelvis to allow for vaginal delivery even under optimal circumstances. Relative CPD is where the fetus is too large for the bony pelvis because of malpresentation (brow, compound presentation).

Technical considerations

• Elective caesarean can be performed after 39 weeks' gestation.
• Regional is preferred over general analgesia.
• Routine use of prophylactic antibiotics will decrease the incidence of postoperative febrile morbidity.
• Skin incision may be either Pfannenstiel (low transverse incision, muscle separating, strong, but limited exposure), midline vertical (offers the best exposure, but is weak), or paramedian (vertical incision lateral to rectus muscles, rarely used). Pfannenstiel incisions may rarely be modified to improve exposure by dividing the rectus muscles horizontally (Maylard incision) or lifting the rectus off the pubic bone (Cherney incision).
• Types of hysterotomy are reviewed opposite.
• Elective surgery (such as myomectomy) should not be performed at the time of caesarean, because of the risk of bleeding.

Puerperal (caesarean) hysterectomy
Incidence

Around 1 in 6000 deliveries.

Indications

• Performed primarily as an emergency procedure when the mother's life is at risk due to uncontrolled haemorrhage (30–40%).
• Other indications include abnormal placentation (Chapter 53), severe cervical dysplasia, and cervical cancer.
• Permanent sterilization is not an acceptable indication for puerperal hysterectomy.

Technical considerations

• A highly morbid procedure usually requiring general anaesthesia. As such, it should be performed only as a last resort.
• Warming blanket, three-way Foley catheter, and blood products should be available.
• Emergency puerperal hysterectomies are associated with a 4-fold increased risk of complications as compared with elective procedures. Blood loss is often excessive (2–4 L) and blood transfusions are usually required (90%). Despite a high morbidity, overall maternal mortality is low (0.3%).

• It may be possible to leave the cervix behind (subtotal or supracervical hysterectomy) thereby minimizing complications, especially blood loss. This may not be possible if the cervix is the source of the excessive bleeding, such as with placenta previa.
• Although women will be amenorrhoeic and sterile, menopausal symptoms will not develop if the ovaries are left in place.

Vaginal birth after caesarean
Background

• 30% of caesarean deliveries are elective repeat procedures.
• Maternal mortality from caesarean delivery is <0.1%, but is 2- to 11-fold higher than that associated with vaginal birth.
• Maternal morbidity (infection, thromboembolic events, wound dehiscence) is markedly higher with caesarean.

Results

• Successful *vaginal birth after caesarean* (VBAC) can be achieved in 65–80% of women.
• Factors associated with successful VBAC include prior vaginal delivery, estimated fetal weight <4000 g, and a non-recurrent indication for the prior caesarean (breech, placenta previa) rather than a potential recurrent indication (such as CPD).

Contraindications

• Absolute contraindications include a prior classical (high vertical) caesarean, 'fetal distress', transverse lie, and placenta previa.
• Relative contraindications include breech presentation, prior full-thickness uterine myomectomy, prior uterine rupture, and (possibly) multiple gestations.

Complications

• *Uterine dehiscence* (subclinical separation of the prior uterine incision) occurs in 2–3% of cases. It is often detected only by manual exploration of the scar following vaginal delivery. In the absence of vaginal bleeding, no further treatment is necessary.
• *Uterine rupture* may be life-threatening. Symptoms and signs include acute onset of fetal bradycardia (70%), abdominal pain (10%), vaginal bleeding (5%), haemodynamic instability (5–10%), and/or loss of the presenting part (<5%). Epidural anaesthesia may mask some of these features. Risk factors include:

   (i)   type of prior uterine incision (<1% for lower segment transverse incision, 2–3% for lower segment vertical, and 4–8% for high vertical);
   (ii) ≥2 prior caesareans (4%);
   (iii) prior uterine rupture;
   (iv) 'excessive' use of oxytocin (although 'excessive' is poorly defined);
   (v) dysfunctional labour pattern (especially prolonged second stage or arrest of dilatation).

Factors NOT associated with an increased risk for rupture include epidural anaesthesia, unknown uterine scar, fetal macrosomia, and indication for prior caesarean.

Clinical considerations

• Continuous intrapartum fetal monitoring is recommended.
• Follow labour curve carefully for evidence of labour dystocia.
• The capacity to perform an emergency cesarean should be at hand.

HAEMOSTASIS OF THE UTERUS

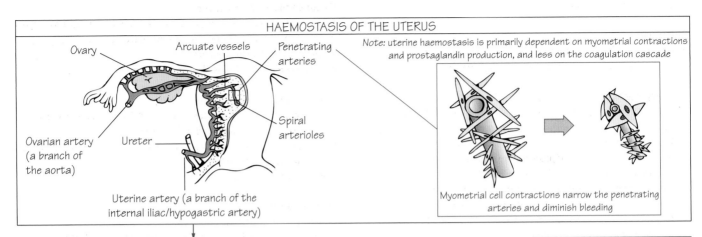

Ovary

Arcuate vessels

Penetrating arteries

Ovarian artery (a branch of the aorta)

Ureter

Spiral arterioles

Uterine artery (a branch of the internal iliac/hypogastric artery)

Note: uterine haemostasis is primarily dependent on myometrial contractions and prostaglandin production, and less on the coagulation cascade

Myometrial cell contractions narrow the penetrating arteries and diminish bleeding

INITIAL MANAGEMENT OF POSTPARTUM HAEMORRHAGE (PPH)

- early recognition of PPH, monitor vital signs, O_2
- establish intravenous access, place urinary catheter
- baseline laboratory values, alert anaesthesia and blood bank
- correct hypovolaemia with crystalloid
- central haemodynamic monitoring (if indicated)
- correct anaemia/coagulation disorders with blood products

DETERMINE UNDERLYING CAUSE OF PPH

- examine placenta, genital tract, uterus
- aetiology will determine further management

RETAINED PLACENTAL FRAGMENTS

- manual exploration and removal
- curettage

COAGULOPATHY

- replace red blood cells
- replace platelets
- replace coagulation factors (with fresh frozen plasma and/or cryoprecipitate)

UTERINE RUPTURE

- laparotomy
- repair of scar and/or hysterectomy

LOWER GENITAL TRACT LACERATIONS

- include cervical, vaginal or perineal tears
- identify sources of bleeding, establish surgical haemostasis
- evacuate haematoma (if necessary)
- if unresponsive to local repair, consider further surgical management (such as uterine packing, hypogastric artery ligation, uterine artery ligation, hysterectomy, embolization)

ABNORMAL PLACENTATION

- most commonly placenta accreta
- attempt conservative surgery (curettage, local repair)
- may require further surgical management (laparotomy, uterine or hypogastric artery ligation, hysterectomy)
- consider angiography and embolization if time permits

UTERINE ATONY

- bimanual massage and/or compression
- exclude retained placental fragments, uterine rupture
- medical uterotonic therapy as follows:
(i) rapid oxytocin infusion (10–40 units in 1 L or may be given intramuscularly or intramyometrially)
Note: IV boluses of oxytocin can cause hypotension
(ii) methylergonovine 0.2 mg IM q.2 h a maximum of 3 doses (avoid in hypertension)
(iii) 15-methyl-prostaglandin $F_{2\alpha}$ (Hemabate) 0.25 mg IM or intramyometrial q.15–20 min for a maximum of 8 doses (avoid in asthma)
(iv) ? dinoprostone (PGE_2) 20 mg or misoprostil (PGE_1)
- 1000 mg rectally
If no response to above management, consider:
(i) uterine packing (rarely used)
(ii) angiography and embolization
(iii) explorative laparotomy with surgical options including uterine/utero-ovarian/infundibulopelvic vessel ligation, hypogastric artery ligation, hysterectomy (see below)

Hypogastric (internal iliac) artery ligation

- always perform bilaterally
- decreases uterine perfusion pressure by 50%

Superior gluteal artery

Hypogastric artery ligation site

External iliac

Uterine artery

Obturator artery

Hysterectomy (removal of uterus)

- usually for uterine atony, accreta, rupture

Uterine artery ligation (O'Leary stitch)

- perform bilaterally
- doesn't ligate descending cervical branch of uterine artery

Ureter

Uterine artery

Bladder

Third stage of labour

Definition
- Begins with delivery of the fetus and ends with delivery of the placenta and fetal membranes.

Duration
- Median duration of the third stage of labour is 6 minutes.
- 3–5% of women have a third stage lasting ≥30 minutes.

Management
- The third stage of labour is usually managed expectantly. Uterine contractions result in cleavage of the placenta between the zona basalis and zona spongiosum.
- The three clinical signs of placental separation include:
  (i) a sudden gush of blood ('separation bleed');
  (ii) apparent lengthening of the umbilical cord;
  (iii) elevation and contraction of the uterine fundus.
- Placental separation can be encouraged by 'controlled cord traction' using either the Brandt–Andrews manoeuvre (where the uterus is secured and controlled traction is applied to the cord) or the Credé manoeuvre (where the cord is secured and the uterus is elevated). Care should be taken to avoid placental inversion.

Complications
- Postpartum haemorrhage (*below*).
- Retained placenta is defined as failure of the placenta to deliver within 30 minutes. If there is excessive bleeding, manual removal may be required earlier. Failed manual removal of the placenta suggests abnormal placentation (Chapter 53).

Postpartum haemorrhage

Definition
- Postpartum haemorrhage (PPH) has traditionally been defined as an estimated blood loss of ≥500 mL. However blood loss is underestimated clinically by 30–50%. The average blood loss following vaginal delivery is 500 mL, with 5% of women losing >1000 mL. Blood loss following caesarean averages 1000 mL.
- More recently, PPH has been defined as a 10% drop in haematocrit from admission or bleeding requiring blood transfusion.

Incidence
10–15% (4% after vaginal delivery, 6–8% after caesarean delivery).

Classification
Early PPH
- Defined as PPH ≤24 hours after delivery.
- Causes include uterine atony, retained placental fragments, lower genital tract lacerations, uterine rupture, uterine inversion, abnormal placentation, coagulopathy.

Late or delayed PPH
- Defined as PPH >24 hours but <6 weeks post-delivery.
- Causes include retained placental fragments, infection (endometritis), coagulopathy, and placental site subinvolution.

Aetiology and Management of PPH (*opposite*)
Uterine atony
- *Risk factors* include uterine overdistension (due to polyhydramnios, multiple pregnancy, fetal macrosomia), high parity, rapid or prolonged labour, infection, prior uterine atony and use of uterine-relaxing agents.
- *Management* is reviewed opposite.

Retained placental fragments
- May result from retention of a cotyledon or succenturiate lobe (seen in 3% of placentae). Examination of the placenta may identify defects suggestive of retained products.
- *Management*: D & C possibly under ultrasound guidance.

Lower genital tract lacerations
- *Risk factors* include assisted vaginal delivery, fetal macrosomia, precipitous delivery, and use of episiotomy.
- *Diagnosis* should be considered when vaginal bleeding continues despite adequate uterine tone.
- *Management*: primary repair.

Uterine rupture
- *Incidence:* 1 in 2000 deliveries.
- *Risk factors* include prior uterine surgery, obstructed labour, 'excessive' use of oxytocin, abnormal fetal lie, grandmultiparity, and uterine manipulations in labour (forceps delivery, breech extraction, and intrauterine pressure catheter insertion).
- *Treatment*: laparotomy with repair or hysterectomy.

Uterine inversion
- *Incidence:* 1 in 2500 deliveries.
- *Risk factors* include uterine atony, excessive umbilical cord traction, manual removal of placenta, abnormal placentation, uterine anomalies, and fundal placentation.
- *Symptoms* include acute abdominal pain and shock (30%). The uterus may be visibly extruding through the vulva.
- *Treatment:* immediate manual or hydrostatic replacement.

Abnormal placentation
- Includes abnormal attachment of placental villi to the myometrium (accreta), invasion into the myometrium (increta), or penetration through the myometrium (percreta).
- Placenta accreta is the most common type (1 in 2500 deliveries).
- *Risk factors* include prior uterine surgery, placenta previa, smoking, and grandmultiparity. Placenta previa alone is associated with a 5% incidence of accreta, which increases to 10–25% with placenta previa and one prior caesarean and >50% with placenta previa and two or more prior caesareans.
- *Management:* D & C or hysterectomy.

Coagulopathy
- *Congenital coagulopathy* complicates 1–2 per 10,000 pregnancies. The most common diagnoses are von Willebrand's disease and ITP.
- *Acquired* causes include anticoagulant therapy and consumptive coagulopathy resulting from obstetric complications (such as pre-eclampsia, sepsis, abruption, amniotic fluid embolism).
- *Management:* stop on-going bleeding and replace blood products (including platelets, coagulation factors, and red blood cells).

PHYSIOLOGY OF LACTATION

Development of the mammary gland

Mammogenesis refers to growth and development of the mammary gland which begins at puberty. Pregnancy is required for final alveolar growth. Lactogenesis refers to production of breast milk which begins during pregnancy. Full milk synthesis, however, only occurs after delivery when oestrogen levels decline thereby allowing prolactin to act unopposed to promote milk production.

Neuroendocrine reflexes initiated by suckling

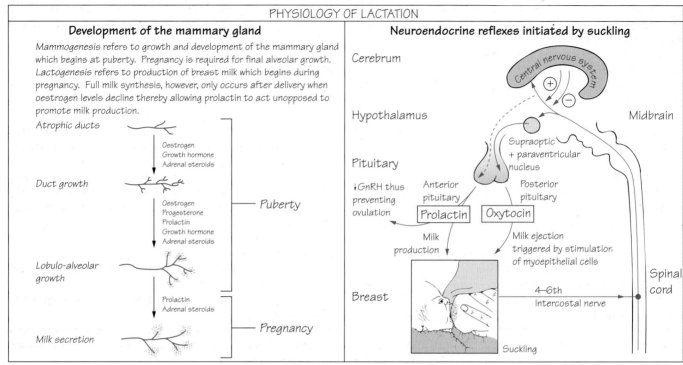

COMPLICATIONS OF THE PUERPERIUM

Breast engorgement

Caused by vascular and lymphatic stasis

Breasts are heavy, painful, warm, firm and tender to palpation

Mastitis

Well-defined zone of induration, 10% will go on to abscess formation

Endometritis and possible sequelae

The inflammatory process often extends to the parametrium and may cause pelvic cellulitis and peritonitis

Endometritis with necrotic yellow-green endometrium extending into the wall of the uterus

Involvement of the adjacent blood vessels can result in septic pelvic thrombophlebitis

Severe induration may develop into a parametrial phlegmon

Walled-off infection can develop into a pelvic abscess

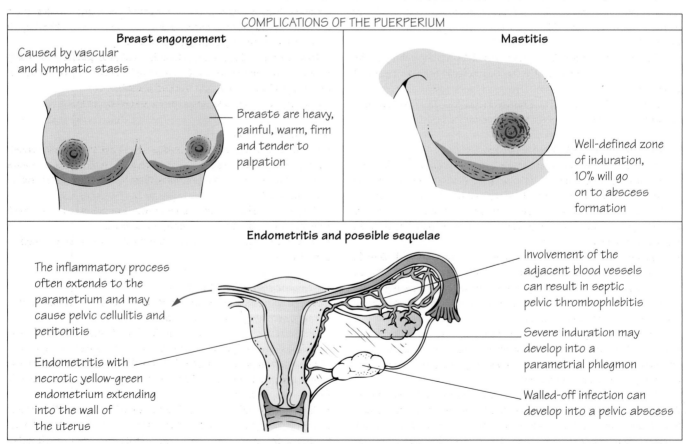

Physiology

- The *puerperium* is the 6-week period following delivery when the reproductive tract returns to its non-pregnant state.
- Immediately following delivery, the uterus shrinks down to the level of the umbilicus. By 2 weeks postpartum, it is no longer palpable above the symphysis. By 6 weeks, the uterus has returned to its non-pregnant size.
- Decidual sloughing after delivery results in a physiological vaginal discharge, known as *lochia*.
- The abdomen will resume its prepregnancy appearance, with the notable exception of *abdominal striae* ('stretch marks'). These fade with time.
- Most women will experience the return of menstruation by 6–8 weeks postpartum.

Postpartum care

- In the *immediate postpartum period*, maternal vital signs should be taken frequently, the uterine fundus should be palpated to ensure it is well contracted and the amount of vaginal bleeding should be noted.
- Early ambulation is encouraged regardless of route of delivery. Adequate pain management is essential.
- Shortly after birth, neonates should receive topical ophthalmic prophylaxis (to prevent ophthalmia neonatorum) and vitamin K (to prevent haemorrhagic disease of the newborn due to a physiological deficiency of vitamin K-dependent coagulation factors).
- Prior to discharge, skilled nursing staff should be made available to prepare the mother for care of the newborn. The mother should receive anti-D immunoglobulin (if she is Rh-negative and her baby Rh-positive) and MMR vaccine (if she is rubella non-immune).
- Coitus can be resumed 2–3 weeks after delivery depending on the patient's desire and comfort. Contraception is necessary to prevent conception.
- A *routine visit* is recommended 6 weeks postpartum. Contraceptive counselling and breast-feeding should be addressed.

Lactation and breast-feeding *(opposite)*

- *Advantages.* Breast-fed infants have a lower incidence of allergies, gastrointestinal infections, otitis media, respiratory infections, and (possibly) higher intelligence quotient (IQ) scores. Women who breast-feed appear to have a lower incidence of breast cancer, ovarian cancer and osteoporosis. Breast-feeding is also a bonding experience between infant and mother.
- *Contraindications:* HIV, cytomegalovirus, chronic hepatitis B or C. Most drugs given to the mother are secreted to some extent into breast milk, but the amount of drug ingested by the infant is typically small. There are some drugs, however, in which breast-feeding is contraindicated (radioisotopes, cytotoxic agents).
- *Physiology.* Prolactin is essential for lactation. Women with pituitary necrosis (Sheehan syndrome) do not lactate. Cigarette smoking, diuretics, bromocriptin, and combined oral contraceptives (not the progestin-only pill) decrease milk production.
- *Colostrum* is a lemon-coloured fluid secreted by the breasts during the first 4–5 days postpartum. It contains more minerals and protein than mature milk, but less sugar and fat. *Mature milk* production is established within a few days. It contains high concentrations of lactose, vitamins (except vitamin K), immunoglobulins, and antibodies.

Complications of the puerperium

Breast engorgement *(opposite)*

- May occur on days 2–4 postpartum in women who are not nursing or at any time if breast-feeding is interrupted.
- Conservative measures (tight-fitting brassiere, ice packs, analgesics) are usually effective. Bromocriptine may be indicated in refractory cases.

Mastitis *(opposite)*

- Refers to a regional infection of the breast parenchyma, usually by *Staphylococcus aureus*.
- Uncommon. >50% of cases occur in primiparas.
- Mastitis is a *clinical diagnosis* with fever, chills, and focal unilateral breast erythema, oedema, and tenderness. It usually occurs during the 3rd or 4th week postpartum.
- *Treatment:* overcome ductal obstruction (by continuing breast-feeding or pumping), symptomatic relief, and oral antibiotics (usually flucloxacillin). 10% of women will develop an abscess requiring surgical drainage.

Endometritis *(opposite)*

- Refers to a polymicrobial infection of the endometrium that often invades the underlying myometrium.
- *Incidence:* <5% after vaginal delivery, but 5- to 10-fold higher after caesarean delivery.
- *Risk factors:* caesarean delivery, prolonged rupture of membranes, multiple vaginal examinations, manual removal of the placenta, and internal fetal monitoring.
- Endometritis is a *clinical diagnosis* with fever, uterine tenderness, a foul purulent vaginal discharge, and/or increased vaginal bleeding. It occurs most commonly 5–10 days after delivery.
- *Treatment:* broad-spectrum antibiotics (until the patient is clinically improved and afebrile for 24–48 hours) and dilatation and curettage (if retained products of conception are suspected).
- *Complications:* abscess, septic pelvic thrombophlebitis.

Necrotizing fasciitis

- Refers to necrotic infection of the superficial fascia that spreads rapidly along tissue planes to the abdominal wall, buttock, and/or thigh leading to septicaemia and circulatory failure. Maternal mortality approaches 50%.
- *Diagnosis:* skin oedema, blue-brown discolouration, or frank gangrene with loss of sensation or hyperaesthesia.
- *Treatment:* early diagnosis, antibiotics, aggressive surgical debridement.

Psychiatric complaints (Chapter 45)

- A mild *transient depression* ('postpartum blues') is common after delivery, occurring in >50% of women.
- *Postpartum depression* occurs in 8–15% of women. Risk factors include a history of depression (30%) or prior postpartum depression (70–85%). Symptoms develop 2–3 months postpartum and resolve slowly over the following 6–12 months. Supportive care and monthly follow-up is necessary.
- *Postpartum psychosis* is rare (1–2 per 1000 live births). Risk factors include young age, primiparity, and a personal or family history of mental illness. Symptoms typically start 10–14 days postpartum. Hospitalization, pharmacological and/or electroconvulsant therapy (ECT) may be necessary. Recurrence of postpartum psychosis is high (25–30%).

66 Circumcision

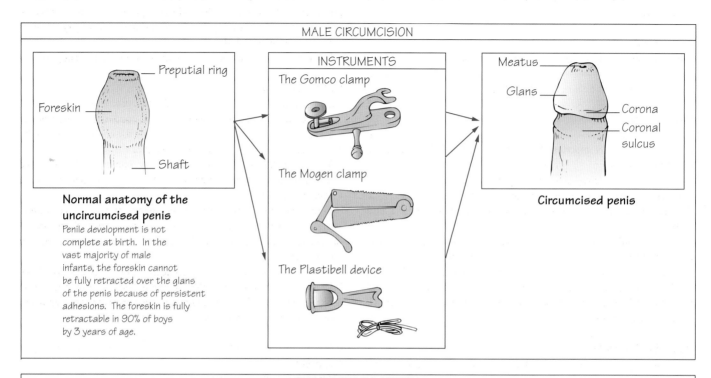

MALE CIRCUMCISION

Normal anatomy of the uncircumcised penis

Labels: Preputial ring, Foreskin, Shaft

Penile development is not complete at birth. In the vast majority of male infants, the foreskin cannot be fully retracted over the glans of the penis because of persistent adhesions. The foreskin is fully retractable in 90% of boys by 3 years of age.

INSTRUMENTS

The Gomco clamp

The Mogen clamp

The Plastibell device

Circumcised penis

Labels: Meatus, Glans, Corona, Coronal sulcus

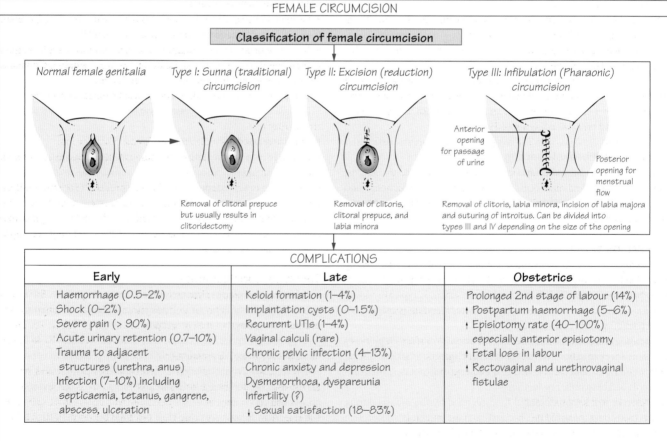

FEMALE CIRCUMCISION

Classification of female circumcision

Normal female genitalia

Type I: Sunna (traditional) circumcision
Removal of clitoral prepuce but usually results in clitoridectomy

Type II: Excision (reduction) circumcision
Removal of clitoris, clitoral prepuce, and labia minora

Type III: Infibulation (Pharaonic) circumcision
Anterior opening for passage of urine
Posterior opening for menstrual flow
Removal of clitoris, labia minora, incision of labia majora and suturing of introitus. Can be divided into types III and IV depending on the size of the opening

COMPLICATIONS

Early	Late	Obstetrics
Haemorrhage (0.5–2%)	Keloid formation (1–4%)	Prolonged 2nd stage of labour (14%)
Shock (0–2%)	Implantation cysts (0–1.5%)	↑ Postpartum haemorrhage (5–6%)
Severe pain (> 90%)	Recurrent UTIs (1–4%)	↑ Episiotomy rate (40–100%)
Acute urinary retention (0.7–10%)	Vaginal calculi (rare)	especially anterior episiotomy
Trauma to adjacent	Chronic pelvic infection (4–13%)	↑ Fetal loss in labour
structures (urethra, anus)	Chronic anxiety and depression	↑ Rectovaginal and urethrovaginal
Infection (7–10%) including	Dysmenorrhoea, dyspareunia	fistulae
septicaemia, tetanus, gangrene,	Infertility (?)	
abscess, ulceration	↓ Sexual satisfaction (18–83%)	

Male circumcision (*opposite*)

Definition

Circumcision refers to the surgical removal of all or part of the foreskin of the male penis.

Incidence

• It is the most common surgery performed on males.
• Circumcision rates vary from country to country: 90–95% in Israel, 60–90% in the USA, 50% in Canada and UK.

Indications

• The most common indications are religious traditions and/or social beliefs. Cultural traditions also often dictate the timing of the procedure and the person responsible for performing it.
• Newborn (male) circumcision has potential medical benefits and advantages as well as disadvantages and risks. It is generally accepted that there is no medical indication for routine circumcision of newborn males.
• Medical indications are rare. These include persistent non-retractability (especially if associated with urinary obstruction), phimosis and paraphimosis (acute onset of pain and swelling of the glans due to obstruction of venous return resulting from a persistent retracted foreskin), and possibly recurrent urinary tract infections and/or sexually transmitted diseases.

Potential benefits

• Facilitates genital cleanliness. It does not eliminate the need for proper genital hygiene; it simply makes it easier.
• May reduce the incidence of urinary tract infections from 1% in uncircumcised to 0.1% in circumcised males.
• May reduce the risk of transmission of some sexually transmitted diseases (such as HIV and HPV).
• Penile carcinoma is a disease of the elderly with an incidence of around 1 in 600 uncircumcised males. It can be almost completely prevented by circumcision. However, poor genital hygiene may be equally important in the pathogenesis of this disease.
• May prevent cervical cancer in the partners of uncircumcised males infected with HPV.
• Will avoid circumcision later in life where the procedure may be more complicated and more traumatic for the patient. Of all uncircumcised males, up to 10% will require circumcision later in life for medical indications.

Contraindications

• *Absolute contraindications* include a documented or family history of a bleeding disorder or a structural defect of the penis (such as hypospadias in which the foreskin is used as a surgical graft to repair the defect). Circumcision is an elective procedure. It should be performed only in healthy, stable infants.
• *Relative contraindications* include prematurity, infants <24 hours old, and a very small appearing penis ('micropenis') that may result from webbing or tethering of the glans to the scrotum.

Technical considerations

• Informed consent should be obtained from the parent(s).
• Examination of the external genitalia should be performed.
• The infant is temporarily restrained.
• Infants do experience pain and discomfort with the procedure. Analgesia is not universally used, but is highly recommended. The preferred method of analgesia has not been determined. Swaddling, sucrose by mouth, and acetaminophen may reduce stress. Local infiltration (dorsal penile block or ring block) is effective. Epinephrine should not be given. Topical anaesthesia (5% lidocaine/prilocaine (Emla)) may be effective, but should be applied 1 hour prior to the surgery. General anaesthesia is not justified.
• Instruments available for male circumcision are detailed opposite.

Complications

• Complications occur in 0.2–0.6% of procedures. The most common complication is excessive bleeding. Other immediate complications include postoperative infection, haematoma formation, injury to the penis, and excessive skin removal (denudation).
• The Plastibell device is left in place over a number of days until the foreskin separates by infarction and falls off. It is associated with a higher incidence of infection.
• Long-term complications are rare and include stenosis of the urethral meatus. As regards future sexuality, Masters and Johnson found no difference in sexual experience and sensitivity between circumcised and uncircumcised men.
• More serious complications are exceptionally rare and invariably involve breach of protocol (such as complete destruction of the penis by electrocautery or ischemia following the inappropriate use of epinephrine containing local anaesthetics).

Female circumcision (genital mutilation)
(*opposite*)

General considerations

• Despite universal condemnation, this practice persists in many countries with prevalence rates ranging from <1% to 99%.
• It is practiced on all continents, across socioeconomic classes, and among different ethnic and cultural groups, including Christians, Muslims, Jews, and indigenous African religions.
• There are at least 100 million circumcised women worldwide.

Indications

• There is no medical indication for female circumcision.
• In many cultures, female circumcision is looked upon as an initiation into womanhood.
• Reasons given for the procedure include prevention of immorality, to make a woman eligible for marriage, to make intercourse more enjoyable for the man, and to promote cleanliness. In reality, it symbolizes social control of a woman's sexual pleasure (clitoridectomy) and reproductive capacity (infibulation).

Technical considerations

• Techniques of female circumcision are detailed opposite. Sunna (the Arabic word for 'traditional') circumcision is the least mutilating procedure with removal of the clitoral prepuce alone. It is said to be analogous to male circumcision; however, it invariably results in severe clitoral damage and/or amputation.
• Circumcision is generally performed by untrained operators without anaesthesia or sterilized instruments. Haemostasis is achieved by the application of cow dung or mud, by pressure with dirty clothes, or by crude suturing. A girl's legs may be tied together for weeks to facilitate healing.

Complications

The complications of female circumcision (early, late and intrapartum) and their respective incidence are detailed opposite.

Index

Italic indicates figures, **bold** indicates tables.